Health at Home™

Your Complete Guide to Symptoms, Solutions, & Self-Care

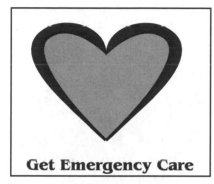

Get Emergency Care

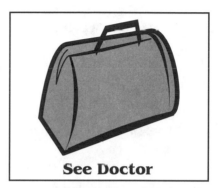

See Doctor

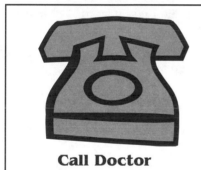

Call Doctor

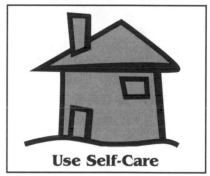

Use Self-Care

Written by

Don R. Powell, Ph.D.

and the

American Institute for Preventive Medicine

Published by

American Institute for Preventive Medicine Press
Farmington Hills, Michigan

Acknowledgements:

The material in this book has undergone an extensive process in order to ensure medical accuracy and present the latest medical research. We are indebted to the physicians and other health professionals who served on our clinical review team.

Richard S. Lang, M.D., M.P.H., Head, Section of Preventive Medicine, Department of Internal Medicine, Cleveland Clinic Foundation, Cleveland, OH

Richard N. Matzen, M.D., Physician, retired, the Cleveland Clinic Foundation, Adjunct Assistant Professor of Medicine, Epidemiology Biostatistics, Case Western Reserve School of Medicine, Cleveland, OH

Susan Schooley, M.D., Chairperson, Department of Family Practice, Henry Ford Health System, Detroit, MI

Edward Adler, M.D., S.A.C.P., Attending Physician, Division of Geriatric Medicine, William Beaumont Hospital, Royal Oak, MI; Clinical Assistant Professor of Medicine, Wayne State University School of Medicine, Detroit, MI

Richard Aghababian, M.D., President, American College of Emergency Physicians, Washington, D.C.

Sarah D. Atkinson, M.D., Child & Adolescent Psychiatry; General Psychiatry, Menninger Clinic, Topeka, KS

Mark H. Beers, M.D., Senior Director of Geriatrics and Associate Editor, Merck Manual, West Point, PA

Joseph Berenholz, M.D., F.A.C.O.G., Diplomate, American College of Obstetrics and Gynecology, Faculty and Staff Physician, Detroit Medical Center, Detroit, MI

Dwight L. Blackburn, M.D., Medical Director, Anthem Blue Cross/Blue Shield, Louisville, KY

Douglas D. Blevins, M.D., Departments of Infectious Disease, Internal Medicine, Lewis-Gale Clinic, Salem, VA

Frances B. DeHart, R.N., B.S.N., Health Management Specialist, HealthFirst, Greenville, SC

Lynn DeGrande, A.C.S.W., CEAP, DeGrande & Associates, Senior Consultant, General Motors EAP, Detroit, MI

Peter Fass, M.D., Medical Director, KeyCorp, Albany, NY

Elaine Frank, M.Ed., R.D., Vice President, American Institute for Preventive Medicine, Farmington Hills, MI

Gerald Freidman, M.D., Medical Director, Physicians Health Plan, Kalamazoo MI

Abe Gershonowicz, D.D.S., Family Dentistry, Sterling Heights, MI

Gary P. Gross, M.D., Dermatologist, Lewis-Gale Clinic, Salem, VA

J. Bruce Hagadorn, M.D., Otolarygologist, Lewis-Gale Clinic, Salem, VA

Donald Hayes, M.D., Medical Director, Sara Lee Corporation, Winston-Salem, NC

William Hettler, M.D., Director, University Health Service, University of Wisconsin, Stevens Point, WI

Ronald Holmes, M.D., Director, Division of General Pediatrics, Professor, Department of Pediatrics, University of Michigan Medical Center, Ann Arbor, MI

William J. Kagey, M.D., Pediatrician, Lewis-Gale Clinic, Salem, VA

Jeanette Karwan, R.D., Director, Product Development, American Institute for Preventive Medicine, Farmington Hills, MI

Telephone Numbers & Information

Emergency Medical Service (EMS): _____

Fire: _____ Police: _____

Poison Control Center: _____ Suicide Prevention Center: _____

Health Care Providers:

Name	Specialty	Telephone Number
_____	_____	_____
_____	_____	_____
_____	_____	_____

Hospital: _____ Pharmacy: _____

Employee Assistance Program (EAP): _____

Health Insurance Information:

Company: _____ Phone Number: _____

Address: _____

Policyholder's Name: _____ Policy Number: _____

What to Tell Your Health Care Provider

(Photocopy as needed)

Use this summary when you call or visit a provider. See pages 13 to 15 and 30 to 31 for more information.

Symptoms:

- ❏ Pain
- ❏ Fever/chills
- ❏ Skin problems
- ❏ Stomach problems
- ❏ Nausea/vomiting
- ❏ Breathing problems
- ❏ Eye, ear, nose, throat problems
- ❏ Muscle or joint problems

Other problems: _____

Specific questions I have now: _____

What I need to do: _____

Medications:

	Name/Dose	Name/Dose
Medications I take now:	_____	_____
	_____	_____
Medications I'm allergic to:	_____	_____

Note: This book is not meant to substitute for expert medical advice or treatment. The information is given to help you make informed choices about your health. Follow your doctor's or health care provider's advice if it differs from what is given in this book.

Please know that many of the designations used by manufacturers and sellers to distinguish their products are claimed as trademarks. Where those designations appear in this book and the American Institute for Preventive Medicine was aware of a trademark claim, the designations have been printed in initial capital letters (e.g., Tums).

This guide is one of a series of publications and programs offered by the American Institute for Preventive Medicine designed to help individuals reduce health care costs and improve the quality of their lives. Other booklets in the series include:

HealthyLife® Self-Care Guides – Each booklet discusses the most common health problems and teaches when to see the doctor or provide self-care. Addressing specific needs, the titles are: *Self-Care Guide; Women's Self-Care Guide; Children's Self-Care Guide; Seniors' Self-Care Guide; Prenatal Self-Care Guide; Emergency/First Aid Guide;* and *Mental Fitness Guide.* Some guides are also available in a low literacy format and Spanish. The books *Seniors' Health at Home* and *HealthySelf* are also available.

The Wise consumer series includes: *All the Right Questions; Being a Wise Health Care Consumer; Healthy Savings; Toll-Free Hotlines to Health; Minding Your Mental Health;* and *Glossary of Medical & Health Terms.*

For more information, call or write:

American Institute for Preventive Medicine
30445 Northwestern Hwy., Suite 350
Farmington Hills, MI 48334-3102
(248) 539-1800 / FAX (248) 539-1808
e-mail: aipm@healthy.net

Web Site Information

For information on 365 health topics, access the American Institute for Preventive Medicine's web site: www.aipm.healthy.net and double click on "365 Health Topics".

ISBN 0-9635612-8-6

James Kohlenberg, M.D., Internal Medicine, John R. Medical Clinic, Madison Heights, MI

Martin Levinson, M.D., Chairman, Department of Pediatrics, Sinai Hospital, Detroit, MI

Julie T. Lusk, M.Ed., Director of Health Management, Lewis-Gale Clinic, Salem, VA

Herb Martin, Ph.D., CEAP Director, Employee Assistance Program, Vista Health Plans, San Diego, CA

Dan Mayer, M.D., Associate Professor, Emergency Medicine, Albany Medical College, Emergency Department, Albany Medical Center, Albany, NY

Tony Mendes, Ph.D., Manager, Training and Development, AT&T Health Promotion, Basking Ridge, NJ

Myron Miller, M.D., Vice Chairman and Professor, Department of Geriatrics and Adult Development, The Mount Sinai School of Medicine, New York, NY

Alonzo H. Myers, Jr., M.D., Orthopaedic Surgeon, Lewis-Gale Clinic, Salem, VA

Joseph L. Nelson, III, M.D., Gastroenterologist, Lewis-Gale Clinic, Salem, VA

E. Blackford Noland, M.D., Department of Internal Medicine, Lewis-Gale Clinic, Salem, VA

Thomas C. Overhold, M.D., Department of Internal Medicine and Pediatrics, Henry Ford Hospital, Detroit, MI

William A. Pankey, M.D., Senior Vice President, Corporate Medical Director, D.C. Chartered Health Plan, Inc., Washington, D.C.

Anthony Pelonero, M.D., Associate Professor of Psychiatry, Medical College of Virginia-Virginia Commonwealth University and Medical Director, Mental Health Care, Trigon Blue Cross Blue/Shield, Richmond, VA

J. Courtland Robinson, M.D., M.P.H.; Associate Professor, Dept. Gynecology and Obstetrics, Johns Hopkins School of Medicine, Baltimore, MD; joint appointment in the Department of Population Dynamics at the Johns Hopkins School of Hygiene and Public Health, Baltimore, MD

Edward J. Roccella, Ph.D., M.P.H., Coordinator, National High Blood Pressure Education Program, Office of Preventive Education and Control, National Heart, Lung and Blood Institute, Bethesda, MD

Lee B. Sacks, M.D., President, Advocate Health Partners, Oak Brook, IL

Mark A. Schmidt, M.D., Urologist, Lewis-Gale Clinic, Salem, VA

Joel Schoolin, D.O., Medical Director, Lutheran General Health Plan, Mt. Prospect, IL

Ian Shaffer, M.D., Executive Vice President and Chief Medical Officer, Value Behavioral Health, Falls Church, VA

E.A. Shaptini, M.D., Vice President and Medical Director, American Natural Resources Company, Detroit, MI

Steven Starr, D.P.M., Director, Birmingham Foot Care, Birmingham, MI

Bruce Stewart, M.D., Department of Internal Medicine, Lewis-Gale Clinic, Salem, VA

J. Steven Strosnider, M.D., Director of Psychological Counseling, Lewis-Gale Clinic, Salem, VA

David J. Thaler, D.O., Internal Medicine, Lewis-Gale Clinic, Salem, VA

Neill D. Varner, D.O., M.P.H., Medical Director, Saginaw Steering Division, General Motors Corporation, Member of the UAW-GM Health Promotion Task Force, and Medical Director, Saginaw County Department of Public Health, Saginaw, MI

Mark Werner, M.D., Obstetrics and Gynecology, Staff Physician, William Beaumont Hospital, Royal Oak, MI

Yael Zoldan, Manager, Graphic Design, American Institute for Preventive Medicine, Farmington Hills, MI

Table of Contents

Section III
Emergencies

Section IV
Major Medical Conditions

Section V
Health Resources

SECTION I
Wise Medical Consumerism

Introduction

Section I helps you learn to be a wise medical consumer. Chapters 1 through 6 give many tips and guidelines to help you use the health care system wisely. Chapter 7 offers information on what you should do about basic dental health. Chapter 8 lists mental health facts and reasons to seek help for mental health problems. Ways to stay well and prevent disease are presented in Chapter 9. This section combines important information and a common sense approach to make it easier for you and your family to take responsibility for your own health and well-being.

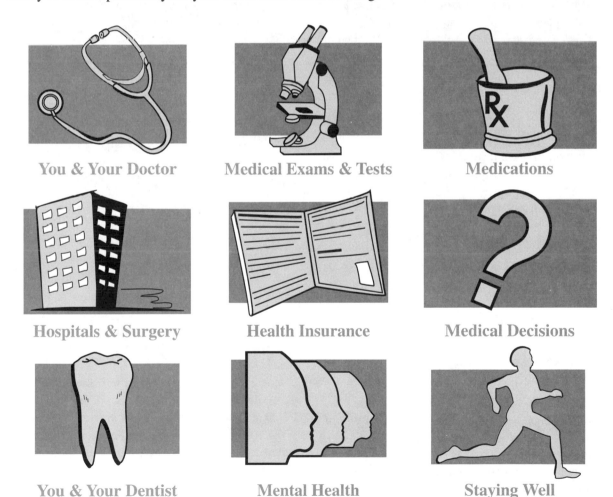

You & Your Doctor   Medical Exams & Tests   Medications

Hospitals & Surgery   Health Insurance   Medical Decisions

You & Your Dentist   Mental Health   Staying Well

1. You & Your Doctor

Choosing a Doctor

- Look for a doctor who accepts your health insurance. Read the materials provided by your carrier and/or talk to your Employee Assistance Program (EAP) representative.

- If you belong to a managed care plan, get a list of doctors who work with the plan. Health Maintenance Organizations (HMOs) and Preferred Provider Organizations (PPOs) are two types of managed care plans. The doctor(s) you see now may be on your HMO or PPO list.

When Looking for a New Doctor

- Make a list of things you want in a doctor, such as location, gender, age, etc.

- Ask relatives and friends for doctors that have given them good medical care and whom they trust.

- Find out if the doctor is licensed by the state he or she practices in. Check with your local medical society. Find out, too, if the doctor is board-certified or board-eligible in the specialty in which he or she practices. To find out, call the American Board of Medical Specialists (ABMS) at 1-800-776-2378.

- Find out if a doctor is taking new patients. Check with your health plan or call the doctor's office.

- Interview several doctors before you decide on the one you want. Look for a doctor whom you can relate to, communicate with, and who meets your expectations of how medical decisions are made (the doctor alone, you alone, you and the doctor together).

- Ask about office hours, staffing, and how long you must wait for an appointment. Find out how many patients the doctor schedules to see in one hour.

- Ask about the office policy regarding payment. Ask whether you must pay a certain amount for your visit at that time or whether you can be billed and pay later.

- Find out what other doctors serve as backups when the doctor is away. Ask who cares for you after office hours.

- Find out which hospital the doctor sends patients to and if your health insurance is accepted there.

- Ask if prevention services such as exercise and nutrition programs are covered by the health plan the doctor accepts.

See Your "Primary" Doctor Before You See a Specialist

Internists, family doctors, and pediatricians are examples of primary care doctors. They manage your medical care. If you are a member of a Health Maintenance Organization (HMO), your primary care doctor is the doctor you select from the HMO plan to coordinate your medical care. This person could be a family doctor, internist, obstetrician/ gynecologist, etc. Whether or not you belong to an HMO, call or see your primary care doctor before you see a specialist. If your primary care doctor cannot take care of your health problem, he or she can refer you to a specialist.

Talking With Your Doctor/Provider Checklists

(Photocopy as needed. Use the lines given to fill in the information.)

Checklist 1 – Before You Call Or See Your Doctor/Provider

A. Find out these things in advance:

❑ What are the doctor's office hours _____

❑ What is the best time to call? _____

❑ What is the doctor's policy for returning calls? _____

❑ Whom should you speak with (i.e., physician's assistant, nurse, etc.) if the doctor can't come to the phone? _____

❑ What is the phone number for emergency calls or calls when the office is closed?
_____

❑ Whom can you call if your doctor is out of town? _____

B. Be ready to tell your doctor these things:

❑ What do I think the problem is and when did it start? _____

❑ What makes it better and worse? _____

❑ What are my signs and symptoms? Be specific. If you have pain, be able to say where the pain is, how much it hurts, and if it is dull, aching, stabbing, throbbing, etc. _____
_____

❑ Results of home testing such as your temperature, blood pressure, pulse rate per minute, etc.
_____

❑ Medicines you take. Know the name(s), dose(s), etc. Include over-the-counter ones, vitamins, etc.
_____

❑ Allergies to medicines, food, etc.
_____

❑ Other medical conditions you have _____

❑ Medical conditions that run in your family _____
_____

❏ Your lifestyle: Eating, drinking, sleeping, exercising habits, etc. _____
_____

❏ Concerns you have about your health _____

❏ What you would like the doctor to do for you _____

❏ Your pharmacist's phone number _____

Note: If needed, have your medical records, results of lab tests and x-rays, etc. from other health care providers sent to your doctor before your visit.

Checklist 2 – During the Doctor/Provider Visit Or Call

A. Tell the doctor the answers to the questions and the information you wrote down in Checklist 1. Take the list with you to the doctor's office. Make sure you have your eyeglasses and hearing aid, if you need them.

B. Ask your doctor these questions:

❏ What do you think the problem or diagnosis is? If you are confused by medical terms, ask for simple definitions. Repeat in your own words what the doctor has told you. Use simple phrases like, "Do I hear you say that…?" Or "My understanding of the problem is…" _____
_____

❏ Do I need any tests to rule out or confirm your diagnosis? If so, what tests do I need? Where do I go for the test(s) and how and when will I get the test results? _____
_____

❏ What do I need to do to treat the problem? How can I prevent it in the future? Are any changes needed in my activities? _____
_____

❏ Do I need to take any medicine? If so, what is the name of the medicine, how often do I take it, and how long do I take it? What side effects should I be aware of? Which ones should I let you know about? _____
_____

❏ When do I need to call or see you again? _____

❏ How are costs handled for this visit and tests? _____

Checklist 3 – After the Doctor/Provider Visit or Call

❑ Follow your doctor's advice. If you can't remember what to do, call the doctor's office. Ask, again, what it is you should do. _____

❑ Tell your doctor if you feel worse, have additional problems, or have bad side effects from medicines your doctor told you to take. _____

❑ Keep return visit appointments. If you need to cancel or reschedule an appointment, call your doctor's office at least 24 hours ahead of time.

Rating Your Doctor

In order to feel good about your medical care, you should feel good about your doctor, too. Ask the following questions to evaluate your physician.

■ Does your doctor listen to you and answer all your questions about the causes and treatment of your medical problems? Or, is he or she vague, impatient, or unwilling to answer?

■ Are you comfortable with your doctor? Can you openly discuss your feelings and talk about personal concerns, including sexual and emotional problems?

■ Does your doctor take a thorough history? Your doctor should ask about past physical and emotional problems, your family medical history, medications you take, and other matters that affect your health.

■ Does your doctor address the root causes of your medical problems or simply prescribe medications to treat the symptoms?

■ Are you satisfied with the doctor's substitute when he or she is not available?

■ Do you feel at ease asking your doctor questions that may sound "silly"?

■ Does your doctor explain things in simple terms?

■ Is the office staff friendly? Do they listen to you?

■ Does your doctor answer your telephone calls promptly?

■ Are you generally kept waiting for a long time when you have an appointment?

■ Does the doctor have hospital privileges at a respected hospital?

If you are not satisfied with your answers to these questions, discuss your concerns with your doctor. If, after this discussion, you are still not satisfied, consider looking for another doctor.

Having a Routine Checkup

The routine physical exam from a doctor or at a health clinic is a way to find out about the state of your health. It allows you to ask your doctor questions. It helps you find out if you have a health problem you don't know about. Some diseases like high blood pressure and some cancers may not have any symptoms in the early stages. Tests your doctor does can help detect these. Check the chart on page 17 for when health tests and checkups are recommended.

The basic parts of a checkup are:

- A complete medical history (questions on family health history, previous illnesses, emotional well-being)

- A check on how well body organs are functioning (eyes, ears, heart, skin, bowels, etc.)

- Checking the vital signs (blood pressure, pulse, breathing rate, temperature)

- Actual body examination (listening, thumping and looking at specific body parts)

- Routine diagnostic tests (blood tests, X-rays, etc.)

- A check of specific health concerns

Tests & What They Are For

Blood Pressure Test – Checks 2 kinds of pressure within the blood vessels. The higher number (systolic blood pressure) gauges the pressure when your heart is pumping. The lower number (diastolic blood pressure) gauges the pressure between heartbeats. High blood pressure is a symptomless disease that can lead to a heart attack and/or a stroke.

Vision – Checks for marked changes or degeneration of eye functioning

Pap Test – Checks for early signs of cervical cancer, uterine cancer and genital herpes

Mammography – An X-ray to detect breast tumors or problems

Professional Breast Exam – A physician or nurse examines the breasts for signs of abnormalities

Digital Rectal Exam – Checks for early signs of colorectal and/or prostate abnormalities including cancer

Stool Blood Test – Checks for early signs of colorectal abnormalities, including cancer

Sigmoidoscopy – Checks for early signs of colorectal abnormalities and cancer

Cholesterol Blood Test – Checks the levels of fatty deposits (cholesterol) in the blood. High cholesterol levels are linked to heart disease.

Glaucoma Screening – Checks for increased pressure within the eye. Glaucoma can result in blindness if not treated.

Common Health Tests & How Often to Have Them

Health Test		Ages 20-29	Ages 30-39	Ages 40-49	Age 50 and older
Physical Exam					
Blood Pressure					
Vision					
Pap Test[1]	**W**				
Mammogram[2]	**O**				
Breast Self-Examination*	**M**	Monthly	Monthly	Monthly	Monthly
Professional Breast Examination	**E**				
	N				
Testicular Self-Exam**	**M E N**		Monthly		
Digital Rectal Exam					
Stool Blood Test					
Sigmoidoscopy					
Cholesterol Blood Test[3]					
Glaucoma Screening[4]					
Regular Dental Checkup					
Diabetes Screening[5]					

■ Every year　　▥ Every 1–2 years　　▨ Every 2–3 years　　▧ Every 3–5 years

Note: Recommendations for routine medical exams may vary. These apply only to healthy people who do not have symptoms of illnesses. If you have an increased risk of a particular illness, testing may need to be done sooner or more often. Extra tests may also need to be done. Follow your doctor's advice. Also, check with your insurance company to see if and when tests are covered.

1. Pap tests should start at age 18, or under age 18 if sexual activity has begun. They should be given every year until tests are normal 3 years in a row. Thereafter, pap tests should be given at least every 3 years. {*Note:* The American College of Obstetricians and Gynecologists recommends an annual pap test.}

2. As recommended by The National Cancer Institute. Women who are at higher risk for breast cancer should seek expert medical advice about whether to have mammograpms before age 40 and how often to get mammograms in their 40s.

3. The National Cholesterol Education Program (NCEP) recommends a blood cholesterol test at least once every 5 years and that high-density lipoprotein (HDL) be part of the initial cholesterol testing.

4. Glaucoma screening is recommended earlier for African Americans. Screening should begin every 2 to 3 years between the ages of 40 and 49.

5. Diabetes screening should be done every 3 years starting at age 45.

* See "How to Examine Your Breasts" on pages 222 and 223.
** See "Testicular Self-Exam (TSE)" on page 221.

2. Medical Exams & Tests

Immunization Schedule & Record

Age ▶ Vaccine[1] ▼	Birth	1 month	2 months	4 months	6 months	12 months	15 months	18 months	4–6 years	11–16 years	14–16 years
Hepatitis B[2,3]	Hep B-1										
		Hep B-2			Hep B-3					Hep B-3[3]	
Diphtheria Tetanus Pertussis[4]			DTaP	DTaP	DTaP				DTaP	Td[4]	
H. Influenzae type b[5]			Hib	Hib	Hib	Hib					
Polio[6]			IPV	IPV		Polio			Polio		
Measles, Mumps, Rubella[7]						MMR			MMR[7]	MMR[7]	
Varicella[8]						Var				Var[8]	
Rotavirus[9]			RV	RV	RV						

Approved by the Advisory Committee on Immunization Practices (ACIP), the American Academy of Pediatrics (AAP), and the American Academy of Family Physicians (AAFP), for January – December 1999.

1. This shows what vaccines your child should get and when. Some vaccines may be given with others.
2, 3. The type, timing, and dose of Hepatitis B vaccine that an infant gets is based on the mother's Hepatitis B status. Hepatitis B should also be given to children and teenagers who have not had 3 doses of the vaccine.
4. The 4th dose can be given as early as 12 months, if the 3rd dose was given 6 months sooner. Td (tetanus and diphtheria) is recommended at 11 to 12 years of age, if at least 5 years have gone by since the last dose of DTP, DTaP, or DT. After that, Td boosters should be given every 10 years.
5. There are 3 brands of Hib vaccines. With one brand, the 6 month dose is not given.
6. Two forms are used: IPV and OPV. The first 2 doses should be IPV followed by 2 doses of OPV or 2 doses of IPV.
7. The 2nd dose of MMR is recommended at 4 to 6 years of age, but may be given during any visit if at least 1 month has gone by since the 1st dose. The 2nd dose should be given no later than 11 to 12 years of age.
8. Children who have not had chickenpox should get the VAR vaccine at 11 to 12 years of age. Children 13 years of age or older should get 2 doses, at least 1 month apart.
9. Rotavirus is a common virus in children under age 5 that causes diarrhea and vomiting. The 1st dose of the vaccine should not be given before 6 weeks of age. All 3 doses should be given by the first birthday.

Adult Immunizations

Td[4]	Tuberculin Tests	Influenza Vaccine (A&B)	Pneumococcal Vaccine
Every 10 years after 11-16 years of age	Upon exposure	Annually at age 65 and older	Once at 65 years

Home Medical Tests

Medical self-testing kits are easy to use, relatively inexpensive, and readily available. They can be used without a visit to the doctor. It's no wonder that Americans are buying them more and more, spending over $500 million annually. Home tests can offer you a sense of self-reliance that can assist, though not take the place of, the service of your doctor.

Self-testing kits can be grouped into two categories:

- Those that diagnose when conditions are or are not present. These include the popular self-testing kits for pregnancy, cholesterol, and kits that test for blood in the stool.

- Those that monitor an ongoing condition. These include blood sugar testing for diabetes and blood pressure kits for high blood pressure.

The U.S. Public Health Service and the Food and Drug Administration (FDA) offer some suggestions for safe and proper use of self-testing kits. (Each of these does not necessarily apply to all tests.)

- For test kits that contain chemicals, note the expiration date. Beyond that date, chemicals may lose potency and affect results. Don't buy or use a test kit after the expiration date.

- Check whether the product needs protection from heat or cold. If so, don't leave it in the car trunk or by a sunny window on the trip home. At home, follow storage directions.

- Study the package insert. First, read it through to get a general idea of how to perform the test. Then, go back and review the instructions and diagrams until you fully understand each step.

- Be sure you understand what the test is intended to do and what its limitations may be. Remember, the tests are not 100 percent accurate.

- If the test results rely on color comparison and you're color-blind, ask someone who is not color-blind to help you interpret the results.

- Note special precautions, such as avoiding physical activity or certain foods and medications before testing.

- Follow instructions exactly, including the specimen collection process, if that is a part of the test. Sequence is important.

- Don't skip a step.

- When collecting a urine specimen (unless you use a container from a kit), wash the container thoroughly and rinse out all soap traces, preferably with distilled water.

- When a step is timed, be precise. Use a stopwatch, or at least a watch with a second hand.

- Note what you should do if the results are positive, negative, or unclear.

- If something isn't clear, don't guess. Call the "800" number on the package or call a pharmacist for information.

- Keep accurate records of results.

- As with medications, keep test kits that contain chemicals out of the reach of children. Throw away used test materials as directed.

Report any malfunction of a self-test to the manufacturer or to the FDA through the agency's reporting system:

U.S. Pharmacopeia, Practitioner's Reporting Network, 12601 Twinbrook Parkway, Rockville, MD 20852. Phone: 1-800-638-6725.

Taking Medications Safely

Medications can be harmful if not used properly. The tips below will help to reduce medicine-related problems:

- Tell your doctor if:
  - You've ever had an allergic reaction, and to what
  - You are pregnant or breast-feeding
  - Another doctor is also treating you
  - You have diabetes or kidney or liver disease
  - You use alcohol, tobacco, or "street drugs"

- Have your doctor keep a record of all the medicines you take. This includes over-the-counter (OTC) items like vitamins, aspirins, laxatives, etc., as well as any medicine another doctor has prescribed.

- Ask your doctor to tell you what a medicine is for, when you should take it, and for how long. Find out, too, if it should be taken in a special way, i.e., with food or plenty of water. Write these things down so you don't forget what the doctor says.

- Use the same pharmacy to buy prescriptions as well as over-the-counter medications. This way, a complete record of your medicines can be kept in one place. This is especially important if more than one doctor has been writing your prescriptions. Your pharmacist can also spot possible harmful combinations of medicines, and food-and-medication interactions.

- Ask your pharmacists to clearly mark each vial with all necessary instructions.

- Always keep medicines in their original containers.

- Let your doctor know about your past reactions to certain medicines. Tolerance levels may change with age. For instance, as some people age, they may show greater sensitivity to some medications such as painkillers or tranquilizers.

- Ask about the possible side effects of a medication. If you do experience some, call your physician and find out what you should do. Often, just a change in dosage is all that is needed.

- Don't drink alcohol while on a medication if you don't know its effect. Regular alcohol use can speed up the metabolism of certain medicines, reducing their intended effectiveness. Some medicines, such as sedatives, can become deadly when used with alcohol.

- Never take someone else's medication.

- Throw away all medications that have expired.

- Try to reduce the need for medications, such as sleeping pills or laxatives. For example, a hot bath and a glass of milk might help you sleep at night. Changing your diet to increase your fiber intake might replace the need for a laxative. Check with your doctor for non-medical alternatives.

- Don't stop taking medications your doctor has prescribed, even if you feel better. Check with your doctor first.

3. Medications

Questions to Ask about Medications

Make sure you get clear answers to these questions before you take any medications.

- What is the name of the medicine and what will it do?
- When should I take it and for how long?
- Are there side effects?
- Is there anything I should avoid while taking it? (Examples: alcohol, sunlight, etc.) Should I take it with meals?
- Is there a generic equivalent?
- Will it interfere with other medicines I am taking?
- Should I stop taking it if I feel better?

Over-the-Counter (OTC) Medications

Over-the-counter (OTC) medicines are ones that you can get without a doctor's prescription. They are generally less potent than prescription medicines. When taken in large amounts, though, an OTC medicine might equal or exceed the dose of a prescription medicine. Follow the directions on the label or package insert.

Use OTC medicines wisely

Follow these tips:

- Ask your doctor what OTC products you should avoid and which ones are safe for you to use. For example, find out what your doctor prefers you to take for pain and fever. (See "Your Home Pharmacy" on pages 22 and 23.)
- Do not exceed the dosages on the labels or take OTC medicines on a regular basis unless your doctor tells you to.
- Read the package labels or look up the name of the medicine in the *Physician's Desk Reference for Nonprescription Drugs*. Information and warnings listed can help you decide whether or not the product is safe for you to take. If you are unsure whether or not a particular OTC medication will help or harm you, check with your doctor or pharmacist.
- Don't take any OTC product if you are pregnant or nursing a baby unless your doctor says it is okay.
- Be sure to store medicines in a convenient dry place, but out of children's reach.
- Don't ever tell children that medicine is candy.
- Check the expiration dates periodically. Discard and replace as needed.
- If you have an allergy to a medicine, check the list of ingredients on all other medicines to see if what you are allergic to is in them. Some labels will warn you not to take that medicine if you are allergic to a certain medicine or ingredient.

3. Medications

Your Home Pharmacy

Basic Over-the-Counter (OTC) Medications that Can Help with Self-Care

Medicines	Common Uses	Side Effects/Warnings
Activated charcoal	To absorb some poisons	Call Poison Control Center before using
Antacids ex: Tums, Rolaids, Mylanta	Stomach upset, heartburn	Don't use for more than 2 weeks without your doctor's advice. Don't use high-sodium ones if on a low-salt diet. Don't use if you have chronic kidney failure.
Antidiarrheal medicine ex: Kaopectate, Imodium A-D, Pepto-Bismol	Diarrhea	Don't give Pepto-Bismol to anyone under 19 years of age because it contains salicylates, which have been linked to Reye's Syndrome. Pepto-Bismol can cause black stools.
Antihistamines ex: Chlor-Trimeton, Benadryl	Allergies, cold symptom relief, relieves itching	May cause drowsiness, agitation, dry mouth, and/or problems with urinating. Don't use with alcohol, when operating machines, or when driving. Don't use if you have glaucoma or an enlarged prostate or problems passing urine.
Cough suppressant ex: Robitussin-DM or others with dextromethorphan	Dry cough without mucus	May cause drowsiness. People with glaucoma, or problems passing urine should avoid ones with diphenhydramine.
Decongestant ex: Sudafed, Dimetapp	Stuffy and runny nose, post-nasal drip, allergies, fluid on the ears	Don't use if have high blood pressure, diabetes, glaucoma, heart disease, history of stroke, or an enlarged prostate.
Expectorant ex: Robitussin or others with guaifenesin	Cough with mucus	Don't give with an antihistamine.
Laxatives ex: Ex-Lax, Correctol (stimulant-types), Metamucil (bulk-forming type)	Constipation	Long-term use of stimulant-type can lead to dependence and to muscle weakness due to potassium loss.
Pain relievers		
Acetaminophen ex: Tylenol, Anacin-3, Datril, Liquiprin Panadol, Tempra	Pain relief, reduces fever (does not reduce inflammation)	More gentle on stomach than other OTC pain relievers. Can result in liver problems in heavy alcohol users. Large doses or long-term use can cause liver or kidney damage.

Chart continued on next page

Your Home Pharmacy, *Continued*

Chart continued

Medicines	Common Uses	Side Effects/Warnings
Aspirin ex: Bayer, Bufferin	Pain relief, reduces fever and inflammation	Can cause stomach upset (which is made worse with alcohol use). May contribute to stomach ulcers and bleeding. Avoid if you: Take blood-thinning medicine, have an ulcer, have asthma, are under 19 years of age (due to its association with Reye's Syndrome), and/or are having surgery within 2 weeks. High doses or prolonged use can cause ringing in the ears.
Ibuprofen ex: Advil, Medipren, Motrin, Pamprin-IC, Children's Advil, Children's Motrin	Pain relief, reduces fever and inflammation, especially good for menstrual cramps	Can cause stomach upset and ulcers. Take with milk or food. Can make you more sensitive to the effects of the sun. Don't use if allergic to aspirin. Don't use if have ulcers, blood clotting problems, kidney disease.
Ketoprofen (adult) ex: Actron, Orudis KT	Pain relief, reduces fever and inflammation	Can cause stomach upset and ulcers. Take with milk or food. Can make you more sensitive to the effects of the sun. Don't use if allergic to aspirin. Don't use if have ulcers, blood clotting problems, kidney disease.
Naproxen Sodium (adult) ex: Aleve	Pain relief, reduces fever and inflammation	Can cause stomach upset and ulcers. Take with milk or food. Can make you more sensitive to the effects of the sun. Don't use if allergic to aspirin. Don't use if have ulcers, blood clotting problems, kidney disease.
Syrup of Ipecac	To induce vomiting for some poisons	Call Poison Control Center before giving.
Throat anesthetic ex: Sucrets, Chloraseptic spray	Minor sore throat	Don't give throat lozenges to children under age 5.
Toothache anesthetic ex: Anbesol	Toothache, teething	Check with doctor before use with babies under 4 months old.

3. Medications

Your Home Pharmacy, *Continued*

Basic Supplies that Can Help with Self-Care

Supplies , Etc.	Common Uses
Adhesive bandages, sterile gauze, first aid tape, scissors	Minor wounds
Antiseptic preparation ex: Betadine	Abrasions, cuts
Eye drops and artificial tears ex: Murine	Minor eye irritations
Heating pad/hot water bottle	Minor pains, strains, menstrual cramps
Hemorrhoid preparation ex: Preparation H, Hemorid	Hemorrhoids
Humidifier, vaporizer ("cool-mist")	Add moisture to the air
Hydrocortisone cream ex: Cortaid	Minor skin irritations, itching and rashes
Ice pack/heat pack or heating pad	Minor pain and injuries
Petroleum jelly ex: Vaseline	Chafing, diaper rash, dry skin
Rubbing alcohol	Topical antiseptic, clean thermometer
Sunscreen - look for ones with a Sun/Protection Factor (SPF) of 15 or more	Prevents sunburn, protects against skin cancer
Thermometer (mercury-containing, digital, etc.)	Measure temperature
Tongue depressor, flashlight	Check for redness or infection in throat
Tweezers	Remove splinters

Overhauling Your Medicine Cabinet

Inventory your medicine cabinet at least once a year:

- Take everything out of the medicine cabinet.
- Check expiration dates. Throw out all out-dated medicine. If you're not sure about a certain item, call your pharmacist and ask what the shelf life is.
- If medications are not in original containers and labeled clearly, throw them away. It's danger-ous to store medicines in anything but their original containers. Some medicines come in tinted glass, for example, because exposure to light may cause them to deteriorate.

- Discard old tubes of cream that have become hardened or cracked. Throw out any liquid medicines that appear cloudy or filmy.
- Every medication is a potential poison. If there are children in the house, keep all medicines and vitamins locked in a high cabinet, well out of their reach.
- Stock a container of syrup of ipecac to induce vomiting for some poisons. {*Note:* Call the poison control center before giving syrup of ipecac.}

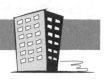

Ambulatory Surgery

Can you have surgery without being admitted to a hospital? Yes, and it's recommended in many cases. Ambulatory surgery can be done on an out-patient basis at a hospital or at facilities that perform out-patient surgeries. Procedures that best qualify for ambulatory surgery:

- Do not require opening a primary body section, like the chest or skull
- Do not require blood transfusions
- Require very little or no general anesthesia
- Do not require specialized postoperative care
- Do not require hours on the operating table
- Pose little risk of complication or additional surgery

The most common types of surgeries performed in an ambulatory care center include:

- Hernia repair
- Some plastic surgeries
- Tubal ligation
- Dilation and curettage (D & C)
- Breast biopsy
- Tonsillectomy
- Cataract removal
- Orthopedic procedures (such as setting a broken bone)
- Varicose vein surgery
- Glaucoma procedures

Ambulatory or outpatient surgery has many advantages:

- Hospitalization poses the risk of exposure to infections and may also keep patients bedridden longer than is necessary.
- Ambulatory surgery gets you in and out quickly.
- The patient has a good deal of choice as to when the surgery will occur. The surgery is scheduled by appointment for patient convenience.
- Most people prefer healing at home in their own beds to staying in a hospital. The home can be a more comfortable place in which to heal than a hospital with its hectic schedules.
- Medical bills are much lower if you don't have to stay in a hospital overnight.

Things to consider:

- Many procedures need special preparation ahead of time. Follow your doctor's orders exactly.
- You may need someone to drive you home and stay with you as you recover.
- Do not bring valuables with you when you have outpatient surgery.

Hospital Admissions

The golden rule here is to arrange as much as you can before being admitted. Ask the following questions:

- Can you have the needed forms mailed to your home before being admitted? This will give you more time to review and complete them. Can you be "preadmitted" over the telephone?

- Is your insurance coverage well understood by both the billing department and you?

- Can you reserve a private or semiprivate room with your coverage?

- What identification will you need to have?

- Do you need special foods? If so, how can you arrange for them?

Saving Money in the Hospital

Don't stay in the hospital unless you need to! The daily hospital rate in some sections of the country is now as high as $1,000. And that doesn't include the costs for treatments, medicines, or doctor's fees. The hospital should never be viewed as a place to get a good rest. Consider these tips:

- Choose outpatient services whenever you can. Many routine lab tests, diagnostic tests and surgeries can be done for less money as an outpatient. You avoid the cost of an overnight stay in a hospital.

- As an inpatient, stay only the prescribed time that is necessary. Ask your doctor about home health care, which can provide a wide range of services at less cost than in a hospital.

- Beware of duplication of tests. Be sure to ask the doctor about what blood tests, X-rays, and medical procedures you can expect.

- Be sure you know when checkout time is and make plans to observe it; otherwise, you're likely to be charged for an extra day's stay.

- If your health problem isn't an emergency, avoid being admitted to a hospital on a weekend. The hospital staff is reduced then, and testing will usually not begin until Monday.

- Same-day or ambulatory surgery is a big moneysaver when compared to inpatient surgery. It can be used for minor procedures such as biopsies, cataract removal, etc.

- Keep a list of all services you receive in the hospital. Ask for an itemized bill so you can make sure you are billed correctly.

Types of Surgery

It's funny. People think of surgery as "major" when it happens to them and "minor" when it's being done to someone else! In reality, surgery is thought to be major when it involves any vital organs and/or requires a long time period to perform. The following words classify various surgeries:

Curative – A procedure that rids the body of a problem or corrects a condition

Diagnostic – A procedure that helps in making a diagnosis about a suspected problem

Elective – A procedure that may or may not be done, depending upon the patient's wishes

Emergency – An immediate operation to save a life or maintain the use of a body part

Exploratory – A surgery that explores a body organ or body area for a suspected disorder

Palliative – A surgery that eases bodily pain but doesn't cure the problem

Planned – A surgery set up well in advance of the actual operation date

Urgent – An operation that must be done within a matter of hours

Patient Rights

What rights and privileges can you expect from a hospital when you become a patient? According to the American Hospital Association (AHA), there are specific standards of care that all patients are entitled to. The AHA has developed a voluntary code, The Patient's Bill of Rights, which presents guidelines for both staff and patients.

■ You have the right to considerate and respectful care.

■ You have the right to obtain from your physician complete, current information concerning your diagnosis, treatment, and prognosis in terms you can reasonably be expected to understand.

■ You have the right to receive from your physician information necessary to give informed consent prior to the start of any procedure and/or treatment.

■ You have the right to refuse treatment to the extent permitted by law, and to be informed of the medical consequences of your action.

■ You have the right to privacy concerning your own medical care program, including all communications and records pertaining to your care.

■ You have the right to expect that within its capacity a hospital must make a reasonable response to your request for services.

■ You have the right to obtain information about any relationship of your hospital to other health care and educational institutions insofar as your care is concerned.

■ You have the right to be advised if the hospital proposes to engage in or perform human experimentation affecting your care or treatment.

■ You have the right to expect reasonable continuity of care.

■ You have the right to examine and receive an explanation of your bill regardless of the source of payment.

■ You have the right to know what hospital rules and regulations apply to your conduct as a patient.

Informed Consent

Every patient should be aware of the policy of informed consent, an ethical standard in medicine that implies that you have been given an explanation and fully understand your treatment. You should be able to explain in your own words what your treatment is about. You should know what the likelihood is that the medical procedure will accomplish what it's supposed to. The benefits and the accompanying risks should always be identified clearly. You should also be notified if your treatment is experimental in nature.

The physician should review any alternatives that are available in lieu of surgery or other procedures. There are no guaranteed outcomes in medicine, but informed consent enables YOU to make a rational and educated decision about your treatment. It is also a tool that promotes greater understanding between you and your doctor and encourages joint decision making.

Three principles of informed consent that involve your responsibility as a patient are:

■ You cannot demand services that go beyond what are considered "acceptable" practices of medicine or that violate professional ethics.

- You must recognize that you may be faced with some uncertainties or unpleasantness.

- You should, if competent, be responsible for your choices. Don't have others make decisions for you.

Advance Directives

There is a federal law called the Patient Self-Determination Act. It requires hospitals and nursing homes to give you information about your rights as a patient under their care. Advance directives are a legal way for you to declare your wishes regarding the withholding or removal of life-sustaining care if you:

- Suffer from a terminal illness, or

- Are in an incurable or irreversible mental or physical condition with no reasonable expectations of recovery

There are two types of advance directives:

- Living Will – A document that spells out what medical treatment you would want or not want if you were unable to state it yourself. Most states have their own living will form, or you can make up your own. You should discuss your living will with your family and physician.

- Durable Power of Attorney (Health-Care Proxy) – A document that names a person who would make treatment decisions for you if you are not able to make them yourself. Generally, it is a person who knows you and your values well, and is in a good position to represent your wishes to your physician.

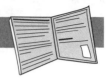

Insurance Terms

Coinsurance – Means you pay a certain percentage (usually 20%) of the costs of a service after a yearly deductible is met.

Copayment – The percentage of or preset fee for the cost of an office visit or covered service

Covered Benefits – Medical expenses that are paid for under the terms of a policy

Deductible – The cost for medical expenses that you pay before the company pays anything

Exclusion – A service the health insurance company will not cover or pay for

Health Maintenance Organization (HMO) – A type of managed care plan. With an HMO, you pick a primary doctor who manages all of the medical services you receive. HMOs cover the costs of many preventive services.

Indemnity Plan – A traditional type of health plan. With this type of plan, also called fee-for-service, you can use any medical provider. You pay a yearly deductible. After that, you pay a percentage of the cost of services until an out-of-pocket maximum is met.

Managed Care – A health care system that finances and delivers care. The goal is to provide health care that is cost effective and of high quality.

Point-Of-Service (POS) – An HMO that gives you the option to go to providers outside of the plan's network of providers and still get some of the cost paid for by the plan.

Pre-existing Condition – A health problem you had when the insurance took effect

Preferred Provider Organization (PPO) – A managed care plan in which a network of providers contracts with an organization to give medical services at a discount to its members. With a PPO, you can choose one or more providers from a list of those who participate with the health plan.

Prior Authorization – Approval ahead of time is needed from the health plan for certain services to be covered

Consider Your Needs

Policies vary; so do costs and what is covered. Ask your employee benefits person or Employee Assistance Program (EAP) representative for information on the health insurance your company offers. Before you choose one plan over another get answers to these questions:

- Is my whole family covered?
- Are most services covered?
- Are routine checkups covered?
- Are well-care visits covered?
- Are immunizations covered?
- Is maternity care covered?
- Are there deductibles? What are they?
- Are there limits if my problem is chronic?
- How many days are covered in the hospital?
- Are psychological services covered?
- Can I choose my provider? Can I be seen by the same provider at each visit?
- Are specialist visits covered?

Compare the answers you get from the insurance plans you are considering. Decide what is important to you and your family. Choose the plan that best meets your needs.

At some point in your life (maybe it's right now), you or a loved one may be faced with making a medical decision that could affect your quality of life. You can deal with this issue with greater ease when you have all the information you need. One way to get this information is to ask your doctor all the right questions. This section will teach you what to ask.

Key Questions Checklist

(Photocopy as needed)

The following is a summary of the key questions and recommendations that will help you make medical decisions. Use them as a guide when you visit your doctor or health care provider. Check off the items you wish to discuss with your doctor or health care provider as the need arises.

1. **Description – What is my current complaint?**
   - ❑ What do I think the problem is?
   - ❑ When did it start?
   - ❑ What makes it better?
   - ❑ What makes it worse?
   - ❑ What are my signs and symptoms?
   - ❑ What daily habits are affected (i.e., eating, sleeping, activity, etc.)? Is it constant or does it only occur at certain times?

2. **Diagnosis – What is my diagnosis?**
   - ❑ Can you explain the diagnosis to me in detail?
   - ❑ Is my condition chronic or acute?
   - ❑ If it is chronic, how will it affect my life?
   - ❑ Is my condition one that will be with me all of the time or will it come and go?
   - ❑ If it will come and go, how often should I expect it?
   - ❑ Is there anything I can do to help prevent it?
   - ❑ Is my condition contagious? If yes, what should I do?
   - ❑ Is my condition genetic? If yes, what can I do?
   - ❑ How certain are you about this diagnosis?
   - ❑ Do you have any literature about my condition?
   - ❑ Is there a support group available?

3. **Treatment – What is the recommended treatment plan?**
   - ❑ Write down a description of the recommended treatment plan.
   - ❑ What results do you expect?
   - ❑ When can I expect to see results?

If you are discussing surgery:
   - ❑ Give me a step-by-step account of the procedure, including anesthesia and recovery. Also, consider getting a second opinion.

If you are discussing a test:
   - ❑ What is the test called, and how will it help identify what is wrong?
   - ❑ Will it give us specific or general information?
   - ❑ If the answer is general, where do we go from here?
   - ❑ Will more tests be necessary?
   - ❑ How accurate and reliable is the test?
   - ❑ Is the test invasive or noninvasive?
   - ❑ What will I have to do to prepare for the test?
   - ❑ Where do I go for the test?
   - ❑ How and when will I get the test's results?

(Also see "Questions to Ask about Medications" on page 21.)

4. **Benefits – What are the benefits of the treatment?**

   ❑ What will be the specific benefits if I go ahead with the treatment?

   ❑ To what extent will the treatment improve my condition?

   ❑ Is there documented evidence that shows the recommended treatment will have a positive outcome?

5. **Risks – What are the potential risks of the treatment?**

   ❑ List the possible risks and complications.

   ❑ Do the benefits outweigh the risks, or vice-versa?

   ❑ Make a list of the risks and benefits, rating each between 1 and 5 to aid in your decision-making process. (1 being not as important, and 5 being very important).

6. **Success – What is the success rate for the treatment?**

   ❑ What is the national success rate?

   ❑ What is the success rate at the hospital/medical facility where my treatment is planned?

   ❑ What is the surgeon's success rate and experience with the surgery?

   ❑ How many procedures are the above success rates based on?

   ❑ Are there any personal factors that will affect my odds either way?

   ❑ How long will the results of my surgery/treatment last?

7. **Timing – When should I begin the treatment?**

   ❑ When is the best time to get started with the treatment plan?

   ❑ Do I have to undergo treatment right away? If not, how long can I safely wait?

   ❑ Determine the best time for you to begin the treatment plan.

8. **Alternatives – What are my options?**

   ❑ What will happen if I decide to do nothing?

   ❑ What are my other options? Include non-surgical and outpatient alternatives if you are discussing surgery.

   ❑ If you are not satisfied with your options, discuss this with your doctor. If you are still not satisfied, you may consider consulting another physician.

   ❑ Look into every option which you are considering as thoroughly as the original treatment plan.

9. **Cost – How much will the treatment cost?**

   ❑ What is the cost of the recommended treatment plan?

   ❑ Check with your insurance company to see what portion will be covered and whether you need to do anything to receive maximum coverage, i.e., seeking a second opinion, getting preauthorization, etc.

   ❑ What related costs do I need to consider, i.e., time off work, child care, transportation, etc.?

10. **Decision – What do I decide to do?**

    ❑ You are now in a better position to make an intelligent, informed decision.

    ❑ Remember, you are ultimately responsible for your body and have the right to choose or refuse treatment.

    ❑ If you feel rushed or uncomfortable when you discuss this information with your doctor, tell him or her how you feel.

6. Medical Decisions

Medical Decision Comparison Chart

(Photocopy as needed)

Use this chart to help you compare different medical options that are available to you.

Diagnosis _____

	Option One		Option Two		Option Three	
Treatment						
Benefits						
Risks						
Success						
Timing						
Alternatives						
Cost						
Decision	Yes ❑	No ❑	Yes ❑	No ❑	Yes ❑	No ❑

6. Medical Decisions

Wallet-Size Checklist

1. Diagnosis
- ❑ What is my diagnosis?
- ❑ Is my condition chronic or acute?
- ❑ Is my condition one that will be with me constantly?
- ❑ Is there anything I can do to help prevent it?
- ❑ Is my condition contagious or genetic?
- ❑ How certain are you about this diagnosis?

2. Treatment
- ❑ What is the recommended treatment?
  If you are discussing medications:
- ❑ What will the medicine do for my particular problem?
- ❑ When, how often, and for how long should I take the medicine?
- ❑ How long before the medicine starts working?
- ❑ Will there be side effects?
- ❑ Will there be interactions with other medications I am taking?
  If you are discussing a test:
- ❑ What is the test called, and how will it help identify the problem?

- ❑ Will it give us specific or general information?
- ❑ Will more tests be necessary?
- ❑ How accurate and reliable is the test?
- ❑ How should I prepare for the test?
- ❑ Where do I go for the test?
- ❑ How and when will I get the test's results?
  If you are discussing surgery:
- ❑ Will you give me a step-by-step account of the procedure, including anesthesia and recovery?

3. Benefits vs. Risks
- ❑ What are the benefits if I go ahead with the treatment?
- ❑ What are the possible risks and complications?
- ❑ Do the benefits outweigh the risks or vice-versa?

4. Success
- ❑ What is the success rate for the treatment?
- ❑ Are there any personal factors that will affect my odds either way?

- ❑ How long will the results of my treatment last?

5. Timing
- ❑ When is the best time to begin the treatment?
- ❑ When can I expect to see results?

6. Alternatives
- ❑ What will happen if I decide to do nothing?
- ❑ What are my other options?

7. Cost
- ❑ What is the cost of the recommended treatment?
- ❑ What related costs should I consider, i.e., time off work, child care, travel, etc.?

8. Decision
- ❑ You can now make an informed decision.
- ❑ Remember, you have the right to choose or refuse treatment.
- ❑ If you feel rushed or uncomfortable when talking with your doctor, tell him or her how you feel.

©1994, American Institute for Preventive Medicine

Overall health includes proper dental care and good oral hygiene. A family dentist who is knowledgeable and prevention oriented is a valued part of everyone's health care team.

The Dental Checkup

A proper dental checkup should include these things:

- A visual check of the soft tissues (tongue, cheek, throat, and gums) for redness and puffiness, or white discoloration
- A check of the bite and jaw joints
- Measuring any pockets which may have developed between the teeth and the gums. (This is a check for gum [periodontal] problems.)
- A full set of X-rays (if they haven't been taken recently)
- Asking the patient about any areas of concern

When to Visit Your Dentist

- Every 6 months for a cleaning and checkup
- If your gums bleed easily or are swollen, reddened, or soft
- If you notice a change in your bite
- If you have an injury to a tooth or it is dislodged due to an accident. (It can often be replanted if you are seen by a dentist immediately.)
- If you have any discomfort from a tooth
- If you have a tendency to grind your teeth, experience pain near the jaw joint, or have chronic headaches

Dental Specialties

The American Dental Association recognizes a number of different dental specialties:

Endodontics – disease prevention and treatment of root pulp (the living tissue that conveys sensation to the tooth)

Oral Surgeon (Maxillofacial Surgeon) – surgical treatment of jaw and mouth injuries, diseases or tooth extraction

Orthodontics – correcting mouth deformities or tooth irregularities, often through braces or functional appliances

Pedodontics – care of children's teeth

Periodontics – preventive care and treatment of structures that surround and support the teeth (Example: gums)

Prosthodontics – rehabilitation of oral problems with such devices as bridges, crowns, or dentures

Public Health Dentistry – control of dental disease through community dental programs

All of these specialties require at least 2 additional years of advanced training after dental school

7. You & Your Dentist

People who are mentally healthy feel good about themselves and comfortable with others. They are also able to deal with the demands, challenges, and changes in everyday life.

Everyone, regardless of age, race, sex, or economic status, is subject to emotional upsets. You can feel down, angry, or anxious in response to a variety of things. Feelings like these can come and go quite often. When these feelings are disturbing, interfere with daily life, and/or linger for weeks or months, they may signal a problem that requires professional assistance. According to the National Institute for Mental Health (NIMH), at any given time, approximately 40 million Americans (about 1 in 6) experience a mental disorder that interferes with employment and/or daily life.

Mental Health Facts

- About 25% of the people who seek medical help for physical problems actually have troubled emotions.

- The most common reasons people seek mental health treatment are for depression and anxiety.

- Between 8 and 14 million Americans suffer from depression each year.

- Approximately 80 to 90% of all depressed people respond to treatment.

- Approximately 10% of Americans have phobias.

- 12.5 million Americans are drug abusers or are chemically dependent.

- 13 million are dependent on alcohol. (This includes 3 million children.)

- Nearly 25% of the elderly who are thought to be senile actually suffer some form of mental illness that can be treated effectively.

- Therapy does not have to take a long time. Almost one-half of the people who enter therapy will complete it in 7 sessions or less.

It's Smart to Ask for Help

Many people are reluctant to seek mental health services because of the "stigma" of having an "emotional" problem. Society has a tendency to view mental health issues differently from medical ones. When someone breaks a leg, has chest pains, or needs to get a prescription, they'll see a doctor. When they experience depression, excessive fears, or a problem with alcohol, though, they may be embarrassed to seek help. Many people view these conditions as "weaknesses" that they should be able to handle themselves. Unfortunately, this view keeps them from getting professional care that can help them deal with and/or treat these conditions.

To recognize a problem and receive psychological help is not a sign of weakness. To do so is a sign of strength. Also, taking part in your company's Employee Assistance Program (EAP) or seeing a therapist is completely confidential. No information will be given to anyone without your permission.

Reasons to Seek Help

The following symptoms usually signal the need for professional help. Only a trained professional can diagnose and determine the treatment needed.

- Thinking or talking about suicide
- Seeing or hearing things that aren't actually present
- Suspiciousness or paranoia
- Strange or grandiose ideas
- Crippling or excessive anxieties (fears or phobias)
- Wide mood swings (extreme highs and lows)
- Prolonged depression and apathy (a sense of hopelessness, loss of pleasure in life, confusion or constant frustration)
- Marked personality change
- Compulsive behaviors (i.e., over spending, overeating, excessive exercising)
- Marked changes in eating or sleeping patterns

- Excessive anger or hostility; destructive, abusive, or violent behavior
- Problems with the law
- Difficulty with authority
- Abuse of alcohol and/or other drugs
- Difficulty interacting with other people (spouse, parents, children, coworkers, and friends)
- Denial of obvious problems; strong resistance to receiving help
- Social withdrawal and isolation
- Inability to cope with the loss of a loved one
- Extreme jealousy
- Preoccupation with physical illness
- Overall decline in job performance
- Problems on the job
- A feeling that you've lost control of your life
- Inability to cope with problems or daily activities such as school, job or personal needs
- Sexual problems

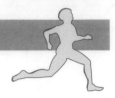

A new interest is taking hold today: The interest people have in making themselves healthy. The American public, in greater numbers than ever before, wants to do those things that will promote health, and longevity, and increase the quality of life. Exercise gyms are booming. Health foods are common. Cigarette smoking is the exception and not the rule. You can hardly go anywhere without seeing walkers or joggers. We have come a long way from Mark Twain's philosophy that "the only way to keep your health is to eat what you don't want, drink what you don't like and do what you'd rather not."

It's encouraging to see people's desire to make their lifestyle the best it can be! There is a shift from traditional medicine, which is designed to treat illness, to doing those things that prevent sickness from occurring in the first place. People want to become better health consumers as well. We recognize warning signs. We read labels. We know when a doctor is or is not needed. We are opening our eyes to the risk factors for conditions such as heart disease, diabetes, and cancer.

This chapter deals with 7 topics that are important to good health as well as to preventing disease.

Cigarette Smoking – Packing It In

It is not easy to quit smoking cigarettes. Why? Nicotine is a physically addictive substance. After an initial rejection by the body, a tolerance level develops in the smoker, and withdrawal symptoms occur when nicotine is withheld. Cigarettes also produce a psychological dependence. The desire to smoke is "triggered" by certain situations, emotions, and a need to inhale and exhale on something.

Smoking Facts

- Cigarette smoking is our nation's number 1 preventable cause of illness and premature death. Over 420,000 people in the U.S. die from the effects of smoking each year.

- After inhaling, 70–90% of the chemical compounds in a cigarette stay in the smoker's lungs.

- Cigarette smokers are 15 times more likely to get lung cancer, 16 times more likely to have emphysema, 10 times more likely to have bronchitis, and twice as likely to have a heart attack than nonsmokers.

- Nonsmokers who inhale secondhand smoke from a burning cigarette have an increased risk of lung cancer and heart disease as well.

- Children of smokers have twice the incidence of respiratory ailments as the children of nonsmokers.

- According to the American Cancer Society, 8 out of 10 smokers would like to quit.

The "Warm Pheasant" Plan to Quit Smoking

You've heard of quitting cigarettes cold turkey, all at once. Well, that works for some, but not all, smokers. In fact, there are as many ways to quit smoking as there are brands of cigarettes for sale. If you're like Mark Twain, who said, "Quitting smoking is easy. I've done it over a hundred times," you might want to try the "warm pheasant" method. Unlike the cold turkey approach, this three-phase plan allows you to continue to smoke while you prepare to quit, psychologically and physically.

Phase I: Preparing to Quit

This phase takes approximately 1 week.

- Mark a "quit" date on your calendar 1 week in advance.

- Keep track of each cigarette you smoke by making a slash mark on a piece of paper tucked in the wrapper of your cigarette pack.

- Every time you have an urge to light up, wait 10 minutes.

- Collect your cigarette butts in a "butt bottle." (The mere sight of so many spent cigarettes will graphically demonstrate just how much you really smoke in a week.)

Phase II: Quitting

This phase takes approximately 1–2 weeks.

- Throw away all your cigarettes and hide all smoking paraphernalia, like matches, lighters, ashtrays, and so forth.

- Whenever you have an urge to smoke, take a deep breath through your mouth and slowly exhale through pursed lips. Repeat 5–10 times.

- Change your routine to eliminate familiar smoking cues. If you always light up when driving to work, take a different route. Or substitute a walk for your usual coffee-and-cigarette break. Or sit in a chair you don't customarily use when relaxing or watching television at home.

- Take up activities you don't normally associate with smoking. Enroll in a cooking class, visit a nonsmoking friend, or go swimming at your local Y, for example.

- Keep your hands busy by holding something, such as a pen, Nerf Ball, or binder clip.

- In place of cigarettes, substitute other things that will provide oral gratification, like sugarless gum or mints, toothpicks, or coffee stirrers.

- Avoid drinking coffee and alcohol or eating foods high in sugar, like candy and pastries. They cause biochemical changes in the body that increase your desire for a cigarette.

- Create a "piggy bank" and put the money you used to spend on cigarettes in a jar. Watch it add up.

- Place a rubber band on your wrist and snap it every time you get an urge to smoke.

Phase III: Staying off Cigarettes

Allow 3 months for this final phase.

- Always remember that the craving to smoke will pass, whether you smoke or not.

- Renew your commitment to stay off cigarettes each day.

- Beware of saboteurs, usually other smokers, who may try to encourage you to light up. Assert your right to not smoke.

- Talk to a nonsmoking buddy for support.

- Make a list of good things you've noticed since you quit, e.g., food tastes better, you cough less, your clothes don't smell bad, and so forth.

- Continue to practice the behavior modification techniques listed in the quitting phase.

SOURCE: *The Smokeless Program*, American Institute for Preventive Medicine, Farmington Hills, Michigan, 1994.

9. Staying Well

Stress – Learning to Cope

Do you know what stress is?

- Stress is the body's nonspecific response to any increased demand placed upon it.
- Stressors are those events, objects, or thoughts that will cause the stress response to occur.

Keeping Track of Stress Signals

Many of us have symptoms of stress every day without realizing it. To recognize the signals your body is sending you, read this partial list of stress symptoms. Make a mental note or place a check next to those symptoms that you've experienced when under stress. Place 2 checks if you experience this symptom frequently. Write in any other symptoms you experience when feeling stressed. {*Note:* Symptoms of stress could indicate a physical problem and should be checked out before assuming you are not coping well.}

Symptoms of Stress

- ❏ Backache
- ❏ Clearing throat
- ❏ Clenching hands
- ❏ Constipation
- ❏ Crying
- ❏ Depression
- ❏ Diarrhea
- ❏ Drinking
- ❏ Dry mouth and throat
- ❏ Faintness or dizziness
- ❏ Feeling fearful
- ❏ Feeling lonely
- ❏ Foot tapping
- ❏ Forgetfulness
- ❏ Frequent urination
- ❏ Gritting teeth
- ❏ Headache
- ❏ Insomnia
- ❏ Irritability
- ❏ Lack of concentration
- ❏ Lack of interest
- ❏ Loss of appetite
- ❏ Low energy level
- ❏ Neckache
- ❏ Negative thoughts
- ❏ Nervous tic

- ❏ Nightmares
- ❏ Overeating
- ❏ Pacing
- ❏ Rapid heartbeat
- ❏ Sexual difficulties
- ❏ Skin rash
- ❏ Smoking
- ❏ Sweating
- ❏ Temper outbursts
- ❏ Queasy stomach
- ❏ _____
- ❏ _____
- ❏ _____
- ❏ _____

Conditions Related to Stress

Research has revealed a clear link between physical illness and stress. In some cases, stress plays an important part in the nature and severity of the illness. In fact, the American Academy of Family Physicians states that approximately two-thirds of all visits to the family doctor are for stress-related disorders. Read the list below. Make additions if you feel that stress contributes to a condition that is not listed.

Conditions Associated with or Made Worse by Stress

- ❏ Acne
- ❏ Alcoholism
- ❏ Allergies
- ❏ Arthritis
- ❏ Asthma
- ❏ Backaches
- ❏ Cancer
- ❏ Common cold
- ❏ Coronary heart disease
- ❏ Eating disorders
- ❏ Eczema
- ❏ Gout
- ❏ Headaches
- ❏ High blood pressure
- ❏ Insomnia
- ❏ Low back pain
- ❏ Lowering of the body's immune system
- ❏ Nervous breakdown
- ❏ Neurosis
- ❏ Premenstrual syndrome (PMS)
- ❏ Stroke
- ❏ Temporomandibular joint syndrome (TMJ)
- ❏ _____
- ❏ _____
- ❏ _____

Life Events Questionnaire

Is there a connection between the number of major life events a person experiences in a year and the likelihood of illness? Drs. Thomas Holmes and Richard Rahe think so. They reached this conclusion after questioning 7,000 people about the number of life events they went through in 1 year. The people who scored highest on this questionnaire experienced the highest amount of physical illness in the year following the test. Since major life changes can produce stress-induced illness, take a look at how the past year's life events add up for you.

Instructions – Place a check mark in the column labeled "Happened" for those events that occurred in the past 12 months. Then record your score with the event value for each. Total the score for each column, and then add those totals to get a grand total.

Event Rank	Event Value	Hap-pened	Your Score	Life Event	Event Rank	Event Value	Hap-pened	Your Score	Life Event
1	100	___	___	Death of a spouse	24	29	___	___	In-laws trouble
2	73	___	___	Divorce	25	28	___	___	Outstanding personal achievement
3	65	___	___	Marital separation	26	26	___	___	Spouse beginning or ceasing work outside the home
4	63	___	___	Jail/institution term					
5	63	___	___	Death of close family member	27	26	___	___	Going back to school
6	53	___	___	Major personal injury or illness	28	25	___	___	Major change in living condition (building, remodel-ing or deterioration of home)
7	50	___	___	Marriage					
8	47	___	___	Being fired at work					
9	45	___	___	Marital reconciliation	29	24	___	___	Revision of personal habits
10	45	___	___	Retirement from work	30	23	___	___	Troubles with supervisor, boss, or superiors
11	44	___	___	Major change in the health or behavior of a family member					
					31	20	___	___	Major change in working hours or conditions
12	40	___	___	Pregnancy					
13	40	___	___	Sex difficulty	32	20	___	___	Change in residence
14	39	___	___	New family member through birth, adoption or remarriage	33	20	___	___	Change to a new school
					34	19	___	___	Major change in type or amount of recreation
15	39	___	___	Major business readjustments					
16	38	___	___	Major change in financial state	35	19	___	___	Major change in church activities
17	37	___	___	Death of close friend	36	18	___	___	Major change in social activities
18	36	___	___	Change to a different line of work	37	17	___	___	Major purchase (car, etc.)
					38	16	___	___	Major change in sleeping habits
19	35	___	___	Major increase in the number of arguments with spouse	39	15	___	___	Major change in the number of family get-togethers
20	31	___	___	Taking on a mortgage	40	15	___	___	Major change in eating habits
21	30	___	___	Foreclosure on mortgage/loan	41	13	___	___	Vacation
22	29	___	___	Major change in responsibili-ties at work (promotion, demotion, transfer)	42	12	___	___	Christmas or holiday observances
					43	11	___	___	Minor violations of the law (traffic tickets)
23	29	___	___	Son or daughter leaving home					Total _____

1976, Thomas Holmes, M.D., and Richard Rahe, Ph.D.

9. Staying Well

Scoring

- People who score 100–199 have a very mild risk.

- People who score 200–299 have a more moderate risk of developing physical illness in the next 12 months.

- People who score 300 or more have a strong risk of developing physical illness in the next 12 months.

{*Note:* These scores only represent a likelihood of getting sick and are not a definite prediction.}

Tips for Stress Management

- Maintain a regular program of healthy eating, good health habits, and adequate sleep.

- Exercise regularly. This promotes physical fitness and emotional well-being.

- Don't let your emotions get "bottled up" inside. Share your feelings with others.

- Learn to manage your time efficiently.

- Avoid unnecessary arguments or quarrels.

- Do a "stress rehearsal." Prepare for stressful events by imagining yourself feeling calm and handling the situation well.

- Minimize your exposure to things that cause distress.

- Practice a relaxation technique daily.

- Several times a day, do a "body check" for tensed muscles and let them relax.

- Do deep breathing exercises.

- Be a good Samaritan. Spend time helping others.

- Balance work and play.

- Plan some "me" time daily.

- Engage in activities you enjoy and look forward to.

- Discover the "elf' in yourself. Learn to have fun.

- He or she who laughs, lasts. Improve your laugh life.

- Participate in activities with people who share your interests.

- Reward yourself with little things that make you feel good.

- Challenge yourself to do something new.

- Surround yourself with cheery people. Avoid stress-carriers.

- Shun the "superman" or "superwoman" syndrome. No one is perfect.

- Set realistic goals for yourself.

- Be flexible in dealing with people and events. Avoid "psychosclerosis" – a hardening of the attitudes.

- Accept the things you cannot change in yourself or others.

- Forgive yourself for mistakes.

- Take satisfaction in your accomplishments. Don't dwell on your shortcomings.

- Develop and maintain a positive attitude. View changes as positive challenges, opportunities, or blessings.

- Seek professional help if needed.

Fitness – Get Fit, Stay Fit

Physical fitness has many benefits:

- Stress, boredom, and depression are minimized, as exercise seems to take the edge off daily tension.
- Skin tone is improved through fitness, giving that healthy glow!
- When our bodies demand more oxygen, such as for climbing stairs, it's no problem!
- Muscle tone is revitalized; strength, endurance, and even posture can improve.
- Fitness allows your heart to function with less strain placed upon it.
- Our self-esteem tends to improve as we see good things in the mirror!
- Blood circulation gets better and better.
- We sleep better.
- Our appetite for food is more manageable and our digestive process works better.
- Greater flexibility and ease are seen in the joints. Fewer creaks!
- Physical exercise increases the number of calories that are burned. In fact, calories are burned at a 15% higher rate for up to 6 hours after activity.

Beginning an Exercise Program

There are some basic points to keep in mind when beginning an exercise program:

- Before beginning to exercise, consult your physician, especially if you have been inactive for an extended period of time, are overweight, are over 35 years old, and/or have a medical problem.

- Choose an activity plan that is right for you. Consider where it will be done, what equipment is needed, whether it will be done with others, if it can be done in bad weather, what it will cost, and most importantly, whether you will enjoy it.

- Ease into your exercise program. Start off with activities of low intensity, frequency, and duration. Then build up your pace over the next several weeks. A good rule to follow is this: If you can't talk while exercising, you're overdoing it.

- Do warm-up exercises before the activity. Loosen up your muscles by stretching and/or walking for 5 minutes. When the activity is done, cool down with 5 more minutes of walking and/or stretching.

- Select an appropriate time and place to do your exercise. Get into a routine where the activity is done at the same time each day. Wait at least 2 hours after eating before doing a strenuous activity. If you exercise before a meal, wait about 25 minutes before you eat.

- For good results you should exercise at least 3 times a week for at least 20 minutes.

- Be in tune with your body while exercising. If muscles or joints start to hurt, ease up. It is usually not necessary to stop all activity for minor soreness. Be aware of the warning signs of serious health problems.

- Don't overdress. There is no benefit to excessive sweating, and it can even be dangerous.

- Read about fitness and exercise.

- Talk about good fitness habits with persons who stay fit.

- The first step is the hardest, but also the most important. Get up and start!

Four Popular Physical Activities to Consider

Walking

Walking is the most popular form of physical activity. If done on a regular basis, walking can not only help you to lose weight, but will relax you as well. There are some other advantages to walking: It can be done anywhere and anytime; it's free; you already know how to do it; and it can be done by almost anyone. Body posture is important to make your walking as efficient as possible. Keep these pointers in mind when walking:

- Hold your head erect.
- Keep your back straight.
- Point your toes straight ahead.
- Keep your abdomen flat.
- Swing your arms loosely at your sides.
- Land on your heel and roll forward off the ball of your foot.
- Wear shoes that are cushioned and provide support.
- If you become breathless, you're walking too fast.
- Don't compete with others – you're not in a race.
- Make your walk a pleasant experience.

Jogging

Jogging is perhaps the most ideal fitness activity to improve our overall fitness level. People who are unaccustomed to exercise can, with proper progression, advance from being walkers, to walk-joggers (woggers), to joggers, with little difficulty. Correct posture, pace, number of times you jog per week, and wearing the proper attire are all factors in its effectiveness.

Swimming

Swimming has long been a popular exercise for people who suffer from orthopedic problems or obesity because it reduces pressure on muscles and bones. Swimming has been found to produce relaxation and sound sleep patterns. In comparing swimming to jogging, 100 yds. of swimming is roughly equivalent to 400 yds. of jogging.

Bicycling

Bicycling is a good exercise to do with others and is a method of transportation as well. It provides wonderful conditioning for the legs and can improve cardiovascular fitness. Safety precautions are important when bicycling outdoors. (Make sure you wear a bicycle helmet.) To improve cardiovascular fitness, cycling should be done at least 3 times a week for 40–60 minutes each time. A stationary bicycle that has a resistance adjuster is good for regular exercise. It's certainly convenient, since you can read or watch TV while you pedal away and the weather doesn't interfere with your exercising.

Nutrition – Eating for Life

The old saying "You are what you eat" seems to be more true now than ever before. Eating right plays a pivotal role in good health and in disease prevention. The foods you "chews" can help lower your risk for heart disease, stroke, diabetes, osteoporosis, and certain cancers.

The United States Department of Agriculture (USDA) and Department of Health and Human Services (HHS) have stated what defines eating well in their "Dietary Guidelines for Americans."

These guidelines cover the most up-to-date advice from nutrition scientists and are the basis of federal nutrition policy.

Dietary Guidelines for Americans

- **Eat a variety of foods.** To make sure you get all of the nutrients and other substances needed for health, choose the recommended number of daily servings from each of the 5 major food groups displayed in the Food Guide Pyramid. (See the Food Guide Pyramid on page 44.) Vary your choices from each of the food groups.

- **Balance the food you eat with physical activity – maintain or improve your weight.** Many Americans gain weight in adulthood, increasing their risk for high blood pressure, heart disease, stroke, diabetes, certain types of cancer, arthritis, breathing problems, and other illnesses. Therefore, most adults should not gain weight. If you are overweight and have one of these problems, you should try to lose weight, or at the very least, not gain weight.

- **Choose a diet with plenty of grain products, vegetables, and fruits.** These foods provide vitamins, minerals, complex carbohydrates (starch and dietary fiber), and other substances that are important for good health. They are also generally low in fat, depending on how they are prepared and what is added to them at the table.

- **Choose a diet low in fat, saturated fat, and cholesterol.** High levels of saturated fat and cholesterol in the diet are linked to increased blood cholesterol levels and a greater risk for heart disease. Also, fat contains over twice the calories of an equal amount of carbohydrate or protein. A diet low in fat can help you maintain a healthy weight.

- **Choose a diet moderate in sugars.** Because maintaining a nutritious diet and a healthy weight is very important, sugars should be used in moderation by most healthy people and sparingly by people with low calorie needs. Avoid eating sugars in large amounts and frequent snacks of foods and beverages containing sugars that supply unnecessary calories and few nutrients.

- **Choose a diet moderate in salt and sodium.** A high salt intake is associated with higher blood pressure. Most evidence suggests that many people at risk for high blood pressure reduce their chances of developing this condition by consuming less salt.

- **If you drink alcoholic beverages, do so in moderation.** Moderation is defined as no more than 1 drink per day for women and no more than 2 drinks per day for men. When you drink alcoholic beverages, do so with meals, and when consumption does not put you or others at risk.

What Is the Food Guide Pyramid?

An easy way to follow the Dietary Guidelines for Americans is to choose foods daily, using the Food Guide Pyramid. The pyramids of Egypt have withstood the passage of time. Likewise, the Food Guide Pyramid can be used throughout a lifetime as a good foundation of what Americans should eat every day. It is not a rigid prescription but a general guide that lets you choose a healthful diet that's right for you and members of your family.

The pyramid calls for eating a variety of foods from each group to get the nutrients you need. At the same time, you can get the right amount of calories (and grams of fat) you need to lose or gain weight or maintain a healthy weight by adjusting the number of servings you eat from each group.

> *Note:* Fat and added sugars come mostly from fats, oils, and sweets, but can be part of or added to foods from the other food groups as well.

Fats, Oils, & Sweets
Use sparingly

Milk, Yogurt, & Cheese Group
2-3 servings

Meat, Poultry, Fish, Dry Beans, Eggs, & Nuts Group
2-3 servings

Vegetable Group
3-5 servings

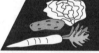

Fruit Group
2-4 servings

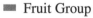

Bread, Cereal, Rice, & Pasta Group
6-11 servings

What Counts as a Serving?

- Bread, Cereal, Rice, and Pasta Group
  - 1 slice of bread
  - 1 ounce of ready-to-eat cereal
  - 1/2 cup of cooked cereal, rice, or pasta
- Vegetable Group
  - 1 cup of raw, leafy vegetables
  - 1/2 cup of other vegetables – cooked or chopped raw
  - 3/4 cup of vegetable juice
- Meat, Poultry, Fish, Dry Beans, Eggs, and Nuts Group
  - 2–3 ounces of cooked, lean meat, poultry or fish
  - 1/2 cup of cooked dry beans or 1 egg counts as 1 ounce of lean meat. Two tablespoons of peanut butter or 1/3 cup of nuts count as 1 ounce of meat.

- Fruit Group
  - 1 medium apple, banana, or orange
  - 1/2 cup of chopped, cooked, or canned fruit
  - 3/4 cup of fruit juice
- Milk, Yogurt, and Cheese Group
  - 1 cup of milk or yogurt
  - 1 1/2 ounces of natural cheese
  - 2 ounces of processed cheese

FYI – Key Nutrition Issues

Balance is the key. Know what to say yes to, what to moderate, and what to go easy on. Say yes to 5 or more servings of fruits and vegetables a day to get vitamins, minerals, dietary fiber, and anticancer substances.

Say Yes to Dietary Fiber

Dietary fiber comes from plant foods only. (The part that goes undigested and unabsorbed.) Animal foods have no fiber. Aim to get between 20 and 35 grams of dietary fiber per day. Food labels list the grams of dietary fiber per serving. Read them.

Say Yes to Calcium

Why? It is needed to strengthen bones and teeth, to help guard against osteoporosis, and to help your heart beat, your blood clot, your muscles flex, and your nerves react. Health experts recommend 1000–1500 milligrams of calcium a day for adults. Good food sources are:

- Milk, yogurt, cheese (choose nonfat and low-fat ones)
- Broccoli, collard greens, kale, spinach
- Legumes, dried beans and peas
- Tofu (if calcium is used in processing)
- Salmon, sardines (with bones)
- Calcium-fortified juices, cereals, breads, etc.

Use Sugar, Salt, Sodium, and Alcohol in Moderation

- Sugar – Many foods that contain large amounts supply calories, are limited in nutrients, and can contribute to tooth decay.
- Salt and sodium – Most Americans eat more salt and sodium than they need. (Salt contains 40% sodium, 60% chloride.) The recommended amount of sodium is 2400–3000 milligrams per day.

- Alcohol – Moderate use means no more than 1–2 drinks per day, 1 per day for women, 2 per day for men. 1 drink = 12 oz. regular beer, 4–5 oz. wine, 1½ oz. distilled spirits (80 proof). {*Note:* Women who are trying to conceive or are pregnant should not drink alcoholic beverages.}

Say No to Too Much Fat

Why? Populations with diets high in fat have more obesity and certain types of cancer (breast, colon, prostate). How much is too much? It is recommended that you get less than 30% of total calories from fat.

To figure out how to get less than 30% of calories from fat:

- Take 30% of total calories.
  Example: .30 x 1200 calories = 360 calories.
- Divide the answer by 9 calories/gram (fat contains 9 calories per gram) to get the upper limit of grams of fat per day.
  Example: 360 calories ∏9 calories/gram of fat = 40 grams of fat.

Max. Grams of Fat / Day			
For this many Calories	30% of Calories	25% of Calories	20% of Calories
1500	50 grams	42 grams	34 grams
1800	60 grams	50 grams	40 grams
2000	67 grams	56 grams	44 grams

Read food labels to find out how many grams of fat a food item contains per serving.

Say No to Saturated Fat

Why? Saturated fat raises blood cholesterol more than anything else in the diet. Saturated fats are generally solid at room temperature. Examples of foods that are high in saturated fat:

- Coconut oil
- Palm oil
- Animal fats
- Cocoa butter
- Dairy foods with fat

Say No to Too Much Dietary Cholesterol

Why? Dietary cholesterol in excess can contribute to hardening of the arteries.

About Cholesterol

Cholesterol is an odorless, white, waxy substance. Cholesterol is made only by animals. It is present in every cell in all parts of the body, including the brain and nervous system, muscle, skin, liver, intestines, heart, and skeleton. There are 2 sources of cholesterol: The cholesterol our body makes (mostly in the liver) and the cholesterol that is found in animal foods (dietary cholesterol). Plant foods have no cholesterol. Examples of foods with cholesterol are:

- Organ meats, such as liver and kidneys
- Eggs yolks, meats, poultry, and fish
- Dairy products that contain fat

It is recommended that we eat no more than 300 milligrams of dietary cholesterol per day. Your blood cholesterol can be measured using a blood sample taken from your finger or arm. The U.S. government has established the following guidelines for individuals:

Total blood cholesterol

Less than 200 mg/dl .... Desirable
200–239 mg/dl .... Borderline High
More than 240 mg/dl .... High

A fasting blood test is not needed to measure total blood cholesterol. A fasting blood test will reveal a more complete "cholesterol profile". It will give measurements of types of lipoproteins – "packages" in which cholesterol travels in the blood. Two types of lipoproteins of interest are:

Low-density lipoproteins (LDL) – carry most of the cholesterol in the blood. LDLs deposit cholesterol in the artery walls. They are called "bad cholesterol."

High-density lipoproteins (HDL) – contain a small amount of cholesterol. HDL's help remove cholesterol from the blood. They are called "good cholesterol."

A **high** LDL-cholesterol and/or a **low** HDL-cholesterol level increases your risk for coronary heart disease. The following guidelines are used today:

LDL-cholesterol

Less than 130 mg/dl .... Desirable
130–159 mg/dl .... Borderline High
More than 160 mg/dl .... High

HDL-cholesterol

Less than 35 mg/dl .... High Risk
More than 55 mg/dl .... Low Risk

Some health care experts use a ratio of total cholesterol divided by HDL-cholesterol to determine risk for heart disease as follows:

Total cholesterol / HDL (ratio)

More than 6.0 .... High Risk
Less than 4.0 .... Low Risk

About Triglycerides

Triglycerides are fatlike substances carried through the bloodstream to the tissues. The bulk of the body's fat tissue is in the form of triglycerides, stored for later use as energy. We get triglycerides from the fat in our foods, both animal and plant sources. Normal fasting blood triglyceride levels range from 40–160 mg/dl. They are thought to be elevated if fasting levels are over 250 mg/dl. To lower elevated triglycerides, do the following:

- Lose weight if you are overweight.
- Exercise regularly; eat a low-fat diet.
- Limit alcohol, sugar, and foods with sugar.

{*Note:* Some people may need medicine to help lower cholesterol and/or triglycerides in addition to dietary measures. Check with your doctor.}

Weight Control – "Chewsing" Well

Millions of Americans are caught up in the daily struggle to shed unwanted pounds. The link between obesity and such medical conditions as diabetes, high blood pressure, and heart disease has been well established. These threats to our health don't always provide the incentives we need to change, however.

Only a small percent of Americans who try to lose weight seem to keep it off long-term. It is not easy to change old habits. Liquid potions, diet pills, powders, and crash or fad diets do not prove successful over the long run, and can even be harmful.

The 3 key ingredients for successful weight loss are:

- Regular, physical activity
- Reduction of caloric intake, especially from fat
- Modification of eating and exercise behaviors

What Should You Do?

- See page 41 to set up a regular exercise program.
- Follow USDA Dietary Guidelines for Americans. (See page 43.)

Use the Food Guide Pyramid, but opt for choices in each level that are low in fat (ones inside the pyramid). Limit choices outside the pyramid.

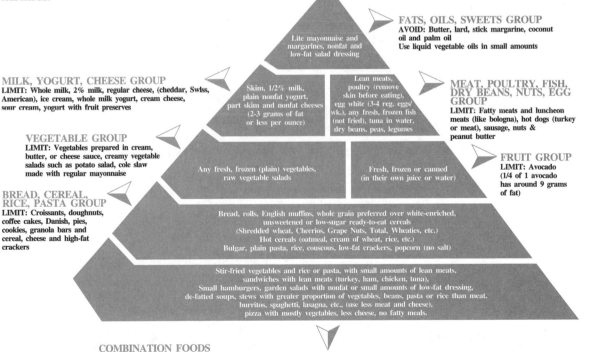

FATS, OILS, SWEETS GROUP
AVOID: Butter, lard, stick margarine, coconut oil and palm oil
Use liquid vegetable oils in small amounts

Lite mayonnaise and margarines, nonfat and low-fat salad dressing

MILK, YOGURT, CHEESE GROUP
LIMIT: Whole milk, 2% milk, regular cheese, (cheddar, Swiss, American), ice cream, whole milk yogurt, cream cheese, sour cream, yogurt with fruit preserves

Skim, 1/2% milk, plain nonfat yogurt, part skim and nonfat cheeses (2-3 grams of fat or less per ounce)

Lean meats, poultry (remove skin before eating), egg white (3-4 reg. eggs/ wk.), any fresh, frozen fish (not fried), tuna in water, dry beans, peas, legumes

MEAT, POULTRY, FISH, DRY BEANS, NUTS, EGG GROUP
LIMIT: Fatty meats and luncheon meats (like bologna), hot dogs (turkey or meat), sausage, nuts & peanut butter

VEGETABLE GROUP
LIMIT: Vegetables prepared in cream, butter, or cheese sauce, creamy vegetable salads such as potato salad, cole slaw made with regular mayonnaise

Any fresh, frozen (plain) vegetables, raw vegetable salads

Fresh, frozen or canned (in their own juice or water)

FRUIT GROUP
LIMIT: Avocado (1/4 of 1 avocado has around 9 grams of fat)

BREAD, CEREAL, RICE, PASTA GROUP
LIMIT: Croissants, doughnuts, coffee cakes, Danish, pies, cookies, granola bars and cereal, cheese and high-fat crackers

Bread, rolls, English muffins, whole grain preferred over white-enriched, unsweetened or low-sugar ready-to-eat cereals (Shredded wheat, Cheerios, Grape Nuts, Total, Wheaties, etc.) Hot cereals (oatmeal, cream of wheat, rice, etc.) Bulgar, plain pasta, rice, couscous, low-fat crackers, popcorn (no salt)

Stir-fried vegetables and rice or pasta, with small amounts of lean meats, sandwiches with lean meats (turkey, ham, chicken, tuna), Small hamburgers, garden salads with nonfat or small amounts of low-fat dressing, de-fatted soups, stews with greater proportion of vegetables, beans, pasta or rice than meat, burritos, spaghetti, lasagna, etc. (use less meat and cheese), pizza with mostly vegetables, less cheese, no fatty meals.

COMBINATION FOODS
LIMIT: Fried meat and fish sandwiches. Large double decker hamburgers, cheeseburgers, taco salad, hot dogs, Coney Island hot dogs, nachos with cheese, pizza with double cheese and high fat meats like pepperoni and sausage.

Follow Behavior Modification Techniques for Weight Control

Use the suggestions below to change the way you eat.

Eating Pace

- Eat slowly. Chances are you will eat less.
- Chew and swallow each bite thoroughly before beginning another.
- Take sips of water between bites.

Eating Mood

- Make a point to eat only when relaxed. (Many people eat to reduce tension.)
- Instead of thinking of "not eating," think of showing respect for your body by refusing to overeat.
- Concentrate on feelings of being bloated or stuffed before you overeat. Be aware of these negative physical sensations. This will help you limit your food intake.

Eating Out

- Choose restaurants where a variety of low-fat foods are available. Decide what you'll eat ahead of time.
- Don't starve yourself all day prior to dining out.
- Avoid "all-you-can-eat" restaurants.
- Consider ordering "a la carte" or "half orders" to keep portions small.

Eating with Others

- Beware of "Saboteurs" who try to undermine your weight-loss efforts. They may feel threatened by your success.
- Tell others about your weight loss goals.
- Meet friends for a walk instead of lunch.

Self Rewards

- Spend some time imagining yourself at your healthy body weight. Visualize in detail how you look, feel and think as the healthier you.
- Give yourself positive reinforcement each day you follow your eating plan. Choose something that's a little special like a stroll in the park, a long distance call, some "me" time.
- Keep saying positive self statements to yourself or in front of a mirror. Say, "I am in control" or "I choose to respect myself." This will go a long way when you find yourself wanting to eat at inappropriate times.

Miscellaneous Techniques

- Know the difference between appetite and hunger. Appetite is a psychological desire for food, while hunger is a true physical need for it.
- Use smaller-sized plates for meals.
- To avoid impulse buying, shop only from a well-planned list and never shop when hungry.
- Blast out your desire for food by yelling the word "STOP."
- Plan your snacks in advance.
- Put on tight clothes if you feel a desire to binge.
- Don't eat just because others are. Wait until you are really hungry.
- Above all, maintain a positive attitude. Commit to being a positive thinker. Focus on what you can do and what rewards come from eating well and exercising. This will result in improved health, a better mental attitude, more energy and improved appearance and performance, etc.

Playing It Safe – Tips for Home

Most accidents happen at home. If you think your house is "home, safe home," take a look around. At first glance it may look orderly, but certain trouble spots can lead to cuts, falls, burns, or other injuries. The following room-by-room checklist can alert you to accidents waiting to happen.

Kitchen

- Cleaners and dangerous chemicals should be stored out of children's reach.
- Scissors, knives, ice picks, and other sharp tools should be stored separately from other utensils and out of the reach of children.
- Towels, curtains, and other flammable materials should hang a safe distance from heat sources like the stove.
- Kitchen fans and stove ventilation exhausts should be clean and in good working order.
- Electrical cords should run a safe distance from the sink or range.
- Electrical outlets should not be overloaded.
- A sturdy step stool should be available to help reach high cabinets.
- Vinyl floors should be cleaned with non-skid wax.
- A nonskid floor mat should be in place in front of the sink.
- The kitchen should be well lit.

Bedroom

- Electrical cords should be in good working order and tucked away from foot traffic.
- Electrical outlets should not be overloaded.
- Electric blankets should not be covered by bedspreads or other blankets when in use.
- Carpeting should be secured to the floor.
- A night light should be put between the bed and the bathroom or hallway.
- The bedroom telephone should be easy to reach, even from the floor, if necessary.
- Ashtrays, irons, electric hair curlers, and other potential fire hazards should be located away from bedding, curtains, or other flammable material.
- Smoke detectors should be located near entrances to rooms, and their batteries should be checked often and replaced when needed.

Bathroom

- Floor mats should have nonskid backing.
- Rubber mats or adhesive-backed strips should be in place in the bathtub or shower stall.
- A support bar should be securely installed in the bathtub or shower stall.
- Hair dryers, electric shavers, or other electric appliances should be kept away from water and unplugged when not in use.
- A light switch should be located near the bathroom entrance or entrances.

Halls and Stairs

- Halls and stairs should be well lit, with a light switch at each end of a stairway.
- If a staircase is dimly lit, the top and bottom steps should be marked with reflective tape.
- Sturdy hand rails should be securely installed on both sides of each stairway.
- Floor covering on stairs and in halls should be skid-proof or carpeted and not creased or frayed.
- Stairways should be clear of shoes, books, toys, tools, or other clutter.
- When young children are in the house, gates should block access to stairways.

Basement and Garage

- To avoid confusion and misuse, all chemicals and cleaners should be kept in their original containers and out of children's reach.
- Hazardous chemicals should be kept under lock and key and out of children's reach.
- Sharp or otherwise potentially hazardous tools should be in good working order and kept off-limits to children.
- Gasoline and other flammable materials should be stored in airtight containers and away from heat sources (outside the home, if possible).
- Buy a radon test kit from your state department of health or department of environmental protection, or contact the Environmental Control Agency, 230 South Dearborn Street, Chicago, IL 60604 for information on radon testing. (Radon is an invisible gas that causes health problems if it builds up in homes and can't escape.) If your home has high radon levels, hire a reliable radon expert to help you reduce levels of this gas in your home.

Elsewhere Around the House

- Outdoor porches and walkways should be kept clear of ice in winter weather.
- Window screens should be securely fastened, especially if small children are around.
- Do not have poisonous plants in your yard or inside your house.
- Do not leave children unattended near swimming pools and playground equipment.
- Plan escape routes in case of fire or other emergencies. Talk about these with household members and practice using them.

Take steps to remedy unsafe situations as soon as possible.

Pregnancy - Planning a Healthy Baby

Healthy moms tend to have healthy babies. If you plan to, or become pregnant, take the following steps to help your pregnancy be a healthy one and to see that your baby gets off to a good start.

- Consider genetic tests or counseling if you or your husband have a family history of genetic disorders, if you are 35 or older, or if your husband is 60 or older.
- Have a complete medical exam, including a gynecological exam. A number of medical problems can cause harm to you and your baby. These include:
  - High blood pressure
  - Diabetes
  - Sexually transmitted disease (STDs)
  - HIV/AIDS

- RH disease (after the first pregnancy, if not treated with Rhogam)
- German measles (Rubella)
- Obesity

▬ Take measures to control and/or treat all medical conditions and take care of your health before you get pregnant and when you are pregnant. If you have a chronic medical condition, ask your doctor how it may affect your pregnancy.

▬ See your health care provider as soon as you know you are pregnant. Get regular prenatal care.

▬ Consult your doctor before taking any medication.

▬ Ask your doctor about prenatal vitamins while trying to get pregnant. These have folic acid, a B-vitamin that may prevent certain birth defects, such as spina bifida. Continue to take vitamin-mineral supplements as prescribed by your doctor throughout your pregnancy.

▬ Ask your doctor or a dietitian for a meal plan that meets the special needs of pregnancy.

▬ Don't drink alcohol, take "street" drugs, or smoke.

▬ Limit your intake of caffeine. Try to do without it completely.

▬ Follow your doctor's advice about weight gain. The amount of weight you gain should depend on your pre-pregnancy weight and health status, as well as your ethnic background. If you're very overweight, plan to lose excess pounds before you get pregnant.

▬ Exercise in moderation 3 times a week with your doctor's okay. Some activities thought safe during pregnancy are walking, golf, swimming, and low-impact aerobics.

▬ Practice relaxation and other stress control techniques.

▬ Enroll in childbirth preparation classes.

▬ If you own a cat, arrange for someone else to empty the litter box. Cat feces can transmit a disease called toxoplasmosis. If you're infected while pregnant, your baby may be stillborn, born prematurely, or suffer serious damage to the brain, eyes, or other parts of the body. It is safe, however, to handle or pet the cat.

▬ Be informed. Know the warning signs of pregnancy complications. These include increasing blood pressure and early labor. Getting treatment early is important.

Preventing Preterm Labor

A pregnant woman who starts to have her baby too soon is in preterm labor. A full-term pregnancy is about 40 weeks. Babies born before 37 weeks are considered preterm and may have health problems because they were born early.

The cause of preterm labor is not completely understood. Any pregnant woman can have preterm labor. The following conditions are associated with an increased risk of having a preterm baby:

▬ Previous preterm birth

▬ Three or more miscarriages in a row

▬ Bleeding problems

▬ Pregnant with more than one baby

▬ Abnormally shaped uterus

▬ Daughter of a mother who took DES (a medication used from the 1940s to 1970s by pregnant women to prevent miscarriage)

9. Staying Well

- Infections of the urinary tract, vagina, cervix, etc.
- Not enough weight gain, poor diet, lack of prenatal care
- Smoking, drinking alcohol, misusing drugs
- Severe emotional stress
- Mother is younger than 18 or older than 35

This is not an all-inclusive list. If you have questions about these conditions, discuss them with your doctor.

Being at an increased risk does not mean a woman will have a preterm baby. Whether you are at risk or not, learn the warning signs and how to feel your uterus (womb) to tell if you are in labor. It is possible to prevent a baby from being born too early, in some cases, if early warning signs are recognized and steps are taken to stop labor.

The following are warning signs of preterm labor:

- Contractions come every 15 minutes or closer and last from 20 seconds to 2 minutes each.
- Contractions come closer together as time goes on.
- Menstrual-like cramps come and go or don't go away.
- Pressure in your pelvis, back, or insides of your thighs. It feels like the baby is pushing down.
- Dull backache below your waist comes and goes or doesn't go away.
- Change in vaginal discharge
- Fluid leaking from the vagina
- A strange feeling that something is not right
- Fever of 100.4°F or higher and/or chills

Remember that preterm labor is usually not painful. If you have any of the signs of preterm labor, do the following:

- Lie down, tilted toward your left side for 1 hour. Do not lie flat on your back.
- Drink 2 to 3 glasses of water or juice during this hour.
- Keep feeling your stomach for uterine contractions. Time your contractions.

If the signs do not go away in 1 hour, or if you have fluid leaking from your vagina, do not wait. Call your health care provider! When you call, tell your nurse or doctor:

- Your name
- When your baby is due
- What signs you are having
- How often you are having contractions

SECTION II
Common Health Problems

Introduction
Getting sick costs more than ever before. All these health care costs are going up:

- Insurance rates
- Co-pays
- Deductibles
- Tests
- Prescriptions
- Doctor office and health clinic visits

You have to make a lot of decisions when you get sick, such as:

- Should I go to the emergency room?
- Should I call my doctor?
- Can I wait and see if the problem gets better?
- Can I take care of it myself?
- What things can I do to take care of myself?

This section can help you answer these questions. It presents common health problems and tells what you can do when you have one of them.

Sometimes you can treat these problems with self-care. Sometimes you need medical help. This section can help you ask the right questions and find the answers to take care of your health.

Each health problem is divided into 3 parts:

- Facts about the problem: What it is, what causes it, symptoms and treatments
- YES or NO questions to help you decide if you should get help fast, call your doctor, see your doctor, or use self-care
- A list of Self-Care Tips to treat the problem

Eye, Ear, Nose & Throat Problems

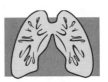
Respiratory Conditions

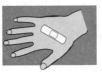
Skin Conditions

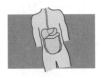
Abdominal Problems

Muscle & Bone Problems

Other Health Problems

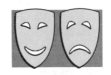
Mental Health Conditions

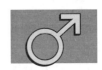
Men's Health Problems

Women's Health Problems

Children's Health Problems

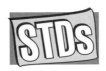
Sexually Transmitted Diseases (STDs)

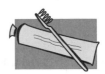
Dental Problems & Injuries

How to Use This Section

■ Find the problem in the table of contents in the beginning of the book and go to that page. The problems are listed in chapters. Each chapter covers certain concerns. Examples are "Eye, Ear, Nose & Throat Problems", "Skin Problems," etc. The topics in each chapter are listed in order from A to Z.

■ Read about the problem, what causes it (if known), it's symptoms and treatments.

■ Ask yourself the "Questions to Ask." Start at the top of the flow chart and answer YES or NO to each question. Follow the arrows until you get to one of these answers:

- Get Emergency Care
- See Doctor
- See Counselor or Call Counselor
- Call Doctor
- Use Self-Care

What the Instructions Mean

Get Emergency Care

You should get help fast. Go to the hospital emergency room or call for emergency medical service (EMS), from your city EMS department or local ambulance service. You may not need a hospital emergency room or EMS service for some emergencies if they do not threaten life or can be taken care of at out-patient centers. Some hospital emergency departments may have "Prompt Care" areas to treat minor injuries or illnesses. An example is a sprained ankle. Ask your doctor ahead of time where you should go for a sprained ankle or similar type of problem that needs prompt care but not necessarily emergency care.

Make sure you know phone numbers for emergency medical help. Write them down near your phone and in the "Emergency Phone Numbers" list on page 1 of this book. If no such numbers are at hand and failing all else you can call 911 where the service is available.

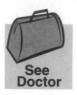

See Doctor

The term "doctor" can be used for a number of health care providers. They include:

■ Your physician

■ Your Health Maintenance Organization (HMO) clinic, primary doctor or other health care provider

■ Walk-in clinic

■ Physician's assistants (P.A.s), or certified nurses (C.N.s) who work with your doctor

■ Home health care provider

■ Your psychiatrist

■ Your dentist

When you see the "See Doctor" symbol, you may need medicine or treatment to keep the problem from getting worse. Call your health care provider and state the problem. Your provider's office staff can evaluate your symptoms and determine how soon you need to be seen.

See Counselor (icon label)

See Counselor or Call Counselor

The term "counselor" can be used for a number of mental health care providers. They include:

- Your counselor or therapist, if you already have one

- A mental health professional provided by your Employee Assistance Program (EAP) at work. Many EAPs are staffed by mental health professionals who do brief treatment.

- A mental health center

- A psychologist. A psychologist has a doctorate degree in psychology or clinical psychology.

- A social worker with a master's degree (M.S.W.)

- Another health care provider in the mental health field, such as a psychiatric nurse

{*Note:* You may need to call your primary physician for a referral to a counselor or other health care provider, including a psychiatrist, if you belong to a Health Maintenance Organization (HMO) or other managed health care plan. Also, a counselor may have you join a self-help/support group.}

Call Doctor (icon label)

Call Doctor

Call your doctor and state the problem. He/she can decide what you should do. He/she may:

- Tell you to make an appointment to be seen

- Send you to a laboratory for tests

- Prescribe medicine or treatment over the phone

- Tell you specific things to do to treat the problem

Use Self-Care (icon label)

Use Self-Care

You can probably take care of the problem yourself if you answered NO to all the questions. Use the Self-Care Tips that are listed. But call your doctor if you don't feel better soon. You may have some other problem.

Earaches

Earaches can be mild or very painful. The most common cause of an earache is plugged eustachian tubes. These tubes go from the back of the throat to your middle ear. When the eustachian tube gets blocked, fluid gathers, causing pain. Things that make this happen include an infection of the middle ear, colds, sinus infections, and allergies. Other things that can cause ear pain include changes in air pressure in a plane, something stuck in the ear, too much earwax, tooth problems, and ear injuries.

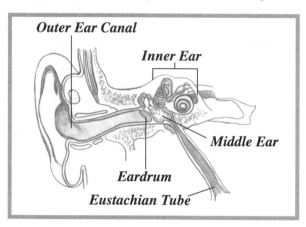

Outer Ear Canal

Inner Ear

Middle Ear

Eardrum

Eustachian Tube

Very bad ear pain should be treated by a doctor. Treatment will depend on its cause. Most often this includes pain relievers, an antibiotic for infection and methods to dry up or clear the blocked ear canal. You can, however, use Self-Care Tips if ear pain is mild and produces no other symptoms. One example is with a <u>mild</u> case of "swimmer's ear", which affects the outer ear. (See "To Treat a Mild Case of Swimmer's Ear" on page 58.)

Prevention

Much can be done to prevent earaches. Heed the old saying, "Never put anything smaller than your elbow into your ear." This includes cotton-tipped swabs, bobby pins, your fingers, etc. Doing so could damage your eardrum. When you blow your nose, do so gently, one nostril at a time. Don't smoke. Smoking and secondhand smoke can increase the risk of blocking the eustachian tube.

Questions to Ask

Did the pain start after a blow to the ear or recent head trauma? **YES** Get Emergency Care

NO

With the earache do you also have all of these symptoms?
• Stiff neck
• Fever
• Drowsiness
• Nausea, vomiting
YES Get Emergency Care

NO

In a child:
Does a child not respond to any sound, even a whistle or a loud clap? **YES** See Doctor

NO

Are there any of the following signs of infection?
• Fever (especially 102°F or higher)
• Sticky, green, or bloody discharge
• Severe ear pain and/or increased pain when wiggling the ear lobe
YES See Doctor

NO

Flowchart continued on next page

Earaches, *Continued*

Flowchart continued

Does a child show these signs of trouble? (These signs are especially important after a respiratory tract infection, a cold, air travel, or if the child has had ear problems before.)
- Constant pulling, touching, or tugging at the ear(s)
- Fever
- Crying that won't stop
- Ear or ears that are hot and hurt when touched
- Acting cranky and restless, especially at night or when lying down

YES **See Doctor**

NO

Is the earache persistent, more than mild and does it occur after any of the following?
- A mild ear injury
- Blowing your nose hard or many times
- Sticking an object of any kind in the ear
- A cold, sinus, or upper respiratory infection
- Swimming, and it is extremely painful when the earlobe is wiggled or touched
- Exposure to extremely loud noises (Examples: rock concerts, heavy machinery)

YES **See Doctor**

NO

Flowchart continued in next column

With the earache do you also have hearing loss, ringing in the ears, dizziness or nausea?

YES **See Doctor**

NO

Has a small object been stuck in the ear that cannot easily be removed or has an insect gotten in the ear that cannot safely be removed?

YES  **See Doctor**

NO

Does the earache occur with jaw pain, headache, and a clicking sound when opening and closing the mouth?

YES **Call Doctor**

NO

 Use Self-Care

Self-Care Tips

To Reduce Pain:

■ Place a warm washcloth or heating pad (set on low, adults only) next to the ear. Some health professionals recommend putting an ice bag or ice in a wet washcloth over the painful ear for 20 minutes.

■ Take an over-the-counter pain reliever. {*Note:* See "Pain relievers" in "Your Home Pharmacy" on pages 22 and 23.}

10. Eye, Ear, Nose & Throat Problems

Earaches, *Continued*

To Open Up the Eustachian Tubes and Help them Drain:

- Sit up.

- Prop your head up when you sleep.

- Yawn. (This helps move the muscles that open the eustachian tubes.)

- Chew gum or suck on hard candy. (Do not give to children under age 5.) This tip is especially helpful during pressure changes that take place during air travel but can also be useful during the middle of the night if you wake up with ear pain.

- Stay awake during take-offs and landings when traveling by air.

- Take a decongestant such as Sudafed, which can dry up the fluid in the ear that causes the pain. But don't use a nasal spray decongestant for more than three days unless directed by your doctor. Take a decongestant:

  - At the first sign of a cold if you have gotten ear infections often after previous colds.

  - One hour before you land when you travel by air if you have a cold or know your sinuses are going to block up.

- Take a steamy shower.

- Use a "cool-mist" vaporizer, especially at night.

- Drink plenty of cool water.

- Gently, but firmly, blow through your nose while holding both nostrils closed until you hear a pop. This will help promote ear drainage. This can be done several times a day.

- Feed a baby its bottle in an upright position, not lying down.

To Treat a Mild Case of "Swimmer's Ear":

The goal is to clean and dry the outer ear canal without doing further damage to the top layer of skin.

- Shake your head to expel trapped water.

- Dry the ear canal. Take a clean facial tissue. Twist each corner into a tip and gently place each tip into the ear canal for 10 seconds. Repeat with the other ear, using a new tissue.

- Use an over-the-counter product such as Swim-Ear. Drop it into the ears to fight infection. Follow package directions.

- Do not remove earwax. This coats the ear canal and protects it from moisture.

To Avoid Getting "Swimmer's Ear":

- Wear wax or silicone earplugs that can be softened and shaped to fit your ears. They are available at most drug stores.

- Wear a bathing cap to help keep water from getting into the ears.

- Don't swim in dirty water.

- Swim on the surface of the water instead of underneath the water.

For an Insect in the Ear:

- Shine a flashlight into the ear. Doing this may cause the insect to come out.

10. Eye, Ear, Nose & Throat Problems

Eyestrain from Computers

Office workers have their share of work-related hazards. People who use video display terminals (VDTs) may often complain of eyestrain, pain, stiffness in their backs and shoulders, and stress. These complaints can be a result of:

- Using a VDT for long periods of time
- Improper positioning of the VDT
- Poor lighting
- Poor posture
- Tight deadlines

Persons can protect themselves from the physical problems that go with using VDTs with the Self-Care Tips listed below.

Questions to Ask

Do you still have eyestrain, or eyestrain with back and shoulder stiffness despite using Self-Care Tips provided?

YES → Call Doctor

NO ↓

Use Self-Care

Self-Care Tips

To Prevent Eyestrain:

- Place the screen so that your line of sight is 10 to 15 degrees (about one-third of a 45-degree angle) below horizontal.
- Dust the screen often.
- Reduce glare. Position the VDT at right angles to a window. Turn off or shield overhead lights. Wear a visor to block overhead lights if necessary.

- Place your paperwork close enough that you don't have to keep refocusing when switching from the screen to the paper. Use a paper document holder placed at the same height as the VDT screen.
- Blink often to keep your eyes from getting dry. Use "artificial tear" eyedrops if needed.
- Tell your eye specialist that you use a VDT. Glasses and contacts worn for other activities may not be good for VDT work. (With bifocals, the near-vision part of the lens is good for looking down, as when you read, but not for looking straight ahead, as when you look at a video display screen. So, you may need single-vision lenses for VDT work.)
- If the image on the VDT screen is blurred, dull, or flickers, have it serviced right away.
- Try to keep the VDT screen 2 feet away from your eyes.

To Prevent Muscle Tension When You Work on a VDT:

- Use a chair that supports your back and can be easily adjusted to a height that feels right for you.
- Take a 15-minute break if you can, for every 2 hours you use a VDT. Get up and go for a short walk, for example.
- Do stretching exercises of the neck, shoulder, and lower back every 1 to 2 hours.
  - Rotate your head in a circular motion, first clockwise, then counterclockwise.
  - Shrug your shoulders up, down, backward, and forward.
  - While standing or sitting, bend at the waist, leaning first to the left, then to the right.

10. Eye, Ear, Nose & Throat Problems

3 Hay Fever

Despite its name, hay fever has nothing to do with hay or fever. A nineteenth-century physician called it this because he began to sneeze every time he entered a hay barn. Hay fever is, actually, a reaction of the upper respiratory tract to anything to which you may be allergic. The medical term for hay fever is "allergic rhinitis." Hay fever is most common in spring and fall (when ragweed is particularly troublesome), but some people have it all year.

Symptoms

- Itchy, watery eyes
- Runny, itchy nose
- Congestion
- Sneezing

Try to avoid things that give you hay fever. Talk to your doctor if that doesn't help. He or she may prescribe any of the following:

- Antihistamines. For best results, take the antihistamine 30 minutes before going outside. {*Note:* Some over-the-counter antihistamines may cause more drowsiness than prescription ones. Also, care should be taken when driving and operating machinery since antihistamines can make you drowsy.}

- Decongestants. These do not usually cause drowsiness.

- Nasal sprays. Use as directed by your doctor.

- Other things, like cromolyn sodium or steroids

- Skin tests to find out what things you are allergic to

- Allergy shots if your hay fever is very bad. First, you have a skin test. Then you get shots that have a tiny bit of the allergen. The shots help your body get used to the allergen, so you won't be so sensitive to it.

It is best to take what your doctor prescribes instead of experimenting with over-the-counter products on your own.

Questions to Ask

Is it so hard for you to breathe that you can't talk (say 4 or 5 words between breaths)? **YES** → Get Emergency Care

NO ↓

Do you have severe breathing difficulties or severe wheezing? **YES** →  Get Emergency Care

NO ↓

Do you have any symptoms of an infection such as:
- Fever
- Nasal discharge or mucus that is green or yellow or bloody-colored
- Headache or muscle aches

YES → See Doctor

NO ↓

Do you still have hay fever symptoms when you avoid hay fever triggers? **YES** → Call Doctor

NO ↓

Flowchart continued on next page

Hay Fever, *Continued*

Flowchart continued

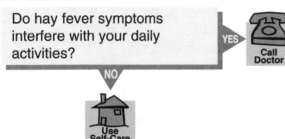

Do hay fever symptoms interfere with your daily activities? → **YES** → Call Doctor

NO → Use Self-Care

Self-Care Tips

Stay Away From Things That Give You Hay Fever:

- Let someone else do outside chores. Mowing the lawn or raking leaves can make you very sick if you are allergic to pollen from grains, trees, or weeds. It's a problem if you are allergic to molds, too.

- Keep windows and doors shut and stay inside when the pollen count or humidity is high. Early morning is sometimes the worst.

- Put an air conditioner or air cleaner in your house, especially in your bedroom. Be sure to clean the filter often.

- To keep dust, mold, and pollen away from you at home and work:
  - Dust and vacuum your home often. Wear a dust and pollen mask if necessary.
  - Wash rugs.
  - Add an electronic air filter to your furnace or use portable air purifiers.
  - Take carpets and drapes out of your bedroom.
  - Cover your mattress with a plastic cover.
  - Do not use a feather pillow.
  - Stay away from stuffed animals. They collect dust.
  - Don't have pets, or keep your pets outside the house.
  - Don't hang sheets and blankets outside to dry. Pollen can get on them.
  - Shower or bathe and wash your hair following heavy exposure to pollen, dust, etc.

- Avoid tobacco smoke and other air pollutants.

10. Eye, Ear, Nose & Throat Problems

4 Hearing Loss

Do people seem to mumble a lot lately? Do you have trouble hearing in church or theaters? Is it hard to pick up what others say at the dinner table or at family gatherings? Does your family ask you to turn down the volume on the TV or radio?

These are signs of gradual, age-related hearing loss called presbycusis. High-pitched sounds are the ones to go first. Hearing loss from presbycusis cannot be restored, but hearing aids, along with the Self-Care Tips listed on page 63 can be helpful.

Hearing loss can also result from other things:

- Acoustic trauma. This may be caused by a blow to the ear or excessive noise. Excessive noise includes that heard from low-flying airplanes when living near an airport, when flying in an airplane, or when working with heavy, loud machines.

- Blood vessel disorders, including high blood pressure

- A blood clot that travels to nerves in the ear

- Earwax that blocks the ear canal

- Chronic middle-ear infections, or an infection of the inner ear

- Ménière's disease – a disease in which there is excess fluid in canals of the inner ear, which results in tinnitus, dizziness, gradual hearing loss etc...

- Multiple sclerosis

- Syphilis

- Brain tumor and small tumors on the auditory nerve

Also, children can be born with hearing loss or a hearing impairment.

Questions to Ask

In a Child:

When your child is awake, does he or she not respond to any sound, even a whistle or loud clap? {*Note:* This may happen after a recent earache or upper respiratory infection, or airplane travel.}

YES → See Doctor

 NO

In a Child or Adult:

Are any of the following present with the hearing loss?
- Discharge from the ear
- Earache
- Dizziness or feeling that things are spinning around you
- Recent ear or upper respiratory infection
- Feeling that the ears are blocked or filled with wax

YES → See Doctor

 NO

Can you <u>not</u> hear a regular (nondigital) watch ticking when held next to the ear?

YES → See Doctor

 NO

Flowchart continued on next page

Hearing Loss, *Continued*

Flowchart continued

Do you hear a ringing sound in one or both ears all of the time?

NO ↓   **YES** →  **See Doctor**

Did you lose your hearing after being exposed to loud noises such as those associated with airplanes, work-or hobby-related loud noises (i.e., heavy machinery, power tools, firearms, etc.), and has this not gotten better?

NO ↓   **YES** → **Call Doctor**

 Use Self-Care

Self-Care/Prevention Tips

For Gradual, Age-Related Hearing Loss (Presbycusis):

- Ask people to speak clearly, distinctly, and in a normal tone.

- Look at people when they are talking to you. Ask them to face you, too. Watch their expressions to help you understand what they are saying.

- Try to limit background noise when having a conversation.

- In a church or theater, sit up front.

- To rely on sight instead of sound, install a buzzer, flasher, or amplifier on your telephone, door chime, and alarm clock. Also, an audiologist (hearing therapist) may be able to show you other techniques for "training" yourself to hear better.

To Clear Earwax:

(Use only if you know that the eardrum is not perforated. Check with your doctor if you are in doubt.)

- Lie on your side. Using a syringe or medicine dropper, carefully squeeze a few drops of lukewarm water into your ear (or have someone else do this). Let the water remain there for 10–15 minutes and then shake it out. Do this again, using only a few drops of hydrogen peroxide, mineral oil, or an over-the-counter cleaner such as Murine Ear Drops or Debrox. Let the excess fluid flow out of the ear.

- After several minutes, follow the same procedure using warm water again, letting it remain there for 10–15 minutes. Tilt the head to allow it to drain out of the ear.

You can repeat this entire procedure again in three hours if the earwax has not cleared.

To Prevent Hearing Loss:

- Don't put cotton-tipped swabs, fingers, bobby pins, etc. in your ear.

- Don't blow your nose with too much force. It is better to do so gently with a tissue or handkerchief held loosely over the nostrils.

10. Eye, Ear, Nose & Throat Problems

Hearing Loss, *Continued*

- Avoid places that have loud noises (airports, construction sites, etc.). Protect your ears with earplugs.

- Keep the volume on low when using radios, stereos, cassette and compact disc (CD) players. If someone else can hear the music when you are listening to one of these devices with earphones, the volume is too loud.

- Wear earplugs when exposed to loud noises from power tools, lawn mowers etc.

- Follow your doctor's advice for disorders that can cause hearing loss. (Examples: Ménière's disease, high blood pressure, etc.)

- Avoid prolonged use of medicines that cause hearing loss, or overdosing on such medications. (Example: heavy use of aspirin, streptomycin, quinine)

Also be aware of things that can help you hear sounds if your hearing is impaired:

- Hearing aids. (See your doctor.)

- Devices made to assist in hearing sounds from the TV and radio

- Special equipment that can be installed in your telephone by the telephone company

- Portable devices made especially to amplify sounds. (These can be used for movies, classes, meetings, etc.)

10. Eye, Ear, Nose & Throat Problems

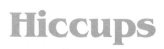 Hiccups

Hiccups are simple to explain: Your diaphragm (the major muscle involved in breathing which sits like a cap over the stomach) goes into spasm. Things that promote hiccups are:

- Eating too fast, which causes you to swallow air along with food

- Doing things to make the stomach full enough to irritate the diaphragm. One example is eating a lot of fatty foods in a short period of time.

One doctor who studies hiccups thinks there is a hiccup center in the brain which triggers a spasm of the esophagus. This, he thinks, is a protective mechanism to keep a person from choking on food or drink. Luckily, hiccups are generally harmless and don't last very long.

Questions to Ask

Do the hiccups occur with severe abdominal pain and spitting up blood or blood in the stools?

YES → **Get Emergency Care**

NO ↓

Have the hiccups lasted longer than 8 hours in an adult or 3 hours in a child?

YES → **Call Doctor**

NO ↓

Have the hiccups started only after taking prescription medicine?

YES → **Call Doctor**

NO ↓

 Use Self-Care

Self-Care Tips

Luckily, there's no shortage of hiccup cures, and better still, most of them work (although some baffle medical science). A study reported in the *New England Journal of Medicine* found that 1 teaspoon of ordinary table sugar, swallowed dry, cured hiccups immediately in 19 out of 20 people (some of whom had been hiccuping for as long as six weeks). If this doesn't stop the hiccups right away, repeat it 3 times at 2-minute intervals. {*Note:* For young children, use a teaspoon of corn syrup.}

Other popular folk remedies worth trying include:

- Hold your tongue with your thumb and index finger and gently pull it forward.

- With your head bent backward, hold your breath for a count of ten. Exhale immediately and drink a glass of water.

- Breathe into and out of a paper (not plastic) bag.

- Swallow a small amount of finely cracked ice.

- Massage the back of the roof of your mouth with a cotton swab. A finger works equally well.

- Eat dry bread slowly.

- Drink a glass of water rapidly. {*Note:* Young children should drink a glass of milk slowly.}

10. Eye, Ear, Nose & Throat Problems

6 Laryngitis

Laryngitis is when your larynx (voice box) is irritated or inflamed. Your voice becomes hoarse, husky, and weak. Air pollution, or spending an evening in a smoky room can irritate the larynx and cause laryngitis. Infections and allergies too, can inflame the larynx. Sometimes laryngitis is painless, but you may get a sore throat, fever, dry cough, a tickling sensation in the back of the throat, or have trouble swallowing. Smoking, drinking alcohol, breathing cold air, and continuing to use already distressed vocal cords can make the situation worse.

Questions to Ask

Is it very hard for you to breathe or swallow or are you coughing up blood? **YES** → **Get Emergency Care**

NO ↓

Do you have a high fever or are you coughing up mucus that is yellow or green or bloody-colored? **YES** → **See Doctor**

NO ↓

Do you have hard, swollen lymph glands in your neck or do you feel like you have a "lump" in your throat? **YES** → **Call Doctor**

NO ↓

Has the hoarseness lasted more than a week in a child or more than a month in an adult? **YES** → **Call Doctor**

NO ↓

Flowchart continued in next column

Do you have two or more of these problems?
- Bothered by the cold more than usual
- Dry hair or skin
- Gaining weight for no reason
- Feeling very tired for no reason

YES → **Call Doctor**

NO ↓

 Use Self-Care

Self-Care Tips

- Don't talk if you don't need to. Use a notepad and pencil to write notes instead. If you must speak, do so softly, but don't whisper.
- Use a "cool-mist" humidifier in your bedroom.
- Drink lots of warm drinks such as tea.
- Gargle every few hours with warm salt water ($\frac{1}{4}$ teaspoon of salt in $\frac{1}{2}$ cup of warm water).
- Take a hot shower or steam bath.
- Don't smoke. Stay away from places with smoke.
- Suck on cough drops, throat lozenges, or hard candy. (Do not give to children under age 5.)
- Take an over-the-counter medicine for pain and/or inflammation. {*Note:* See "Pain relievers" in "Your Home Pharmacy" on pages 22 and 23.}

7 Nosebleeds

Nosebleeds are usually a scary but minor bout with broken blood vessels just inside the nose. They're caused by a cold, frequent nose blowing and picking, allergies, a dry environment, using too much nasal spray, or a punch or other blow to the nose.

A nosebleed is serious, though, when heavy bleeding from deep within the nose is hard to stop. This type usually strikes the elderly. It can be caused by hardening of nasal blood vessels, high blood pressure, medicines to treat blood clots, primary bleeding disorders like hemophilia, or by a tumor in the nose.

Questions to Ask

Did this nosebleed follow a blow to another part of the head or does the nosebleed occur in a person taking blood-thinning medicine, such as Coumadin? **YES** Get Emergency Care

NO

Does the nosebleed last 10–15 minutes or more? **YES** See Doctor

NO

Does the nosebleed start after taking newly prescribed medication? **YES** Call Doctor

NO

Do nosebleeds happen often and/or are they becoming more frequent? **YES** Call Doctor

NO

 Use Self-Care

Self-Care Tips

Although there are lots of ideas about how to treat minor nosebleeds, the following procedure is recommended by the American Academy of Otolaryngology (Head and Neck Surgery).

- Sit with your head leaning forward.

- Pinch the nostrils shut, using your thumb and forefinger in such a way that the nasal septum (the nose's midsection) is being gently squeezed.

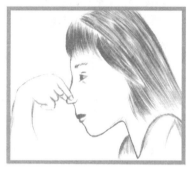

- Hold for 15 uninterrupted minutes, breathing through your mouth.

- At the same time, apply cold compresses (such as ice in a soft cloth) to the area around the nose.

- For the next 24 hours, make sure your head is elevated above the level of your heart.

- Also, wait 24 hours before blowing your nose, lifting heavy objects, or exercising strenuously.

{*Note:* If you are unable to stop a nosebleed by using the Self-Care Tips, call your doctor.}

10. Eye, Ear, Nose & Throat Problems

8 Pinkeye

Pinkeye is an inflammation of the conjunctiva, the underside of both the upper and lower eyelids and the covering of the white portion of the eye. The medical term for pinkeye is conjunctivitis. Some causes of pinkeye and solutions that go with them are:

- Allergic conjunctivitis–a reaction to airborne pollen, dust, mold spores, animal dander, cosmetics, contact lenses, or direct contact with chlorinated water. If you can't avoid the allergens, antihistamines and certain eye drops can help. (Ask your doctor which one(s) to use.)

- Bacterial conjunctivitis–an infection with a puslike discharge. Warm compresses along with an antibiotic ointment or drops prescribed by your doctor can help. When treated right, bacterial conjunctivitis will clear up in two to three days but continue to use the medicine as prescribed by your doctor.

- Viral conjunctivitis–a complication of a cold or flu. This type has less discharge but more tearing than the bacterial form. Antibiotics don't work. Viral conjunctivitis can take 14 to 21 days to clear up.

Questions to Ask

Do you have eye pain or are your eyes sensitive to light? YES **See Doctor**

NO

Do you have a puslike discharge that is yellowish-green in color? YES **See Doctor**

NO

Flowchart continued in next column

Have you tried Self-Care Tips and show no improvement after 24 hours, or are the symptoms worse? YES **Call Doctor**

NO

 Use Self-Care

Self-Care Tips

To relieve the symptoms of pinkeye:

- Don't touch the eye area with your fingers. If you must wipe your eye, use tissues.

- With your eyes closed, apply a washcloth soaked in warm (not hot) water to the affected eye 3–4 times a day for at least 5 minutes at a time. (These soaks also help to dissolve the crusty residue of pinkeye.)

- Use over-the-counter eyedrops. They may soothe irritation and help relieve itching.

- Avoid wearing eye makeup until the infection has completely cleared up. Never share makeup with others.

- Don't cover or patch the eye. This can make the infection grow.

- Don't wear contact lenses while your eyes are infected.

- Wash your hands often and use your own towels. Pinkeye is very contagious and can be spread from one person to another by contaminated fingers, washcloths, or towels.

9 Sinus Problems

Your sinuses are behind your cheekbones and forehead, and around your eyes. Healthy sinuses drain almost a quart of mucus every day. They keep the air you breathe wet.

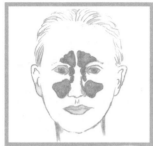

Your sinuses can't drain right if they are infected and swollen. Your chances of getting a sinus infection increase if you:

- Have hay fever
- Smoke
- Have a nasal deformity or sinuses that don't drain well
- Have an abscess in an upper tooth
- Sneeze hard with your mouth closed or blow your nose too much when you have a cold

Symptoms of a Sinus Infection Are:

- Head congestion
- Nasal congestion and discharge (usually yellowish green) with or without foul odor or bad taste
- Pain and tenderness over the facial sinuses
- Pain in the upper jaw
- Recurrent headache that changes with head position and disappears shortly after getting out of bed
- Fever

Sinus complications can be serious. Your doctor can tell if you have a sinus infection with a physical exam, a laboratory study of a sample of your nasal discharge, and X-rays of the sinuses. You may need prescriptions for an antibiotic, a decongestant as well as a nasal spray and/or nose drops. These work to clear the infection and reduce congestion. Severe cases may require surgery to drain the sinuses.

Questions to Ask

Do you have two or more of the following?
- A fever over 101°F
- Greenish-yellow or bloody-colored nasal discharge
- Severe headache which doesn't get better when you take an over-the-counter pain reliever or that is worse in the morning or when bending forward
- Pain between the nose and lower eyelid
- A feeling of pressure inside the head
- Eye pain, blurred vision, or changes in vision
- Cheek or upper jaw pain
- Swelling around the eyes, nose, cheeks, and forehead

YES → See Doctor

NO ↓

 Use Self-Care

See Self-Care Tips on next page

10. Eye, Ear, Nose & Throat Problems

Sinus Problems, *Continued*

Self-Care Tips

A "cool-mist" humidifier can help. Wet air helps make mucus thin. You can put a warm washcloth or compress on your face, too. This can help with the pain. Here are some more tips:

- Drink plenty of water and other liquids.

- Take an over-the-counter medicine for pain. {*Note:* See "Pain relievers" in "Your Home Pharmacy" on pages 22 and 23.}

- Take an over-the-counter decongestant pill or an over-the-counter pill for pain that also has a decongestant, such as Tylenol Sinus. {*Note:* Older men should check with their doctor before taking decongestants. Decongestants that have ephedrine can give older men urinary problems.}

- Use nose drops only for the number of days prescribed. Repeated use of them creates a dependency. Your nasal passages "forget" how to work on their own and you have to continue using drops to keep nasal passages clear. To avoid picking up germs, never borrow nose drops from others. Don't let anyone else use yours, either. Throw the drops away after treatment.

- Add a humidifier to your furnace.

10 Sore Throats

Sore throats range from a mere scratch to pain so severe that even swallowing saliva hurts. They can be caused by heavy cigarette smoking and infections of the throat, tonsils, or nasal passages from a virus, fungus, or bacteria such as streptococcus, the one that causes strep throat.

If an infection is the cause, your doctor may take a throat culture. If streptococcus or any other type of bacteria is the culprit, he or she will prescribe an antibiotic. Be sure you take all of the antibiotic.

If strep throat is left untreated, serious complications, including abscesses, kidney inflammation, or rheumatic heart disease, could arise. An antifungal medicine is used to treat a fungal infection.

Questions to Ask

Is it very hard for you to breathe, are you unable to swallow your own saliva, or are you unable to say more than 3 or 4 words between breaths?

YES → Get Emergency Care

NO ↓

Do the tonsils or the back of the throat look bright red or have visible pus deposits?

YES → See Doctor

NO ↓

Flowchart continued in next column

Do you have any of the following problems with the sore throat?
- Fever
- Swollen, enlarged neck glands
- Headache
- General aching feeling
- Ear pain
- Bad breath
- Skin rash
- Loss of appetite
- Vomiting
- Abdominal pain
- Chest pain
- Dark urine

YES → See Doctor

NO ↓

Does someone else in the family have a strep throat or do you get strep throat often?

YES → Call Doctor

NO ↓

Has even a mild sore throat lasted more than 2 weeks?

YES → Call Doctor

NO ↓

 Use Self-Care

See Self-Care Tips on next page

Sore Throats, *Continued*

Self-Care Tips

■ Gargle every few hours with a solution of $1/4$ teaspoon of salt dissolved in $1/2$ cup of warm water.

■ Drink plenty of warm beverages, such as tea with lemon (with or without honey) and soup.

■ For strep throat, eat and drink cold foods and liquids such as frozen yogurt, popsicles, and ice water.

■ Use a "cool-mist" vaporizer or humidifier in the room where you spend most of your time. If you get a sore throat often consider adding an electronic air filter and humidifier to your furnace system.

■ Don't smoke.

■ Avoid eating spicy foods.

■ Suck on a piece of hard candy or medicated lozenge every so often. (Do not give to children under age 5.)

■ Take an over-the-counter medicine for the pain and/or fever. {*Note:* See "Pain relievers" in "Your Home Pharmacy" on pages 22 and 23.}

■ Do not get in close contact with anyone you know has a sore throat.

11 Sty

A sty is a small boil or bacterial infection in a tiny gland of the eyelid. If the oil-producing glands on the upper or lower rim of the eyelid become infected, they become swollen and painful. A sty is tiny at first, but it can blossom into a bright red, painful sore.

Eventually, a "baby" sty will come to a head and appear yellow, because it contains pus. Generally, the tip will face outward, and the sty will break open and drain on its own.

Questions to Ask

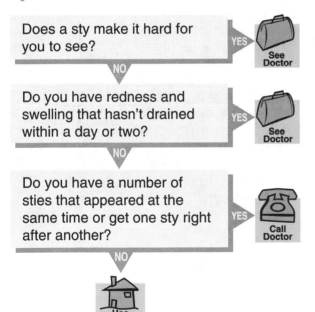

Self-Care Tips

You can relieve the discomfort of a sty by following these steps:

- Apply warm (not hot), wet compresses to the affected area 3–4 times a day for 5–10 minutes at a time.

- Avoid situations that expose your eyes to excessive dust or dirt.

- Don't poke or squeeze the infected area, no matter how tempted you may be to pop the sty. Most sties respond well to home care and don't require further treatment.

10. Eye, Ear, Nose & Throat Problems

12 Tinnitus (Ringing in the Ears)

Imagine hearing a ringing noise in your ears or head that doesn't go away. This maddening noise, called tinnitus, can range in volume from a ring to a roar. It affects nearly 36 million Americans, most of them older adults. Seven million people are bothered so much by tinnitus that living a normal life is not possible. Tinnitus can, in fact, interfere with work, sleep, and normal communication with others.

Causes

Like a toothache, tinnitus isn't a disease in itself, but a symptom of another problem. Examples are:

■ Earwax blocking the ear canals

■ Food allergies

■ Reactions to medications

■ Middle-ear trauma or infections

■ Blood vessel abnormalities in the brain

■ Ear nerve damage due to exposure to loud noise

■ Anemia (see page 148)

■ Ménière's disease – a disease in which there is excess fluid in the canals of the inner ear, which results in tinnitus, dizziness, gradual hearing loss, etc...

■ Diabetes (see page 345)

■ Brain tumors (rarely)

And sometimes tinnitus is simply due to advancing age. It often accompanies loss of hearing. Often, tinnitus is temporary and will not lead to deafness. Treatment is aimed at finding and treating the problem that causes the tinnitus.

Questions to Ask

Do you have severe pain in the ears, forehead or over the cheekbones, a severe headache, dizziness, and/or sudden loss of hearing?

YES Get Emergency Care

NO

Do you have the following problems with ringing in the ears after taking aspirin or other medications that have salicylates, such as Trilisate or Disalcid (which are sometimes used to treat arthritis)?
• Nausea
• Vomiting
• Dizziness
• Rapid breathing
• Hallucinations

YES Get Emergency Care

NO

Flowchart continued on next page

Tinnitus (Ringing in the Ears), *Continued*

Flowchart continued

Along with ringing in the ears, do you have one or more of the following?
- Dizziness
- Vertigo
- Unsteadiness in walking
- Loss of balance
- Vomiting
- Sudden hearing loss

YES → See Doctor

NO ↓

Use Self-Care

Self-Care Tips

- For mild cases of tinnitus, play the radio or a white noise tape (white noise is a low, constant sound) in the background to help mask the tinnitus.

- Biofeedback or other relaxation techniques can help you calm down and concentrate, shifting your attention away from the tinnitus. Relaxation can reduce stress, which can aggravate tinnitus.

- Exercise regularly to promote good blood circulation.

- Ask your doctor or a certified audiologist about a recently developed tinnitus masker, which looks like a hearing aid. Worn on the ear, it makes a subtle noise that masks the tinnitus without interfering with hearing and speech.

- If the noises started during or after traveling in an airplane, try pinching your nostrils and blowing through your nose. Chewing gum or sucking on hard candy may help prevent the popping and ringing sounds in the ear from happening when you do fly. Also, it is prudent to avoid flying when you have an upper respiratory tract or ear infection.

- Limit your intake of caffeine, alcohol, nicotine, aspirin, and aspirin-like medications.

- Wear earplugs when exposed to loud noises such as heavy machinery, etc., to prevent damage to the ear.

10. Eye, Ear, Nose & Throat Problems

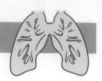

13 Asthma

Asthma cuts down the air flow in the lungs. This makes it hard to breathe and can cause chest tightness and wheezing. {*Note:* Other things can cause wheezing, too. Something may be stuck in the major airways, or there may be an infection. Always tell your doctor about wheezing, especially if your child is wheezing.}

Doctors call asthma an episodic disease because in most asthmatics acute attacks alternate with symptom-free periods. Asthma is a physical problem, not an emotional one (although stress, anxiety, or frustration can cause asthma to worsen), and it can be severe enough to disrupt people's lives. It is a complex disorder which needs to be treated by a doctor who can monitor the person's asthma over time.

A variety of triggers can set off asthma attacks:

- Having an upper respiratory tract infection or bronchitis

- Breathing an allergen like pollen, mold, animal dander, or particles of dust or smoke or other irritants

- Eating certain foods or taking certain medicines

- Exercising too hard

- Breathing cold air

- Experiencing emotional distress

Asthma attacks range from mild to severe, so treatment varies. Generally, asthma is too complex to treat with over-the-counter preparations. A doctor should keep track of how you are doing.

He or she may prescribe one or more of these for your asthma:

- Bronchodilators, in oral, inhaled, or aerosol form, which open airways to make breathing easier

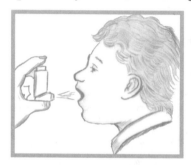

- Steroids, in either oral or aerosol form, to counteract an allergic reaction, and when other medicines do not help your asthma

- Cromolyn sodium to be inhaled before an attack that is triggered by allergies or exercise. This won't work once the attack starts. Used with steroids, or alone, cromolyn sodium may help prevent asthma attacks.

- Peak flow meter for home monitoring of asthma

- Vaccinations for influenza (flu) and pneumonia. (See "Immunization Schedule" on page 18.)

Questions to Ask

Is it so hard for you to breathe that you can't talk (say 4 or 5 words between breaths), or does your chest feel tight, or are you wheezing and can't stop?

YES → Get Emergency Care

NO ↓

Flowchart continued on next page

Asthma, *Continued*

Flowchart continued

Does your asthma attack not respond to home treatment or prescribed medicine? **YES** → **See Doctor**

NO ↓

Do you have signs of an infection such as fever, and/or are you coughing up mucus that is green or yellow, or bloody-colored? **YES** → **See Doctor**

NO ↓

Are your asthma attacks coming more often or getting worse? **YES** →  **See Doctor**

NO ↓

 Use Self-Care

Self-Care Tips

Asthmatics can do a number of things to help themselves.

- Drink plenty of liquids (2–3 quarts a day) to keep secretions loose.

- Find out what triggers your asthma, and get rid of things that bother you at home and at work.

- Make a special effort to keep your bedroom allergen-free.

  - Sleep with a foam or cotton pillow, not a feather pillow.

  - Use a plastic cover on your mattress.

- Wash mattress pads in hot water every week.

- Use throw rugs, not carpeting.

- Don't use drapes.

- Vacuum and dust often. Wear a dust filter mask when you do.

- Avoid using perfumes.

- Don't smoke. Ask other people to not smoke in your home. Try to stay away from air pollution.

- Wear a scarf around your mouth and nose when you are outside in cold weather. Doing so will warm the air as you breathe it in and will prevent cold air from reaching sensitive airways.

- Stop exercising if you start to wheeze.

- Don't eat foods or take medicines that have sulfites. Sulfites are in wine and many shellfish. They bother many people with asthma.

- Sit up during an asthma attack. Don't lie down.

- Put an electronic air filter on your furnace or use portable air purifiers.

- Change and/or wash furnace and air conditioner filters regularly. If you use a portable humidifier or vaporizer, use distilled water, not tap water. Clean and dry the appliance after each use.

- Keep your asthma medicine handy. Take it as soon as you start to feel an attack.

- Some people with asthma are allergic to aspirin. Use acetaminophen instead.

11. Respiratory Conditions

14 Breathing Problems

Some 44 million Americans suffer from allergies and asthma and have trouble breathing during an attack. Also, there are millions of people who have breathing problems because of cigarette smoke and air pollution.

Breathing problems also affect people who are very allergic to some types of shellfish, nuts, medications and insect bites. These people can suffer an allergic reaction called anaphylactic shock. This reaction begins within minutes of exposure to the substance causing the allergy. During this type of allergic reaction, the airways narrow, making it difficult to breathe. Soon, the heartbeat races and blood pressure drops. Anaphylactic shock can be fatal if a person is not treated within 15 minutes.

Breathing problems from some things may require emergency care.

In children they include:

- Wheezing (see page 263)
- Croup, a virus with a "barking cough" common in young children (see page 255)
- Diphtheria, which is a very contagious throat infection
- Heart defects children are born with

In children and adults they include:

- Severe allergic reactions
- A face, head, nose or lung injury
- Carbon monoxide poisoning
- Harsh chemical burns in the air passages

- Epiglottitis, which is inflammation of the flap of tissue at the back of the throat that can close off the windpipe
- Choking (see page 298)
- Drug overdose
- Poisoning (see page 322)
- Asthma (see page 76)
- Bronchitis (see page 81)
- Pneumonia (see page 369)

In adults they include:

- Emphysema (see page 348)
- Congestive heart failure
- Heart attack (see "Chest Pains" on page 150 and "Coronary Heart Disease" on page 343)
- Blood clot in a lung
- Collapse of a lung

Prevention

- Avoid allergic substances or agents that induce asthma, if you have it.
- Do not walk, run or jog on roads with heavy automobile traffic.
- If you have a gas furnace, install a carbon monoxide detector.
- Never leave your car running in a closed garage.
- Make sure immunizations against childhood diseases, especially diphtheria, are up-to-date. This is part of the Diphtheria, Tetanus, Pertussis (DTP) vaccination. (See "Immunization Schedule" on page 18.)
- If you smoke, quit.

11. Respiratory Conditions

Breathing Problems, *Continued*

- Keep small objects a child could choke on out of reach and do not give gum, (especially bubble gum), nuts, hard candy, or popcorn to children under 5 years old.

- Lock up all medications and poisonous substances so small children can't get to them.

Questions to Ask

Has breathing stopped and is there no pulse? **YES** **Get Emergency Care**

{Note: See "CPR" on page 285.}

NO

Has breathing stopped, but there is a pulse? **YES** **Get Emergency Care**

{Note: See "Airway and Breathing" under "CPR" on page 285 and 286.}

NO

Has breathing stopped due to choking on an inhaled object? **YES** **Get Emergency Care**

{Note: See "Choking (Heimlich Maneuver)" on page 289.}

NO

Are there signs of anaphylactic shock?
- Difficulty breathing
- Swollen tongue, eyes, or face
- Unconsciousness
- Difficulty in swallowing
- Dizziness, weakness
- Pounding heart
- Itching, hives

YES **Get Emergency Care**

NO

Flowchart continued in next column

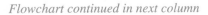

Are any of these problems present with difficulty in breathing?
- Signs of a heart attack such as chest pain, pressure, or tightness; pain that spreads to the arm, neck or jaw; irregular pulse.
- Serious injury to the face, head, or chest
- Signs of a stroke such as blurred or double vision, slurred speech, one-side body weakness or paralysis
- Signs of drug overdose such as drunkenlike behavior, slurred speech, slow or rapid pulse, heavy sweating, enlarged or very small eye pupils

YES **Get Emergency Care**

NO

Is it so hard to breathe that the person can't talk (say 4 or 5 words between breaths) and/or is there wheezing that doesn't go away? **YES** **Get Emergency Care**

NO

Is blood being coughed up? **YES** **Get Emergency Care**

NO

Flowchart continued on next page

11. Respiratory Conditions

79

Breathing Problems, *Continued*

Flowchart continued

Does the difficulty in breathing occur with a cough in a baby and does it make the baby unable to eat or take a bottle? **YES** **Get Emergency Care**

NO

Are any of these signs present?
- Breathlessness at night or at rest
- Pink or frothy phlegm being coughed up and/or
- A high fever along with rapid and labored breathing

YES **Get Emergency Care**

NO

Is a green, yellow, or gray mucus being coughed up? **YES** **See Doctor**

NO

 Use Self-Care

Self-Care Tips

For People Affected by Air Pollution or Pollen:

■ Wear a face mask that covers the nose and mouth, when outdoors. Most hardware stores carry inexpensive ones.

■ Don't smoke. Avoid secondhand smoke. This applies to anyone with breathing difficulties.

■ Install an electronic air filtering system or use an air purifier in your home, especially in the bedroom. Tests show that air filters help clear the air of allergy-causing agents.

For People Allergic to Molds:

Breathing problems can be avoided or lessened if you:

■ Do not rake leaves that have been on the ground for awhile. Molds and mildew grow on leaves after they've been on the ground for a few days.

■ Keep your basement dry, well ventilated, and well lit. Use dehumidifiers and exhaust fans to reduce moisture in the air.

■ Get rid of house plants.

■ Avoid barns, chicken coops, damp basements, and attics.

If you or anyone in your family has serious allergies, it is a good idea to wear a medical identification tag such as ones available at drug stores or ones custom made by MedicAlert Foundation. For more information see "Places to Get Information & Help" under "Medical Identification" on page 376.

See also: "Asthma" on page 76, "Bronchitis" on page 81, "Common Cold" on page 83, "Coughs" on page 85, and "Flu" on page 87.

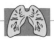

15 Bronchitis

Bronchitis can be either acute or chronic, depending on how long it lasts and how serious the damage.

Acute bronchitis is inflammation of the air passages of the lung. It is generally caused by an infectious agent (like a virus or bacteria) or an environmental pollutant (like smog). These attack the mucous membranes within the windpipe or air passages in your respiratory tract, leaving them red and inflamed.

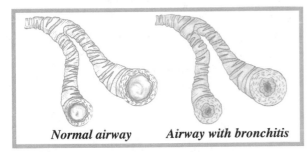

Normal airway   *Airway with bronchitis*

Acute bronchitis often develops in the wake of a sinus infection, cold, or other respiratory infection. It can last anywhere from three days to three weeks.

Signs of Acute Bronchitis Are:

- Cough that has little or no sputum
- Chills, low-grade fever (usually less than 101°F)
- Sore throat and muscle aches
- Feeling of pressure behind the breastbone or a burning feeling in the chest

Treatment for Acute Bronchitis:

A doctor may prescribe:
- Bronchodilators (medicines that open up the bronchial passages)
- Antibiotics

Chronic bronchitis is inflammation and degeneration of the air passages of the lung. The underlying culprit is most often tobacco smoke. **In fact, cigarette smoking is the most common cause of chronic bronchitis.** So quitting is essential and may bring complete relief. Other culprits include pollution and repeated infections of air passages of the lung.

Many people, most of them smokers, develop emphysema (destruction of the air sacs) along with chronic bronchitis. Chronic bronchitis results in abnormal air exchange in the lung and causes permanent damage to the respiratory tract. It's much more serious than acute bronchitis. Chronic bronchitis is not contagious.

Signs of Chronic Bronchitis Are:

- A cough that brings up mucus or phlegm, for as long as 3 months or more, for more than 2 years in a row
- Shortness of breath upon exertion (in early stages)
- Shortness of breath at rest (in later stages)

Treatment for Chronic Bronchitis:

- Not smoking, and avoiding secondhand smoke
- Avoiding or reducing exposure to air pollution, chemical irritants, and cold, wet weather
- Medical treatment for airway infections and heart problems, if present
- Supplemental oxygen

Bronchitis, *Continued*

Questions to Ask

Is the person who has the cough unable to speak more than 4–5 words between breaths or does he or she have purple lips?

YES → **Get Emergency Care**

NO ↓

Does the cough occur in a baby and make the baby unable to eat or take a bottle because he or she has a very hard time breathing?

YES → **Get Emergency Care**

NO ↓

Does the cough occur in an infant less than 3 months old?

YES → **See Doctor**

NO ↓

Does the cough occur in an infant or young child with rapid breathing and sound like a seal's bark?

YES →  **See Doctor**

{*Note:* See "Croup" on page 255.}

NO ↓

Are any of these symptoms also present?
- Fever of 101°F or higher
- Green, yellow, or bloody-colored mucus
- Increase in chest pain
- Shortness of breath at rest and at noncoughing times
- Vomiting

YES → **See Doctor**

NO ↓

Flowchart continued in next column

Have you been exposed to chemicals at work or at home, such as those in new carpet or tobacco smoke, etc.?

YES → **Call Doctor**

NO ↓

 Use Self-Care

Self-Care Tips

■ Breathe air from a "cool-mist" vaporizer or humidifier. Note, though, that vaporizers and humidifiers can harbor bacteria, so clean them after each use. Inhaling bacteria-laden mist may aggravate bronchitis. Use distilled water, not tap water, in the vaporizer.

■ Take an over-the-counter medicine for fever, pain and/or inflammation. {*Note:* See "Pain relievers" in "Your Home Pharmacy" on pages 22 and 23.}

■ Rest.

■ Drink plenty of liquids.

■ Don't smoke. Avoid secondhand smoke.

■ Reduce your exposure to air pollution. (Use air conditioning, air filters, and a mouth and nose filter mask if you have to.) If you develop bronchitis easily, stay indoors during episodes of heavy air pollution.

■ Instead of using cough suppressants, use expectorants. Use bronchodilators and/or take antibiotics as prescribed by your doctor.

11. Respiratory Conditions

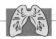

16 **Common Cold**

About 30 million Americans are coughing, sneezing, and blowing their noses while you read this. What's wrong with them? They have the most common illness we know, the common cold. The common cold usually lasts 3 to 7 days and the average person gets 3 or 4 colds a year.

Symptoms
- Sneezing
- Runny nose
- Fever of 101°F or less
- Sore throat
- Dry cough

Causes
Colds are caused by viruses. You can get a cold virus from mucus on a person's hands when they have a cold, such as through a handshake. You can also pick up the viruses on towels, telephones, money, etc. Then someone else picks them up from you. It goes on and on. Cold viruses also travel through coughs and sneezes.

Prevention
- Wash your hands often. Keep them away from your nose, eyes, and mouth.
- Try not to touch people or their things when they have a cold, especially the first 2–3 days they have the cold. This is the most contagious stage.
- Get lots of exercise. Eat and sleep well.

- Use a handkerchief or tissues when you sneeze, cough, or blow your nose. This helps keep you from passing cold viruses to others.
- Use a "cool-mist" vaporizer in your bedroom in the winter.
- Check with your doctor about the use of herbs, such as echinacea, to help prevent colds and to take when you get a cold.
- When you get a cold, check with your doctor about using zinc lozenges. They may shorten the duration of a cold and ease cold symptoms.

Questions to Ask

Are any of these problems present with the cold?
- Chest pain that doesn't go away
- Quick breathing or trouble breathing
- Wheezing

YES See Doctor

NO

Flowchart continued on next page

11. Respiratory Conditions

Common Cold, *Continued*

Flowchart continued

Do you have any of these problems with the cold?
- Earache
- Headache that doesn't go away
- Bright red sore throat, or sore throat with white spots
- Coughing for 10 or more days
- Coughing up mucus that is yellow, green, or gray
- Fever of 104°F in a child under 12 years old
- Fever of over 103°F in an adult under 50 years old
- Fever of 102°F or greater in a person 50–60 years old
- Fever of 101°F or greater in a person over 60 years old
- A bad smell from the throat, nose, or ears

YES → See Doctor

NO ↓

Do you have pain or swelling over your sinuses that gets worse when you bend over or move your head, especially with a fever of 101°F or higher?

YES → See Doctor

NO ↓

 Use Self-Care

Self-Care Tips

Time is the only cure for a cold. Using these Self-Care Tips may make you feel better:

- Rest in bed if you have a fever.
- Drink lots of liquids. They help clear out your respiratory tract. This can help prevent other problems, like bronchitis.
- Take an over-the-counter medicine for muscle aches and pains, and/or fever. {*Note:* See "Pain relievers" in "Your Home Pharmacy" on pages 22 and 23.}
- Use salt water drops to relieve nasal congestion. Mix ½ teaspoon of salt in 1 cup of warm water. Place in a clean container. Put 3 to 4 drops into each nostril several times a day with a clean medicine dropper.
- Use a "cool-mist" vaporizer or humidifier to add moisture to the air.
- Eat chicken soup. It helps clear out mucus.
- Check with your doctor before trying vitamin C. It seems to make some people feel better when they have a cold and may help keep them from getting a cold, even though this has never been medically proven.

For a Sore Throat:

- Gargle every few hours with a solution of ¼ teaspoon of salt dissolved in ½ cup of warm water.
- Drink tea with lemon (with or without honey).
- Suck on a piece of hard candy or medicated lozenge every so often. (Do not give to children under age 5.)

11. Respiratory Conditions

17 Coughs

A lot of things can make you cough:

- An infection
- An allergy
- Asthma (see page 76)
- Tobacco smoke
- Something stuck in your windpipe
- Acid reflux from the stomach (see "Heart-burn" on page 126)
- Dry air
- Certain medications (like some used to treat high blood pressure)
- A collapsed lung

Coughing can be a sign of many ailments. Your body uses coughing to clear your lungs and airways. Coughing itself is not the problem. What causes the cough is the problem. There are 3 kinds of coughs:

- Productive–A cough that brings up mucus or phlegm
- Nonproductive–A cough that is dry. It doesn't bring up any mucus.
- Reflex–A cough that comes from a problem somewhere else, like the ear or stomach

How to treat your cough depends on what kind it is, what caused it, and your other symptoms. Treat the cause and soothe the irritation. Stay away from smoking and secondhand smoke, especially when you have a cough. Smoke hurts your lungs and makes it harder for your body to fight infection.

Questions to Ask

Do you have any of these problems?
- Trouble breathing and not able to say more than 4-5 words between breaths (a baby or small child may be unable to cry, eat, or drink a bottle)
- Chest pain that travels to the neck, arm, or jaw
- Sudden, severe pain in the chest wall followed by a cough and breathlessness without pain
- Fainting
- Coughing up blood

YES Get Emergency Care

NO

Does the cough occur in an infant or a young child with rapid breathing, a fever of 102°F to 103°F, and does it sound like a seal's bark?

YES See Doctor

{*Note:* See "Croup" on page 255.}

NO

Did the cough start suddenly and last an hour or more without stopping? Or do wheezing, shortness of breath, rapid breathing or swelling of the abdomen, legs, and ankles accompany the cough?

YES See Doctor

NO

Flowchart continued on next page

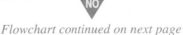

11. Respiratory Conditions

Coughs, *Continued*

Flowchart continued

If the person with the cough is an adult, is there a fever of 102°F or higher? **YES** → **See Doctor**

NO ↓

Do you have any of these problems with the cough?
• Weight loss for no reason
• Feeling tired
• A lot of sweating at night **YES** → **See Doctor**

NO ↓

Does your chest hurt only when you cough and does the pain go away when you sit up or lean forward? **YES** → **See Doctor**

NO ↓

Do you cough up something green, yellow, or bloody-colored, with or without an odor? **YES** → **See Doctor**

NO ↓

Has the cough lasted more than 2 weeks without getting better? **YES** → **Call Doctor**

NO ↓

 Use Self-Care

Self-Care Tips

For Coughs that Bring Up Mucus:

- Drink plenty of liquids such as water and fruit juice. These help loosen mucus and soothe a sore throat.

- Use a "cool-mist" vaporizer, especially in the bedroom. Put a humidifier on the furnace.

- Take a shower. The steam can help thin the mucus.

- Ask your pharmacist for an over-the-counter expectorant. Robitussin is one kind.

- Stop smoking cigarettes, cigars, and/or pipes. Stay away from places where people smoke.

For Coughs that are Dry:

- Drink plenty of liquids. Hot drinks like tea with lemon and honey soothe the throat.

- Suck on cough drops or hard candy. (Don't give these to children under age 5.)

- Take an over-the-counter cough medicine that has dextromethorphan, such as Robitussin-DM.

- Try a decongestant if you have postnasal drip.

- Make your own cough medicine. Mix 1 part lemon juice and 2 parts honey. (Don't give this to children less than 1 year old.)

Other Tips Include:

- Don't give children under age 5 small objects like paper clips, buttons, balloons, or foods like peanuts and popcorn. A small child can easily get something caught in its throat or windpipe. Even adults should be careful to chew and swallow foods slowly so they don't "go down the wrong way."

- Don't smoke. Avoid secondhand smoke.

- Stay away from chemical gases that can hurt your lungs.

11. Respiratory Conditions

18 Flu

"Oh, it's just a touch of the flu," some say, as if they had nothing more than a cold. Yet each year, 20,000 people die from pneumonia and other complications of the influenza virus, or flu.

Cold and flu symptoms resemble each other, but they differ in intensity. A cold generally starts out with some minor sniffling and sneezing, but the flu hits you all at once. You're fine one hour and in bed the next. A cold rarely moves into the lungs. The flu can cause pneumonia. You may be able to drag yourself to work with a cold, but with the flu you may be too ill to leave your bed.

If the following symptoms come on suddenly and intensely, you probably have the flu:

- Dry cough
- Sore throat
- Severe headache
- General muscle aches or backache
- Extreme fatigue
- Chills
- Fever up to 104°F
- Pain when you move your eyes, or a burning sensation in the eyes

Muscle aches and fatigue are the most common signs of the flu. These are normally absent with a cold.

Prevention

An annual flu shot (influenza vaccine) given each fall can help prevent the flu or lessen its severity. Persons who should get a flu shot include: People 65 years of age or older; residents of long term health care facilities; anyone with a chronic medical illness or whose immune system is depressed; and anyone who has close contact with people who are at risk for getting a serious case of influenza. Ask your doctor if you should get an annual flu shot. Also, get plenty of rest, eat well, and exercise regularly to stay strong and fight off the flu.

The antiviral medicines amantadine or rimantadine may be prescribed. {*Note:* In order for rimantadine to be effective, it must be taken within the first 48 hours of the onset of symptoms of the flu.} Antibiotics (to combat any bacterial infection, if also present) may also be prescribed by your doctor.

Questions to Ask

Do you have any of these problems with the flu?
- Inability to speak more than 4 or 5 words between breaths
- Purple lips
- Chest pain that spreads to the neck, jaw, or arm
- Spitting up blood
- Fever, stiff neck, and lethargy

 YES **Get Emergency Care**

NO

Flowchart continued on next page

Flu, *Continued*

Flowchart continued

Do you have any of these problems with the flu?
- Earache
- Sinus pain
- Something thick coming from the nose, ears, or chest

YES → See Doctor

NO ↓

Is your fever and/or other symptoms, like coughing, getting worse?

YES → See Doctor

NO ↓

Have flu symptoms come on 10 days to 3 weeks after a deer-tick bite or exposure to woods or places where deer ticks live?

YES → Call Doctor

NO ↓

Have you had the flu more than a week and not felt better with any Self-Care Tips? Or have new symptoms developed?

YES → Call Doctor

NO ↓

Have you had any side effects from taking any prescribed or over-the-counter medicines?

YES → Call Doctor

NO ↓

 Use Self-Care

Self-Care Tips

There's no cure for the flu. It has to run its course. Generally, if you are in good health, you can treat the flu on your own. Try these tips to minimize discomfort:

- Get plenty of rest.

- Drink lots of hot (not scalding) drinks. They soothe your throat, help unplug your nose, and put back water you lose by sweating.

- Gargle with warm, strong tea or warm salt water. Dissolve $\frac{1}{4}$ teaspoon of salt in $\frac{1}{2}$ cup of water.

- Suck on lozenges or hard candies to lubricate your throat. (Don't give these to children under age 5.)

- Let yourself cough if you are bringing up mucus. Don't suppress a cough that produces mucus. Ask your pharmacist for an over-the-counter expectorant if this is all right with your doctor. Also, if mucus is bloody, yellow, or green, contact your doctor for advice.

- Don't drink milk or eat dairy products for a couple of days. They make mucus thick and hard to cough up in some persons.

- Wash your hands often, especially after blowing your nose and before handling food. This helps you avoid spreading the flu virus to others. It helps to keep you from picking up viruses, too.

- Take an over-the-counter medicine for fever and/or muscle aches. {*Note:* See "Pain relievers" in "Your Home Pharmacy" on pages 22 and 23.}

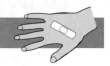

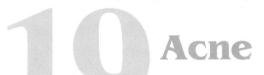

Acne

Acne is a skin condition marked by pimples, such as whiteheads, blackheads, or even raised, red ones that hurt. These pimples show up on the face, neck, shoulders, and/or back. Acne mostly strikes teenagers and young adults. For some, acne, or the scars it can leave, persist into adulthood. Acne results when oil ducts below the skin get clogged with secretions and bacteria. Factors that help cause acne include:

- Hormone changes during adolescence
- Changes in hormone levels before a woman's menstrual period or during pregnancy
- Heavy or greasy lotions or makeup
- Emotional stress
- Nutritional supplements that have iodine
- Cooking oils, tar, or creosote in the air. Creosote is often used as a wood preservative.
- Putting pressure on the face by sleeping on one side of the face or resting your head in your hands
- Birth control pills, steroids, anti-convulsive medications, and lithium (used to treat some forms of depression)

Most cases of acne can be treated with the Self-Care Tips in the next column. When this is not enough, a doctor can prescribe topical ointments, Retin A cream or gel, and/or antibiotics.

Questions to Ask

Is your acne very bad and do you have signs of an infection with it, such as fever and swelling? **YES** → **See Doctor**

NO ↓

Are the pimples big and painful? **YES** → **Call Doctor**

NO ↓

Flowchart continued in next column

Have you tried self-care and it doesn't help or it makes your skin worse? **YES** → **Call Doctor**

NO ↓

 Use Self-Care

Self-Care Tips

Time is the only real cure for acne, but these tips can help:

- Keep your skin clean. Using a clean washcloth every time, work the soap into your skin gently for a minute or two and rinse well.
- Try an astringent lotion, de-greasing pads, or a face scrub.
- Ask your doctor for the name of a good acne soap.
- Leave your skin alone! Don't squeeze, scratch, or poke at pimples. They can get infected and leave scars.
- Use an over-the-counter lotion or cream that has benzoyl peroxide. Follow the directions as listed.
- Wash after you exercise or sweat.
- Wash your hair at least twice a week and keep it off your face.
- For men: Wrap a warm towel around your face before you shave. This will make your beard softer. Always shave the way the hair grows.
- Don't spend too much time in the sun. Don't use a sunlamp.
- Use only water-based makeup. Don't use greasy or oily creams, lotions, or makeups.

20 Athlete's Foot

It smells bad. It's itchy. It's persistent. It's contagious. And it attacks the skin between the toes (usually the third and fourth). What is it? Fungus of the foot, better known as athlete's foot.

People usually get athlete's foot from walking barefoot over wet floors around swimming pools, locker rooms, and public showers that are contaminated with the fungus, which feasts on moisture. Athlete's foot has these signs and symptoms:

- Moist, soft, red or gray-white scales on the feet, especially between the toes
- Cracked, peeling, dead skin areas
- Itching
- Sometimes small blisters on the feet

Questions to Ask

Do you have signs of athlete's foot and are you diabetic or do you have poor leg circulation?

YES → See Doctor

NO ↓

Do you have a fever and/or is the infection spreading or getting worse despite self-treatment described below?

YES →  See Doctor

NO ↓

 Use Self-Care

Self-Care Tips

If you get athlete's foot:

- Wash your feet twice a day, especially between your toes, and dry the area thoroughly. Do not, however, use deodorant soaps.
- Apply an over-the-counter antifungal powder, cream, or spray between your toes and inside of your socks and shoes.
- Wear clean socks made of cotton or wool. (Natural fibers absorb moisture.) Change your socks during the day to help your feet stay dry. Wear shoes that provide some ventilation, like sandals or canvas loafers, whenever you can.
- Alternate shoes daily to let each pair air out.

12. Skin Conditions

21 Burns

Burns can result from dry heat (fire), moist heat (steam, hot liquids), electricity, chemicals, or from radiation, including sunlight. Treatment for burns depends on:

- The depth of the burn (whether it is first, second, or third degree)

- How much of the body area is affected

- The location of the burn

First-degree burns affect only the outer skin layer. The skin area appears dry, red, and mildly swollen. A first-degree burn is painful and sensitive to touch. Mild sunburn and brief contact with a heat source such as a hot iron are examples of first-degree burns. First-degree burns should feel better within a day or two. They should heal in about a week if there are no complications. (See Self-Care Tips on page 92.)

Second-degree burns affect the skin's lower layers and the outer skin. They are painful, swollen, and show redness and blisters. The skin also develops a weepy, watery surface. Examples of second-degree burns are severe sunburn, burns caused by hot liquids, and a gasoline flash. Self-Care Tips can be used to treat many second-degree burns depending on their location and how much area is affected. (See "Questions to Ask" and Self-Care Tips on this page and the next page.)

Third-degree burns affect the outer and deeper skin layers and any underlying tissue and organs. They appear black-and-white and charred. The skin swells, and underlying tissue is often exposed. Third-degree burns may have less pain than first-degree or second-degree burns. There can also be pain when nerve endings are destroyed. Pain may be felt around the margin of the affected area. Third-degree burns usually result from electric shocks, burning clothes, severe gasoline fires, etc. They always require emergency treatment. They may result in hospitalization and sometimes require skin grafts.

Questions to Ask

Is the burn a third-degree burn? (Is there little or no pain; charred, black-and-white skin; and exposure of tissue under the skin?) **YES** → Get Emergency Care

NO ↓

Is the burn a second-degree burn that is on the face, hands, feet, genitals, or on any joint (elbow, knee, shoulder, etc.) or that affects an area larger than 10 inches square? **YES** → Get Emergency Care

NO ↓

Is the burn a second-degree burn that has affected more than the outer skin layer, shows signs of blistering, and covers more than 3 inches in diameter of the skin? **YES** → See Doctor

NO ↓

Flowchart continued on next page

12. Skin Conditions

Burns, *Continued*

Flowchart continued

Is the burn a second-degree burn that covers less than 3 inches of the skin on an infant or a young child?

YES → See Doctor

NO ↓

 Use Self-Care

Self-Care Tips

For Second-degree Burns:

{*Note:* These tips are for second-degree burns that are not extensive and are less than 3" in diameter that occur in an adult or older child.}

■ Immerse the affected area in cold (not ice) water until the pain subsides.

■ Dip clean cloths in cold water, wring them out, and apply them over and over again to the burned area for as long as an hour. Blot the area dry. Do not rub.

■ Do not break any blisters that have formed.

■ Avoid applying antiseptic sprays, ointments, creams.

■ Once dried, dress the area with a single layer of loose gauze that does not stick to the skin. Hold in place with bandage tape that is placed well away from the burned area.

■ Change the dressing the next day and every two days after that.

■ Prop the burned area higher than the rest of the body, if possible.

■ Call your doctor if there are signs of infection (fever, chills, increased redness and swelling, and pus) or if the burn shows no sign of improvement after 2 days.

For First-degree Burns:

■ Cool the area right away. Place the affected area in a container of cold water or under cold running water. Do this for at least 5–10 minutes or until the pain is relieved. (If the affected area is dirty, gently wash it with soapy water first.)

■ Do not apply ice or cold water for too long a time. This may result in complete numbness leading to frostbite.

■ Keep the area uncovered and elevated, if possible. Apply a dry dressing if necessary.

■ Do not use butter or other ointments (for example, Vaseline). You can, though, apply aloe vera gel 3 to 4 times a day. You can buy this at most drug stores.

■ Avoid using local anesthetic sprays and creams. They can slow healing and may lead to allergic reactions in some people.

■ Call your doctor if after 2 days you show signs of infection (fever, chills, increased redness, swelling, or pus in the infected area) or if the burned area is still painful.

■ Take an-over-the-counter medicine for pain. {*Note:* See "Pain relievers" in "Your Home Pharmacy" on pages 22 and 23.}

22 Cold Hands & Feet

Some people wear mittens and heavy socks all year round, even in warm weather, indoors and out. Their hands and feet are always cold. A number of things cause this, such as:

- Poor circulation due to coronary heart disease
- Raynaud's disease (disorder that affects the flow of blood to the fingers and sometimes to the toes)
- Frostbite
- Working with vibrating equipment (like a jackhammer)
- A side effect of taking certain medications
- An underlying disease affecting blood flow in the tiny blood vessels of the skin. (Women smokers may be prone to this last condition.)
- Stress

Symptoms

- Fingers or toes turning pale white or blue, then red, in response to cold
- Tingling or numbness
- Pain during the white phase of discoloration

Questions to Ask

Have your hands or feet had prolonged exposure to sub-freezing temperatures which may have resulted in frostbite? (Frostbite symptoms are tingling and redness followed by paleness – white or bluish appearance – and numbness of affected areas.)

YES → Get Emergency Care

NO ↓

Flowchart continued in next column

Do your hands or feet turn pale, then blue, then red, get painful and numb when exposed to the cold or stress?

YES → Call Doctor

NO ↓

 Use Self-Care

Self-Care Tips

- Stay indoors where it's warm.
- Wear gloves and wool socks.
- Do not wear footwear that is tight-fitting.
- Wiggle your toes. It may help keep them warm as a result of increased blood flow.
- Avoid handling cold objects. Use ice tongs to pick up ice cubes, for instance.
- Don't smoke. It impairs circulation.
- Avoid caffeine. It constricts blood vessels.
- With fingers outstretched, swing your arms in large circles, like a baseball pitcher warming up for a game. This may increase blood flow to the fingers. (Skip this tip if you have bursitis or back problems.)
- Practice a relaxation technique, such as biofeedback.

12. Skin Conditions

23 Corns & Calluses

All too often, corns and calluses are the price we pay for neglecting our feet. Corns and calluses are very much alike; they just differ in where they occur.

Corns show up on the bony area on top of the toes and the skin between the toes. Corns feel hard to the touch, are tender, and have a roundish appearance. A small, clear spot called a hen's eye may form in the center.

Calluses can occur on any part of the body that goes through repeated pressure or irritation. Common places are on the balls or heels of the feet, on the hands, and on the knees. Calluses are flat, painless thickenings of the skin.

Corns and calluses form as a protective response. They are extra cells made in a skin area that gets repeated rubbing or squeezing from such things as:

- Footwear that fits poorly

- Activities that put pressure on the hands, knees, and feet

If Self-Care Tips do not get rid of corns and calluses, a family doctor or foot doctor (podiatrist) may need to be consulted. He or she can scrape away the hardened tissue and peel away the corn with stronger solutions. (Sometimes warts lie underneath corns and need to be treated too.)

Questions to Ask

Do you have any signs of infection (fever, swelling, redness, pus sacs, puffiness)? **YES** → **See Doctor**

NO ↓

Do you have circulation problems or diabetes mellitus? **YES** → **Call Doctor**

NO ↓

Do you have one or both of these problems even after providing self-care?
- Continued or worse pain
- No improvement after 2 to 3 weeks

YES → **Call Doctor**

NO ↓

 Use Self-Care

Self-Care Tips

For Corns:

Never pick at corns or use toenail scissors or clippers, a razor blade, or any other sharp tool to cut off corns. You may injure your skin or trigger an infection. Instead:

- Get rid of shoes that fit poorly, especially if they squeeze your toes together.

- Soak your feet in warm water to soften the corn.

12. Skin Conditions

Corns & Calluses, *Continued*

■ Cover the corn with a protective, nonmedicated pad, usually available in drugstores. (A piece of foam rubber or moleskin will do in a pinch.)

■ If the outer layers of a corn have peeled away, apply a nonprescription liquid of 5 – 10 percent salicylic acid. Gently rub the corn off with cotton gauze.

■ Take your shoe to a shoe repair person and ask that he/she sew a metatarsal bar onto your shoe to use when a corn is healing.

For Calluses:

Never try to get rid of a callus by cutting it with a sharp tool. Instead:

■ Soak your feet in warm water to soften the callus, and pat dry.

■ Rub the callus gently with a pumice stone.

■ Cover calluses with protective pads, available in drugstores.

■ Check for poorly fitting shoes or other sources of pressure that may lead to calluses.

■ Wear gloves if doing a hobby or work that puts pressure on your hands.

■ Wear knee pads for activities that put pressure on your knees.

12. Skin Conditions

Cuts, Scrapes, & Punctures

Cuts, scrapes, and punctures can all result in bleeding.

■ Cuts slice the skin open. Close a cut so it won't get infected.

■ Scrapes hurt only the top part of your skin. They can hurt more than cuts, but they heal quicker.

■ Punctures stab deep. Leave punctures open so they won't get infected.

You can treat most cuts, scrapes, and punctures yourself. But you should get emergency care if you are bleeding a lot, or if you are hurt very badly. Blood gets thicker after bleeding for a few minutes. This is called clotting. Clotting slows down bleeding. Press on the cut to help slow down the bleeding. You may have to apply pressure for 10 minutes or more for a bad cut. Sometimes a cut needs stitches. Stitches help the cut heal.

Questions to Ask

Is the bleeding from the cut, scrape, or puncture severe? Has the victim gone into shock? Does blood spurt from the wound? Has a lot of blood been lost (in an adult, ½ cup or more, less in a child)?

YES **Get Emergency Care**

{*Note:* See "First Aid for Major Bleeding" under Self-Care Tips on page 97.}

NO

Is there still a lot of bleeding, even though pressure has been applied for 10 minutes or more?

YES **Get Emergency Care**

NO

{*Note:* See "First Aid for Major Bleeding" under Self-Care Tips on page 97.}

Flowchart continued in next column

Does the cut or puncture have any of these signs? (If so, the cut will likely need stitches.)

• The cut or puncture is deep (i.e., appears to go down to the muscle or bone) and/or is located on the scalp or face.

• The cut is longer than an inch and located on an area of the body that bends, such as the elbow, knee or finger. (Bending will put pressure on the cut.)

• The skin on the edges of the cut hangs open.

• Bleeding from what seems to be a minor cut continues after 20 minutes of applied pressure.

YES **Get Emergency Care**

{*Note:* Apply pressure to the wound to slow or stop the bleeding.}

NO

Is the cut or puncture from dirty or contaminated objects, such as rusty nails or objects in the soil, or does the puncture go through a shoe, especially a rubber-soled one?

YES **See Doctor**

{*Note:* See your doctor right away for advice on getting a tetanus shot.}

NO

Flowchart continued on next page

Cuts, Scrapes, & Punctures, *Continued*

Flowchart continued

Did any of these signs of infection appear a day or two after the injury?
- Fever of 101°F or higher
- Redness, swelling, tenderness at and around the site of the wound
- Increased pain
- General ill feeling
- Swollen lymph nodes

YES → See Doctor

NO

Use Self-Care

Self-Care Tips

First Aid for Major Bleeding:

■ Monitor for signs of shock. (See "Shock" on page 327.)

■ Put on disposable latex rubber gloves, if available. (See "First-Aid Precautions" on page 284.)

■ Apply direct pressure to the wound using a clean cloth or sterile bandage.

■ Put pressure on the wound for at least 10 minutes. {*Note:* If the cut is large and the edges of it gape open, pinch the edge of the wound while applying pressure.}

■ If bleeding continues before emergency help arrives, put extra cloths or bandages on top of existing ones and reapply pressure.

■ Elevate the wounded area higher than heart level while you apply pressure if there is no broken bone.

■ Do not remove an object that is stuck in a wound. Pack the object in place with padding and put tape around the padding so it doesn't move.

■ If bleeding still continues after 15 to 20 minutes of direct pressure, apply pressure to a "pressure point." Use the pressure point closest to the bleeding site that is between the wound and the heart. (See chart and picture of pressure points.)

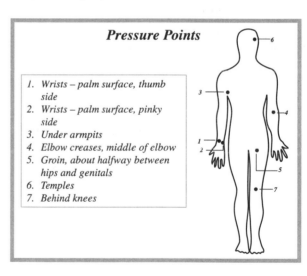

Pressure Points

1. Wrists – palm surface, thumb side
2. Wrists – palm surface, pinky side
3. Under armpits
4. Elbow creases, middle of elbow
5. Groin, about halfway between hips and genitals
6. Temples
7. Behind knees

■ Continue to apply pressure to the bleeding site while you use flat fingers to put pressure on the pressure point. Do this until bleeding stops. Do not apply a tourniquet except to save a life.

■ Continue to monitor for signs of shock.

12. Skin Conditions

Cuts, Scrapes, & Punctures, *Continued*

First Aid for Bleeding from the Scalp:

- Control bleeding by putting pressure around the edges of the wound, not on the wound. Make a ring pad (shaped like a doughnut) with a narrow bandage of narrow but long strips of cloth. Start with one end of the narrow bandage and wrap it around all four fingers on one hand until you form a loop. Leave a long strip of the bandage material to weave in and around the loop so it doesn't ravel. Use this ring pad to apply pressure around the edges of the wound.

- Don't wash the wound or apply an antiseptic or any other fluid to it.

- If blood or pink-colored fluid is coming from the ear, nose, or mouth, let it drain. Do not try to stop its flow.

First Aid for Cuts and Scrapes:

- Clean around the wound with soap and water.

- Press on the cut to stop the bleeding, and continue for up to 10 minutes if you need to. Use a sterile bandage, clean cloth, or, if these are not available, a clean hand. (Try not to use dry gauze. It can stick to the wound.) Don't use a band-aid for applying pressure.

- Press on the cut again if it keeps bleeding. Get help if it is still bleeding after 20 or more minutes. Keep pressing on it while you wait for help.

- Lift the part of the body with the cut higher than the heart. This slows down blood flow to that spot.

- Apply a first-aid cream, such as Neosporin or Johnson & Johnson, on the cut after it has stopped bleeding and when it is clean and dry. Apply it with a sterile cloth or cotton swab.

- Put one or more bandages on the cut. Do it this way:

  - Put the bandage across the cut so it can help hold the cut together.

  - The sides of the cut should touch but not overlap.

  - Don't touch the cut with your hand.

  - You can use a butterfly bandage if you have one.

  - Use more than one bandage for a long cut.

  - For scrapes, make a bandage from gauze and first-aid tape.

- Leave the bandage on for 24 hours. Change the bandage every day or two or more often if you need to. Be careful when you take the bandage off. You don't want to make the cut bleed again. If you have used gauze, wet it before you pull it off.

- Take an over-the-counter medicine for pain. Don't take aspirin every day unless your doctor tells you to, because taking it too much can keep the blood from clotting. {*Note:* See "Pain relievers" in "Your Home Pharmacy" on pages 22 and 23.}

- Call your doctor or local health department if you have not had a tetanus shot in the last 10 years (5 years for a deep puncture).

Cuts, Scrapes, & Punctures, *Continued*

- If the wound is on a child, check with the child's doctor or local health department to find out if the child's DTaP or DTP immunizations are up-to-date. (See "Immunization Schedule" on page 18.)

- Contact your doctor if you notice any signs of infection a day or two after the injury. These include:

  - Fever of 101°F or higher

  - Redness, swelling, tenderness at and around the site of the wound

  - Increased pain

  - General ill feeling

First Aid for Punctures that Cause Minor Bleeding:

- Let the wound bleed to clean itself out.

- Remove the object that caused the puncture. Use clean sterile tweezers. To sterilize them, hold a lit match or flame to the ends of the tweezers. {*Note:* Don't pull anything out of a puncture wound if blood gushes from it or if it has been bleeding badly. Get emergency care.}

- Wash the wound with warm water and soap or take a bath or shower to clean it.

- Leave the wound open. Cover it with a bandage if it is big or still bleeds a little.

- Soak the wound in warm, soapy water 2 to 4 times a day. Then dry it well and apply an antibiotic cream such as Neosporin. Cover it with a bandage.

12. Skin Conditions

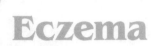 # Eczema

Eczema (atopic dermatitis) is a chronic skin condition that usually appears on the scalp, face, neck, or creases of the elbows, wrists, and knees. The symptoms are small blisters and crusty scales on the skin surface, often accompanied by inflammation. Children and adults alike may be affected, and the condition often runs in families. Asthma is often associated with this skin condition.

A variety of irritants or allergens can aggravate eczema. These include:

- Wearing wool fabric
- Sweating
- Stress
- Exposure to extreme weather conditions (especially high heat and humidity)
- Eating foods such as eggs, milk, seafood, or wheat products
- Contact with cosmetics, dyes, medicines, deodorants, skin lotions, permanent press fabrics, and other allergens

Eczema is quite unpredictable. Usually it's at its worst in childhood and gradually lets up as you get older. Sometimes it goes away for good. Eczema can be a lifetime problem, though.

Questions to Ask

Are there any signs of infection with the eczema, such as fever, or is there a large amount of weeping or crusting present? **YES** →  See Doctor

NO

Flowchart continued in next column

Has the rash lasted for a long time? **YES** → Call Doctor

NO

 Use Self-Care

Self-Care Tips

True eczema needs a doctor's care. You can, however, do much to maintain good skin care and to manage eczema. Follow these tips:

- Don't take baths too often. Sponge bathe in between tub baths. Add bath oil to the water. Or, take quick showers.
- Use warm (not hot) water when you take a bath or shower.
- Use a mild soap or no soap at all on the areas of eczema.
- Stay away from wool clothes and blankets.
- Use a light, nongreasy lotion on your skin after you wash. Pick one that is unscented. Don't use lotions that have alcohol. They can dry the skin.
- Try to keep from sweating. For example, don't wear too many clothes for the weather.
- Wear rubber gloves when you do housework. Put talcum powder or cornstarch inside the gloves. Or, try latex gloves lined with cotton.
- Stay away from foods, chemicals, cosmetics, and other things that make your eczema worse.
- And above all, don't scratch! Scratching eczema only makes it worse. It can get infected. Keep your fingernails cut short.

26 Hair Loss

Most men and women experience hair loss as they get older; indeed, most men have some degree of baldness by age 60. This is quite normal and affects some persons more than others, especially if baldness runs in the family. Sudden or abnormal hair loss could, however, result from:

- Taking certain medications (like some used in treating cancer, circulatory disorders, ulcers or arthritis)

- Following a crash diet

- Hormonal changes such as with menopause

- A prolonged or serious illness

Some medical conditions lead to hair loss. These need treatment. They include:

- Hypothyroidism and ringworm (the latter is a fungal infection that affects the scalp and/or the hairs themselves)

- Areata, which causes areas of patchy hair loss, but does not affect the scalp. This condition improves rapidly when treated, but can even disappear within 18 months without treatment. Doctors may prescribe a topical steroid to be used once or twice a day.

For cosmetic reasons, some older persons wear wigs or toupees. Surgical hair transplant operations and the medication Rogaine are treatment options for both men and women, in very select cases. {*Note*: Wear a hat or use a sunscreen with a sun protection factor (SPF) of 15 or more on the bald parts of your head when your head is exposed to the sun. The risk of sunburn and skin cancer on the scalp increases with baldness.}

Questions to Ask

Do you experience one or more of the following?
- Unexplained fatigue and weight gain
- Feeling cold
- Numbness and tingling of hands and feet
- Slow heartbeat
- Coarse skin and hair
- Deepened or hoarse voice
- Depression
- Decreased sex drive

 YES → **See Doctor**

NO ↓

Has the hair loss occurred suddenly and in patches on the head? Is the scalp affected in any way, such as with red or gray-green scales?

YES → **See Doctor**

NO ↓

Are there signs of infection (e.g., redness, tenderness, swelling and/or pain) at the site of hair loss?

YES → **See Doctor**

NO ↓

Does the hair loss occur from uncontrollably pulling out patches of hair?

YES →  **Call Doctor**

NO ↓

Flowchart continued on next page

12. Skin Conditions

Hair Loss, *Continued*

Flowchart continued

Have you begun losing your hair only after taking prescribed medicine for high blood pressure, high cholesterol, ulcers or arthritis? **YES** Call Doctor

NO

Do you want to find out about hair implants or the medication Rogaine? **YES** Call Doctor

NO

 Use Self-Care

Self-Care Tips

To protect your hair from damage and loss:

 Avoid damaging hair care practices or use them infrequently. These include braiding, cornrowing, bleaching, dyeing, perming, straightening; hot curling irons and rollers, and hair dryers, especially on a high setting.

■ Use gentle shampoos and conditioners.

■ Let your hair dry by patting it with a towel or by air drying.

■ If your hair is damaged, cut it short or change your hairstyle to one that requires less damaging hair care practices.

■ Take measures (e.g., yoga and other relaxation techniques) to reduce anxiety if this results in pulling out patches of hair.

■ Don't be taken in by fraudulent claims for vitamin formulas, massage oils, lotions or ointments that promise to cure baldness. No potion or ointment exists that will produce a full head of hair. The only remedy that comes close is the medication Rogaine, originally developed as a blood pressure medication. Rogaine has shown promising results for some (but not all) cases of baldness. This applies to both men and women. It is available over-the-counter.

■ Ask your doctor for a substitute medication if you are taking one that has caused hair loss. (This is not done, though, for certain medications such as anticancer drugs.)

27 Hives

Hives, or urticaria, are red, raised, itchy welts. They appear, sometimes in clusters, on the face, trunk of the body, and, less often, on the scalp, hands, or feet. Hives can change shape, fade, then rapidly reappear. A single hive lasts less than 24 hours. After an attack, though, new ones may crop up for up to 6 weeks. According to estimates, nearly 20 percent of Americans will get hives at some time in their lives.

Hives can be (but aren't always) an allergic response to something you touched, inhaled, or swallowed. Some common causes of hives include:

- Reactions to medications such as aspirin, sulfa, and penicillin
- Animal dander (especially from cats)
- Cold temperatures
- Emotional or physical stress (including exercise)
- Foods (especially chocolate, nuts, shellfish, or tomatoes)
- Infections
- Inhalants (especially pollen, mold spores, or airborne chemicals)
- Insect bites and stings
- Rubbing or putting pressure on the skin
- Exposure to chemicals
- Malignant or connective tissue disease

Sometimes it is not known what causes hives. But if you can identify the triggers (try keeping a diary), you may be able to prevent future outbreaks.

Questions to Ask

Do you have any of these problems?
- Shortness of breath and breathing difficulties
- Wheezing, dizziness
- Swollen lips, tongue, and/or throat

YES → Get Emergency Care

 NO

Did hives start after recently taking a medication? Or, do you have itching that is constant and severe or do you have a fever?

YES → Call Doctor

NO

 Use Self-Care

Self-Care Tips

Here are some tips for a case of ordinary, non-threatening hives:

- Don't take hot baths or showers. Heat worsens most rashes and makes them itch more.
- Apply cold compresses or take a warm bath.
- Wear loose-fitting clothing.
- Relax as much as possible. Relaxation therapy may help ease the itching and discomfort of hives.
- Ask your doctor whether or not you should take an antihistamine. Have him or her recommend one. Antihistamines can help relieve itching and suppress hives. Take as directed by your doctor, or on the label.
- Avoid taking aspirin, ibuprofen, ketoprofen or naproxen sodium. These may aggravate hives.

12. Skin Conditions

103

28 Ingrown Toenails

An ingrown toenail is one that digs into surrounding skin (usually on the big toe). It can cause discomfort, pain, tenderness, and redness. Sometimes it gets infected.

Causes

Possible causes include:

- Jamming your toes by making sudden stops, especially while playing sports like tennis or basketball
- Wearing tight-fitting shoes or socks
- Clipping toenails too far back, so that the corners penetrate the skin as they grow out
- Having wider-than-average toenails

Home treatment generally is all that is needed for ingrown toenails. If home treatment fails to work, a physician or podiatrist may have to surgically remove the troublesome portion of the nail.

Prevention

- Cut nails straight across. Don't cut the nails shorter at the sides than in the middle.
- File the corners of the nail if they're sharp after clipping them.
- Wear shoes and socks that fit well.

Questions to Ask

Has your toenail shown any signs of infection, such as redness, tenderness, and/or is it filled with pus? **YES** See Doctor

NO

Do you have diabetes mellitus or circulation problems? **YES** Call Doctor

NO

Do you get ingrown toenails frequently? **YES** Call Doctor

NO

 Use Self-Care

Self-Care Tips

Home remedies for a painful ingrown toenail include these steps:

- Soak your foot in warm, soapy water for 5–10 minutes, 1–3 times a day.
- Gently lift the nail away from the reddened skin at the outer corners with the tip of a nail file.
- Place a small piece of cotton soaked in an antiseptic or topical antibiotic, such as Neosporin, just under the outer corners, if you can.
- Repeat the previous 3 steps daily until the nail begins to grow correctly and pressure is relieved. (Wear roomy shoes during this time.)

29 Insect Stings

Insects that sting include:

- Bumblebees
- Honeybees
- Hornets
- Wasps
- Yellow jackets
- Fire ants

Symptoms

Most often, the symptoms that come from these insect stings include:

- Quick, sharp pain
- Swelling
- Itching
- Redness at the sting site
- Hives (see page 103)

Insect stings can even result in a severe allergic reaction. Symptoms of this include:

- Severe swelling, all over and/or of the face, tongue, lips
- Weakness, dizziness
- A difficult time breathing or swallowing
- Airway obstruction or shock

Symptoms of a severe allergic reaction usually happen soon after or within an hour of the sting. A severe allergic reaction can be life-threatening. It needs immediate emergency care.

If you've ever had an allergic reaction to an insect sting in the past, you should carry an emergency kit that has:

- Adrenalin (a medicine called epinephrine that stops the bodywide reaction) and a device with a needle to inject it
- An antihistamine
- An inhaler that contains adrenalin
- Instruction sheet that explains how to use the kit

You have to get this kit from your doctor. You should also wear a medical alert tag that lets others know that you are allergic to insect stings. Persons who have had severe reactions in the past to bee or wasp stings should ask their doctor about allergy shots.

Prevention

Try to avoid getting stung.

- Keep food and drink containers tightly covered. (Bees love sweet things like soft drinks.)
- Don't wear perfume, colognes, or hair spray when you are outdoors.
- Don't wear bright colors. Choose white, or neutral colors like tan. These don't attract bees.
- Wear snug clothing that covers your arms and legs.
- Don't go barefoot.
- If camping, look for insects in your shoes before you wear them.

12. Skin Conditions

Insect Stings, *Continued*

- Wear insect repellants especially if you are sensitive to insect stings.

- Be careful when:

  - Working outdoors

  - Pulling weeds

  - Removing shutters from the house to paint. (Bees often build hives behind shutters.)

  - Mowing tall grass

- If an insect that stings gets in your car, stop the car, roll down the windows and get the insect out of the car.

Questions to Ask

If you are stung by an insect, do you have any of these problems?
- Problems breathing and/or swallowing
- Swelling all over
- Swollen tongue, lips or face
- Throat that feels closed up
- Skin that turns blue
- Seizure
- Wheezing

YES Get Emergency Care

NO {*Note:* Give shot from emergency insect sting kit if there is one. Follow other instructions in kit.}

Were you stung in the mouth or on the tongue?

YES Get Emergency Care

NO {*Note:* Give shot from emergency insect sting kit if there is one. Follow other instructions in kit.}

Flowchart continued in next column

Do you have any of these problems after you are stung by an insect?
- Hives
- Stomach cramps

YES Call Doctor

NO Use Self-Care

Self-Care Tips

- Gently scrape out the stinger as soon as possible. Use a credit card or a fingernail. This applies to bees only. Yellow jackets, wasps, and hornets don't lose their stingers.

- Don't pull the stinger out with your fingers or tweezers. Don't squeeze the stinger. It contains venom. You could re-sting yourself.

- Clean the sting area with soapy water.

- Put a cold compress on the sting. Put ice in a cloth, plastic bag, or plastic wrap. Don't put ice directly on the skin. Hold the cold compress on the site for 15–20 minutes.

- Keep the sting area lower than the level of the heart.

- Take an over-the-counter medicine for the pain. {*Note:* See "Pain relievers" in "Your Home Pharmacy" on pages 22 and 23.}

- Take an over-the-counter antihistamine, such as Benadryl, for the itching and swelling unless you have to avoid this medicine for medical reasons. Look on the label for how much to take.

30 Poison Ivy (Oak, Sumac)

Poison ivy, poison oak, and poison sumac are the most common plants that cause a skin rash. A sap that comes from these plants causes the rash. The name of this sap is urushiol. It is not really a poison but it causes an allergic reaction. Not everyone reacts to urushiol. If you are allergic to it, though, you can get a skin rash when you:

■ Touch poison ivy, poison oak, or poison sumac.

■ Touch clothing, garden tools, or shoes that have the sap on them.

■ Touch pets that have the sap on them.

■ Come in contact with the smoke of these burning plants.

Symptoms

The skin rash comes a day or two after contact with the poisonous plant. Things to look for are:

■ Itching

■ Redness

■ Burning feeling

■ Swelling

■ Blisters

Symptoms can range from mild to severe.

Prevention

■ Know what these plants look like and avoid them:

Poison Ivy

Poison Oak

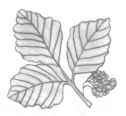

Poison ivy and poison oak both have 3 leaflets per stem. This is why you may have heard the saying, "Leaflets three, let them be."

Poison Sumac

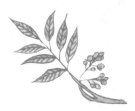

Poison sumac has 7 to 11 leaflets. One leaflet is at the end of the stem. The others are in two rows opposite to each other.

■ Look for an over-the-counter lotion (IvyBlock), which blocks skin contact with the sap from poison ivy, oak, and sumac. You need to apply the lotion before you come in contact with the plants.

If you know you have come in contact with one of the plants, do the things below within 6 hours. You may prevent an allergic reaction if you do.

■ Remove all clothes and shoes that have touched the plant.

Poison Ivy (Oak, Sumac), *Continued*

- Wash your skin with soap and water.

- Apply rubbing alcohol with cotton balls to the parts of the skin that are affected. Or, use alcohol wipes that are prepacked. {*Note:* Carry alcohol wipes with you when you are going to places that have poison ivy, oak, or sumac.} Or, try an over-the-counter product, Tecnu, which removes the poison ivy sap.

- Rinse the affected area with water.

Questions to Ask

Do you have any of these problems?
- Skin that is very bright red
- Severe itching, swelling, or blisters
- Rash on large areas of the body or the face
- Rash that has spread to the mouth, eyes, or genitals
- Pus

YES → See Doctor

NO ↓

Use Self-Care

Self-Care Tips

- Take a cold shower, put the rash area in cold water, or pour cold water over it. Use soap when you shower.

- Take an over-the-counter antihistamine, such as Benadryl, as stated on the label to relieve itching.

- For weeping blisters:
  - Mix 2 teaspoons of baking soda in 1 quart (4 cups) of water.
  - Dip squares of gauze in this mixture.
  - Cover the blisters with the wet gauze for 10 minutes, four times a day. (Do not apply this to the eyes.)

- Make sure you wash all clothes and shoes with hot water and a strong soap. Bathe pets that have come in contact with poison ivy, oak, or sumac. The sap can stay on pets for many days. Also, clean tools etc., that you used to wash your clothes and your pet(s). Wear rubber gloves when you do all these things.

- Keep your hands away from your eyes, mouth, and face.

- Do not scratch or rub the rash.

- Apply any of these to the skin rash:
  - Calamine (not Caladryl) lotion
  - Over-the-counter topical steroid cream, such as Cortaid. {*Note:* Do not apply to the face or genital area.}
  - Paste made with baking soda – mix 3 teaspoons of baking soda with 1 teaspoon of water

- Take baths with lukewarm water and an over-the-counter product called Aveeno colloidal oatmeal

Call your doctor if Self-Care Tips do not bring relief.

31 Shingles

Shingles (herpes zoster) is a skin disorder triggered by the chicken pox virus (varicella zoster) that you had as a child. This virus is thought to lie dormant in the spinal cord until later in life. Shingles most often occurs between the ages of 50 and 70 in both men and women. Even though shingles is not as contagious as chicken pox, infants and people whose immunity is low should not be exposed to it. Besides aging, the risks for getting shingles increases with:

- Hodgkin's disease or other cancer

- Any illness in which infection-fighting systems are below par

- The use of anticancer medications or any medications that suppress the immune system (Example: corticosteroids)

- Stress or trauma, either emotional or physical

Symptoms

Symptoms of shingles include:

- Pain, itching, or tingling sensation before the rash appears

- A rash of painful red blisters which later crust over. Most often, the rash appears on the torso or side of the face. Only one side of the face or body is affected. Shingles is almost never present on both sides of the body. It is serious if it affects the eye, because it can lead to blindness.

- Though rare, fever and general weakness sometimes occur

After the crusts fall off (usually within 3 weeks), pain can persist in the area of the rash. This usually goes away on its own after 1–6 months. Chronic pain can, however, last for months or years. The older you are, the greater the chance that this is the case. The recovery time may also take longer, too.

Most cases of shingles are mild, but shingles can result in chronic, severe pain, blindness or deafness. So, to be on the safe side, let your doctor know if you get shingles.

Treatment

Treatment for shingles includes:

- Pain relief with analgesics. Codeine may sometimes be prescribed.

- Prescription medicines Famvir, Valtrex, and Zovirax can be very effective. The sooner one of these medicines is used, the better the results.

- An antibiotic if the blisters become infected

- Antihistamines

- Corticosteroids

- Tranquilizers for a short time

Questions to Ask

With shingles, are you over 60 years of age, taking anticancer or other immunosuppressive medicines, or do you have a chronic illness?

 YES  See Doctor

NO

Flowchart continued on next page

Shingles, *Continued*

Flowchart continued

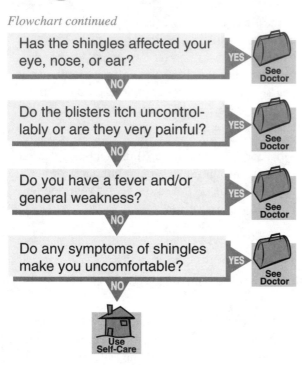

Has the shingles affected your eye, nose, or ear? **YES** → See Doctor

NO ↓

Do the blisters itch uncontrollably or are they very painful? **YES** → See Doctor

NO ↓

Do you have a fever and/or general weakness? **YES** → See Doctor

NO ↓

Do any symptoms of shingles make you uncomfortable? **YES** → See Doctor

NO ↓

Use Self-Care

Self-Care Tips

Following are things you can do (along with your doctor's treatment plan) to help relieve an active outbreak of shingles:

- Unless your doctor has given you prescription pain medicine, take an over-the-counter medicine for pain. {*Note:* See "Pain relievers" in "Your Home Pharmacy" on pages 22 and 23.}

- If possible, keep sores open to the air. Don't bandage them unless you live with or are around children or adults who have not yet had the chicken pox. They could pick up chicken pox from exposure to shingles.

- Don't wear restrictive clothing that irritates the area of the body where sores are present.

- Wash blisters, but never scrub them.

- Apply calamine lotion to the affected area to relieve itching. Or apply a paste made of 3 teaspoons of baking soda mixed with 1 teaspoon of water to the affected area.

- Avoid drafty areas where you can get chilled.

- Put cool compresses on the blisters. You can use several things: a cold cloth or towel dipped in ice water, a bag of frozen vegetables, or an ice pack wrapped in a thin towel. Put the cool compress on the blisters for 20 minutes at a time.

- Drink plenty of liquids.

32 Skin Rashes

Skin rashes come in all forms and sizes. Some are raised bumps; others are flat red blotches. Some are itchy blisters; others are patches of rough skin. Most rashes are harmless and clear up on their own within a few days. A few may need medical attention. The skin is one of the first areas of the body to react when exposed to something you or your child is allergic to.

The chart on page 113 lists information on some common skin rashes.

Questions to Ask

Are you having a lot of trouble swallowing or breathing, especially with wheezing, or is the tongue swollen? **YES →**

Get Emergency Care
{*Note:* Give shot from emergency insect sting kit if there is one. Follow other instructions in the kit.}

NO ↓

Do you have any of these problems with the rash?
- Fever
- Sore throat
- The rash is across the cheeks and forehead and is butterfly shaped
- The rash is a fine, red one that feels rough, like sandpaper
- Joint pain along with a targetlike rash

YES →

See Doctor

NO ↓

Are any large, fluid-filled blisters present or is there pus or swelling around the rash lesions? **YES →**
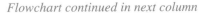
See Doctor

NO ↓

Flowchart continued in next column

With the rash does it look like there is blood or bruising under the skin? **YES →**

See Doctor

NO ↓

Have you recently been exposed to someone with a strep infection? **YES →**

See Doctor

NO ↓

If your child has a diaper rash, is the rash bleeding or are there open, weeping sores? **YES →**

See Doctor

NO ↓

Have you already had the chicken pox and do you now have a rash of painful red blisters on one side of the body? **YES →**

See Doctor

NO ↓

When the rash started, were you taking a new medication or were you stung by an insect? **YES →**

Call Doctor

NO ↓

Is the rash getting worse, keeping you from sleeping and/or do Self-Care Tips not relieve symptoms? **YES →**

Call Doctor

NO ↓

Use Self-Care

See Self-Care Tips on next page

111

Skin Rashes, *Continued*

Self-Care Tips

To Treat Heat Rash:

- Take a bath in cool water, without soap, every couple of hours.
- Let your skin air-dry.
- Stay in a cool, dry area.
- Apply calamine (not Caladryl) lotion to the very itchy spots.
- Put cornstarch in body creases (inside elbows, etc.).
- Don't use ointments and creams that can block the sweat gland pores.

To Treat Diaper Rash in a Child:

- Change diapers as soon as they become wet or soiled (even at night if the rash is extensive).
- Wash your baby with plenty of warm water, not disposable wipes, to prevent irritating the skin. If the skin appears irritated, apply a light coat of zinc oxide ointment after the skin is completely dry.
- Keep the skin dry and exposed to air.
- Before putting on a fresh diaper, keep your baby's bottom naked on a soft, fluffy towel for 10 to 15 minutes.
- Put diapers on loosely so air can circulate under them. If disposable diapers are used, punch a few holes in them. Avoid ones with tight leg bands.
- Don't use plastic pants until the rash is gone.
- Wash cloth diapers in mild soap. Add ¹/₂ cup of vinegar to your rinse water to help remove what's left of the soap.

For Cradle Cap in Babies:

- Use an antidandruff shampoo 2 to 3 times a week, massaging your baby's scalp with a soft brush or washcloth for 5 minutes.
- Before you wash your child's hair, apply mineral oil to the scalp. This will soften the hard crusts. Be sure to wash the oil out completely.

To Protect Yourself from Lyme Disease:

- Wear long pants, tucked into socks, and long-sleeve shirts when you walk through fields and forests or go camping. Light-colored, tightly woven clothing is best. Inspect yourself for ticks after these outdoor activities.
- To remove any ticks found on the skin:
  - Use tweezers to grasp the tick as close to the skin as possible.
  - Pull in a steady upward motion.
  - Try not to crush the tick because the secretions released may spread disease.
  - Wash the wound area and your hands with soap and water after removing ticks.
  - Save any removed ticks in a jar and take them to the doctor to aid in the diagnosis of Lyme disease.

For chicken pox, see "Self-Care Tips" on pages 251 and 252. For eczema, see "Self-Care Tips" on page 100. For hives, see "Self-Care Tips" on page 103. For poison ivy, oak or sumac see "Self-Care Tips" on page 108.

Skin Rashes, *Continued*

Skin Rash Chart				
Condition or Illness	**Causes**	**What Rash Looks Like**	**Skin Area(s) Affected**	**Other Symptoms**
Diaper Rash	Dampness and the interaction of urine and the skin	Small patches of rough skin, tiny pimples	Buttocks, thighs, genitals	Soreness, no itching
Cradle Cap	Hormones that pass through the placenta before birth	Scaly, crusty rash (in newborns)	Starts behind the ears and spreads to the scalp	Fine, oily scales
Heat Rash (Prickly Heat)	Blocked-off sweat glands	Small red pimples, pink blotchy skin	Chest, waist, back, armpits, groin	Itching
[1]Roseola	Herpes virus type-6	Flat, rosy red rash	Chest and abdomen	High fever 2-4 days before rash – child feels only mildly ill during fever
[1]Fifth Disease	Human parvovirus B19	Red rash of varying shades that fades to a flat, lacy pattern (rash comes and goes)	Red rash on facial cheeks, lace-like rash can also appear on arms and legs	Mild disease with no other symptoms or a slight runny nose and sore throat
Eczema	Allergens	Dry, red, cracked skin, blisters that ooze and crust over, sufficient scratching leads to a thickened, rough skin	On cheeks in infants, on neck, wrists, inside elbows, and backs of knees in older children	Moderate-to-intense itching (may only itch first, then rash appears hours to days later)
[1]Chicken Pox[2]	Varicella/herpes zoster virus	Flat, red spots that become raised and look like small pimples. These develop into small blisters that break and crust over.	Back, chest, and abdomen first, then rest of body	Fatigue and mild fever 24 hours before rash appears – intense itching
[1]Scarlet Fever	Bacterial infection (streptococcal)	Rough, bright red rash (feels like sandpaper)	Face, neck, elbows, armpits, groin (spreads rapidly to entire body)	High fever, weakness before rash, sore throat, peeling of the skin afterward (especially palms)
[1]Impetigo	Bacterial infection of the skin	In infants, pus-filled blisters and red skin. In older kids, golden crusts on red sores.	Arms, legs, face, and around the nose first, then most of body	Sometimes fever – occasional itching
Hives	Allergic reaction to food, insect bites, viral infection, medicine, or other substance	Raised red bumps with pale centers (resemble mosquito bites). Shape, size and location of spots can change rapidly.	Any area	Itching – in extreme cases, swelling of throat, difficulty breathing (may need emergency care)
Poison Ivy, Oak, Sumac	Interaction of oily resins of plant leaves with skin	Red, swollen skin rash and lines of tiny blisters	Exposed areas	Intense itching and burning
Lyme Disease	Bacterial infection spread by deer tick bite(s)	Red rash that looks like a bull's-eye: raised edges surround the tick bites with pale centers in the middle. Rash fades after 2 days.	Exposed skin areas where ticks bite, often include scalp, neck, armpit and groin	No pain, no itching at time of bite. Fever-rash occurs in the week following the bite(s).

[1] These conditions are contagious   [2] See pages 250–253 of this booklet for more information on chicken pox

12. Skin Conditions

33 Splinters

Splinters are pieces of wood, glass, metal, or other matter that get caught under the skin. Splinters tend to hurt if they are stuck deep under the skin. Those near the top of the skin are usually painless. Remove splinters so they don't cause an infection.

Prevention

■ Wear shoes out-of-doors at all times and whenever you walk on unfinished floors.

■ Sand, varnish, and/or paint handrails to keep from getting splinters in the hands.

■ Clean up all broken glass and metal shavings around the house. Be careful when you handle broken glass. Wear hard-soled shoes when glass has been broken.

■ Wear work gloves when you handle plants with thorns, sharp tips, or spines.

Make sure tetanus shots are up-to-date. (See "Immunization Schedule" on page 18.) Check with your doctor or health department.

Questions to Ask

For Children and Adults:

Are these signs present?
• Fever, swollen lymph nodes and red streaks spreading from the splinter towards the heart

YES → Get Emergency Care

NO ↓

Flowchart continued in next column

Are any of these signs present?
• The wound shows signs of infection such as pus, puffiness, or redness.
• The splinter is still embedded in the skin, you cannot get it out and it is painful

YES → See Doctor

NO ↓

Is the splinter deeply embedded in the skin, you cannot get it out and you have diabetes?

YES → See Doctor

NO ↓

For Children Only:

Has the child missed any Diphtheria, Tetanus, Pertussis, (DTaP or DTP) vaccinations which should have been given at these times?
• 2 months
• 4 months
• 6 months
• Between 15 and 18 months
• Between 4 and 6 years
• Between 11 and 16 years

YES → 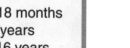 Call Doctor

NO ↓

Is your child running a temperature of 101°F or more?

YES → Call Doctor

NO ↓

Flowchart continued on next page

12. Skin Conditions

Splinters, *Continued*

Flowchart continued

For Adults Only:

Was your last tetanus shot more than ten years ago? If the splinter is deeply imbedded, was your last tetanus shot more than five years ago?

YES → **Call Doctor**

NO ↓

Use Self-Care

Self-Care Tips

■ To remove the splinter:

- Wash your hands, but don't let the area around a wooden splinter get wet. A wooden splinter that gets wet will swell. This will make it harder to remove.

- Sterilize tweezers. Place the tips in a flame. Wipe off the blackness on the tips with sterile gauze if you use a lit match for the flame.

- Use the tweezers to gently pull the part of the splinter that sticks out through the skin. It should slide right out. If necessary, use a magnifying glass to help you see close up.

- If the splinter is buried under the skin, sterilize a needle and gently slit the skin over one end of the splinter. Then, use the needle to lift that end and pull the splinter out with the tweezers.

- Check to see that all of the splinter has been removed. If not, repeat the above step.

- If you still can't get the splinter out, soak the skin around the splinter in a solution made with 1 tablespoon of baking soda mixed in 1 cup of warm water. Do this 2 times a day. After a few days, the splinter may work its way out.

- Once the splinter is removed, clean the wound by washing it with soap and water. Blot it dry with a clean cloth or sterile gauze pad. Apply a sterile bandage.

- To remove a large number of close-to-the-surface splinters, such as cactus spines, apply a layer of hair removing wax, facial gel, or white glue, such as Elmer's, to the skin. Let it dry for 5 minutes. Gently peel it off by lifting the edges of the dried wax, gel, or glue with tweezers. The splinter(s) should come up with it.

- Contact your doctor if you still have the splinter(s) after using Self-Care Tips.

12. Skin Conditions

34 Sunburn

You should never get sunburned! It is not healthy. It leads to premature aging, wrinkling of the skin, and skin cancer.

Sunburn is caused by too much exposure to ultraviolet (UV) light. This can be from the sun, sunlamps, or even from some workplace light sources such as welding arcs. Sunburn results in red, swollen, painful, and sometimes blistered skin. Chills, fever, nausea, and vomiting can occur if the sunburn is extensive and severe.

The risk for sunburn is increased for:

- Persons with fair skin, blue eyes, and red or blond hair
- Persons taking some medications including sulfa medications, tetracyclines, some diuretics and even Benadryl (an over-the-counter antihistamine)
- Persons exposed to industrial UV light sources and/or to excessive outdoor sunlight

Prevention

- Avoid exposure to the midday sun (from 10 a.m. to 2 p.m standard time or from 11 a.m. to 3 p.m. daylight saving time).
- Use sunscreen with a sun protective factor (SPF) of 15–30 or more when exposed to the sun. The lighter your skin, the higher the SPF number should be. Make sure the sunscreen blocks both UVA and UVB rays. Reapply sunscreen every hour and after swimming. Make-up for women is now available with sunscreen protection.

- Wear lip balm with sunscreen protection
- Wear a wide-brimmed hat and long sleeves.
- Wear muted colors such as tan. Brilliant colors and white reflect the sun onto the face. Clothing is now available with sunscreening protection.
- Wear sunglasses that absorb at least 90% of both UVA and UVB rays.

{*Note:* Be aware that severe sunburn can occur even when the skies are overcast.}

Questions to Ask

Are there any of these signs of dehydration?
- Confusion or dizziness
- Very little or no urine output
- Sunken eyes, no tears
- Dry skin that doesn't spring back after being pinched
- Extreme dryness in the mouth
- Extreme thirst

YES → **Get Emergency Care**

NO ↓

Do you have a fever of 102°F or higher or have severe pain or blistering with the sunburn?

YES → **See Doctor**

NO ↓

 Use Self-Care

See Self-Care Tips on next page

12. Skin Conditions

Sunburn, *Continued*

Self-Care Tips

■ Cool the affected area with clean towels, cloths or gauze dipped in cool water, or take a cool bath or shower.

■ Take an over-the-counter medicine for pain and/or fever {*Note:* See "Pain relievers" in "Your Home Pharmacy" on pages 22 and 23.}

■ Apply aloe vera gel to the burned area 2–3 times a day.

■ When you go in the sun again put sunscreen on and cover sunburned skin so you don't get burned more.

■ Rest in a cool, quiet room. Find a comfortable position.

■ Drink plenty of water.

■ Don't use local anesthetic creams or sprays that numb pain, such as Benzocaine or Lidocaine. If you must use them, use only a little because they cause allergic reactions in some people.

Varicose Veins

Varicose veins are swollen and twisted veins that look blue and are close to the surface of the skin. They are unsightly and uncomfortable. Veins bulge and feel heavy. The legs and feet can swell. The skin can itch. Varicose veins may occur in almost any part of the body. They are most often seen in the back of the calf or on the inside of the leg between the groin and the ankle. Hemorrhoids (veins around the anus) can also become varicose.

Causes

Causes and risk factors for varicose veins include:

- Obesity
- Pregnancy
- Hormonal changes at menopause
- Activities or hobbies that require standing or lifting heavy objects for long periods of time
- A family history of varicose veins
- Past vein diseases such as thrombophlebitis (inflammation of a vein before a blood clot forms)
- Often wearing clothing that is tight around the upper thighs
- Body positions that restrict lower leg blood flow for long periods of time. One example is sitting on an airplane, especially in the economy class section, on a long flight.

Treatment

Medical treatment is not required for most varicose veins unless problems result. These include a deep-vein blood clot or severe bleeding, which can be caused by injury to the vein. Problems can occur without an injury, as well. Your doctor can take an X-ray of the vein (venogram) and/or a special ultrasound to tell if there are any problems.

Medical treatment includes:

- Surgery to remove the vein or part of the vein
- Sclerotherapy, which uses a chemical injection into the vein, causing it to close up
- Laser therapy, which causes the vein to fade away

Questions to Ask

Does it look like the varicose vein has broken open and is bleeding a lot under the skin? YES See Doctor

NO

{*Note:* Apply direct pressure on the skin area over the varicose vein.}

Has the varicose vein become swollen, red, very tender or warm to the touch? YES See Doctor

NO

Flowchart continued on next page

Varicose Veins, *Continued*

Flowchart continued

Are varicose veins accompanied by a rash or sores on the leg or near the ankle, or have they caused circulation problems in your feet?

YES → See Doctor

NO ↓

Use Self-Care

Self-Care Tips

To Relieve and Prevent Varicose Veins:

- Don't cross your legs when sitting.

- Exercise regularly. Walking is a good choice. It improves leg and vein strength.

- Keep your weight down.

- Don't stand for long periods of time. If you must do so, shift your weight from one leg to the other every few minutes. Just wiggling your toes can help, too.

- Wear elastic support socks that go up to the knee but do not cover the knee. The top of these socks must not be tight.

- Don't wear tight clothing or undergarments that constrict your waist, groin, or legs.

- Eat high-fiber foods like bran cereals, whole grain breads, and fresh fruits and vegetables. Drink at least 8 glasses of water a day. These things help prevent constipation. (Constipation contributes to varicose veins.)

- To prevent swelling, limit your salt intake.

- Exercise your legs. (From a sitting position, rotate your feet at the ankles, turning them first clockwise, then counterclockwise, using a circular motion. Next, extend your legs forward and point your toes to the ceiling, then to the floor. Then, lift your feet off the floor and gently bend your legs back and forth at the knees).

- Elevate your legs when resting.

- Get up and move about every 35–45 minutes when traveling by air or even when sitting in an all-day conference. (Opt for an aisle seat in such situations.)

- Stop and take short walks at least every 45 minutes when taking long car rides.

12. Skin Conditions

36 Constipation

Constipation is when you have trouble having bowel movements. Signs of constipation are abdominal swelling, straining during bowel movements, hard stools, and the feeling of continued fullness even after a bowel movement. Constipation can be very uncomfortable, but it usually doesn't signal disease or a serious problem.

Causes

A number of things cause or lead to constipation. These include:

- Not drinking enough fluids
- Not eating enough dietary fiber
- Not being active enough
- Using laxatives over a long period of time
- Taking certain medicines (Examples: some heart, pain, and antidepressant medicines, as well as antacids, antihistamines, water pills, and narcotics)
- Taking iron supplements
- Not going to the bathroom when you have the urge to have a bowel movement
- Medical problems such as hemorrhoids or an underactive thyroid gland

It is important to know that it is not necessary to have a bowel movement daily. What is more important is what is normal for you.

The "cure" for constipation generally consists of correcting the things that make bowel habits irregular. (See Self-Care Tips on the next page.) Ask your doctor what you should do if medications and/or health conditions are causing you to be constipated.

Questions to Ask

Is the constipation present with any of the following?
- Fever
- Severe abdominal pain, especially located in the lower left section
- Persistent vomiting
- Abdominal bloating
- Weight loss
- Very thin pencil-like stools or blood seen in the stools

YES See Doctor

NO

Did the constipation occur after taking prescribed or over-the-counter medicines and/or vitamins?

YES Call Doctor

NO

Do you have persistent constipation despite using the Self-Care Tips listed in this section?

YES Call Doctor

NO

 Use Self-Care

See Self-Care Tips on next page

Constipation, *Continued*

Self-Care Tips

■ Eat foods high in dietary fiber, like bran, whole-grain breads and cereals, and fresh fruits and vegetables daily. They serve as natural stool softeners, thanks in part to their fiber content. One type of fiber from these foods absorbs water like a sponge, turning hard stools into large, soft, easy-to-pass masses.

■ Drink at least $1^1/_2$–2 quarts of water and other liquids every day.

■ Drink hot water, tea, or coffee. These may help stimulate the bowel.

■ Get plenty of exercise to help your bowels move things along.

■ Don't resist the urge to eliminate, or put off a trip to the bathroom.

■ Keep in mind that medicines such as antacids (ones with aluminum or calcium), iron supplements, and calcium supplements can be binding. Don't take them if you get constipated easily. Discuss this with your doctor first.

■ If necessary, for occasional constipation you may need an over-the-counter stool softener or mild laxative. Check with your doctor ahead of time so you'll know what is best for you to take if and when you do get constipated.

■ Ask your doctor about the use of "bulk-forming" laxatives such as Metamucil, Perdiem or Fiber Con. You may be able to use these daily, if necessary. Start out slowly and gradually increase how much you take. Also drink plenty of liquids with them. Bloating, cramping, or gas may be noticed at first, but these symptoms should go away in a few weeks or less.

■ Do not use "stimulant" laxatives such as Ex-Lax, Dulcolax, Senokot, or enemas without your doctor's permission. Short-term use of them may be okay, but in the long run they can make you even more constipated. (Your intestines can become lazy and may not work as well on their own.) Long-term use of these laxatives can also:

• Lead to a mineral imbalance

• Make it harder for your body to benefit from medicines

• Lower the amount of nutrients you absorb

37 Diarrhea

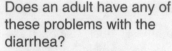

Diarrhea is the frequent passage of watery, loose bowel movements. Almost everyone gets diarrhea once in a while. Usually, it only lasts a day or two and isn't serious.

Causes

Many things can cause diarrhea:

- Infection by viruses, bacteria, or parasites
- Drinking bad water or eating spoiled food
- Allergies
- Emotional upset
- Overuse of laxatives
- Certain medications, including some antibiotics (like tetracycline, clindamycin, and ampicillin)
- Diverticulitis – a disease in the bowel
- Inflammatory bowel disease (usually ulcerative colitis and Crohn's disease)

Questions to Ask

Does the diarrhea occur in an infant or a child and is it present with any of the following?
- Sunken eyes
- Dry skin
- Dry mouth
- Dry diaper for more than 3 hours in an infant
- Passing no urine for more than 6 hours in a child
- Unusual lethargy, weak cry
- Irritability, very upset or cranky

YES → **Get Emergency Care**

NO ↓

Flowchart continued in next column

Does an adult have any of these problems with the diarrhea?
- Blood in the stool
- Severe abdominal or rectal pain
- Dry skin that doesn't spring back after being pinched
- Dry mouth, excessive thirst, and little or no urination

YES → **Get Emergency Care**

NO ↓

In a child or adult, has the diarrhea lasted 48 hours or more and/or is a fever of 101°F or higher present?

YES → **See Doctor**

NO ↓

Is the diarrhea occurring more than 8 times per day in an infant or chronically ill elderly adult?

YES → **Call Doctor**

NO ↓

In a child or adult, are any medicines being taken (this includes regular medicines that the body may not be absorbing due to the diarrhea, or prescribed or over-the-counter ones that might be contributing to diarrhea)?

YES → **Call Doctor**

NO ↓

Flowchart continued on next page

Diarrhea, *Continued*

Flowchart continued

Did diarrhea come on during or shortly after returning from a trip to a foreign country?

YES → Call Doctor

NO

Use Self-Care

Self-Care Tips

■ If vomiting is also present, treat for vomiting first. (See "Vomiting & Nausea" on page 130.)

■ Follow normal diet if there are no signs of dehydration (dry mouth, thirst, muscle cramps, weakness, etc.).

■ If there are signs of dehydration, stop solid foods. Give clear fluids. Fluids of choice are:

• Sport drinks, such as Gatorade. Note: For children under 2, give over-the-counter mixtures, such as Pedialyte and Ricelyte.

• Kool-Aid. This usually has less sugar than juices and soda pop.

• Your own solution made by mixing 4 teaspoons of sugar and 1 teaspoon of salt with 1 quart of water

■ Avoid giving these liquids:

• High "simple" sugar drinks, like apple juice, grape juice, regular colas, other soft drinks, and gelatin. These can pull water into the gut and make the diarrhea persist.

• Boiled milk

■ Adults should have around 2 cups of fluid per hour (if vomiting isn't present). For children under 2, consult their doctor about the amount and type of fluids. For children over 2, give up to $1^1/_2$ quarts of fluid per day.

■ Don't give just clear liquids for more than 24 hours.

■ Start eating normal meals within 12 hours. Good food choices are:

• Starchy foods, like rice; potatoes; cereals (not sugar-sweetened ones); crackers; toast

• Soups with noodles, rice, and/or vegetables

• Vegetables

• Lean meats

• Yogurt, especially with live active cultures of lactobacillus acidophilus

■ Avoid fatty and fried foods.

■ The B.R.A.T. diet: bananas (ripe), rice, applesauce, and dry toast is no longer the diet of choice for diarrhea.

■ Don't exercise too hard until the diarrhea is gone.

■ Adults can try an OTC medication, such as Immodium A-D or Pepto-Bismol. Wait at least 12 hours before taking these medicines, though. Let the diarrhea "run its course" to get rid of what caused it. {*Note:* Do not give aspirin or any medication that has salicylates, such as Pepto-Bismol, to anyone under 19 years of age, unless as doctor tells you to.}

■ Wash your hands after going to the toilet and before preparing food, especially when you have diarrhea which results from an infection in the GI tract. Don't share towels with others. Use disposable paper towels to dry your hands.

13. Abdominal Problems

38 Flatulence (Gas)

Flatulence is passing gas through the anus. For the average adult this happens about 6–20 times per day. What causes gas to be released this way? Often the cause is swallowing air. It also comes from intestinal bacteria that produce carbon dioxide and hydrogen (both odorless, by the way) in the course of breaking down carbohydrates in the food you eat. The tiny amounts of other, more pungent gases gives flatus its characteristic odor. Eating certain foods, like peas, beans, and certain grains produces more gas than eating other foods. All roughages in the diet will produce flatulence. A high-roughage diet, especially, will do this. When increasing dietary fiber in your diet, do so gradually. This will lessen the increase of flatus. Gas may signal a variety of other problems worth looking into. These include:

- Lactose intolerance (inability to properly digest milk, cheese, and other dairy products)

- Bacterial overgrowth in the intestines (often caused by certain antibiotics)

- Abnormal muscle contraction in the colon

Questions to Ask

Is the flatulence accompanied by severe, steady pain in the upper abdomen, nausea and vomiting, or yellowing of the skin or eyes? **YES** See Doctor

NO

Flowchart continued in next column

Has the flatulence occurred only after taking a prescribed antibiotic? **YES** Call Doctor

NO

 Use Self-Care

Self-Care Tips

Eliminate or go easy on food items that often cause gas. Well-known offenders include:

- Apples
- Apricots
- Beans and peas (dried, cooked)
- Bran
- Broccoli
- Brussels sprouts
- Cabbage
- Cauliflower
- Dairy products (for persons allergic to lactose)
- Eggs
- Eggplant
- Onions
- Popcorn
- Prunes
- Raisins
- Sorbitol

{*Note:* Eliminate or go easy on only the foods that affect you personally. With the exception of sorbitol, the foods listed provide nutrients, so should not be cut out altogether.}

Flatulence (Gas), *Continued*

- Keep a list of all of the foods you eat for a few days and note when and the number of times you have gas. If you notice that you have excess gas after drinking milk, for example, try cutting down on it, or eliminate it from your diet. See if the flatulence persists. Do the same for other foods that you think are causing you to have gas.

- If you are lactose-intolerant use lactose-reduced dairy foods or add an over-the-counter lactose-enzyme product such as Lactaid. This can be in drops or tablet form that you add to or take with dairy products to help you digest the lactose they contain.

- Avoid swallowing air at mealtimes.

- Don't drink through straws. Avoid carbonated beverages and chewing gum. These things can cause more air to get into your stomach.

- The medication simethicone may help reduce flatulence by dispersing gas pockets (and preventing more from forming). It has no known side effects. Simethicone is available by prescription as well as over-the-counter under the brand name Mylicon.

- Over-the-counter products (Bean-O and Phazyme 95) may curb flatulence caused by eating some foods such as baked beans.

39 Heartburn

Heartburn has nothing to do with the heart. Rather, it involves the esophagus (the tube that connects the throat to the stomach), and the stomach itself. The esophagus passes behind the breastbone alongside the heart, so the inflammation or irritation that takes place there feels like a burning sensation in the heart.

Causes

Gastric acids from the stomach splash back up into the lower portion of the esophagus, causing pain. The medical term for this is gastroesophageal reflex disease

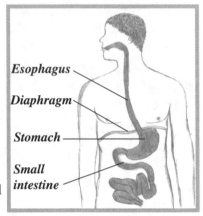

Esophagus

Diaphragm

Stomach

Small intestine

(GERD). The digestive acids don't harm the stomach, thanks to its protective coating, but the esophagus has no such armor, which results in discomfort. The most common heartburn triggers are:

- Taking aspirin, ibuprofen, naproxen sodium, arthritis medicine, or cortisone
- Eating heavy meals or eating too fast
- Eating foods like chocolate, garlic, onions, peppermint, tomatoes, or citrus fruits
- Lying down after a meal
- Smoking after eating
- Drinking coffee (regular or decaffeinated)
- Drinking alcohol
- Being very overweight
- Wearing tight clothing
- Pregnancy

- Swallowing too much air
- Stress
- A weakness or malfunction of the sphincter muscle between the esophagus and the stomach
- A bulging of the upper part of the stomach through the diaphragm. This is commonly known as hiatal hernia.

Questions to Ask

Does the heartburn come with any of the following?
- Chest pressure or pain (may spread to the arm, neck, or jaw)
- Chest discomfort with: Shortness of breath or trouble breathing; sweating; uneven pulse or heartbeat; nausea or vomiting; or sense of doom

YES → **Get Emergency Care**

NO ↓

Are you vomiting something black or red in color?

YES → **Get Emergency Care**

NO ↓

Are your stools tarlike and black in color?

YES → 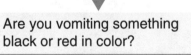 **See Doctor**

NO ↓

Do you also have pain that goes through to your back?

YES → 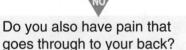 **See Doctor**

NO ↓

Flowchart continued on next page

Heartburn, *Continued*

Flowchart continued

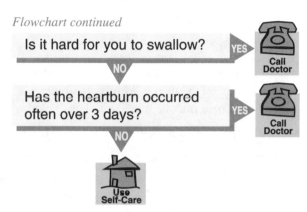

Self-Care Tips

■ Sit straight while eating. Stand up or walk around after you eat. Bending over or lying down after you eat makes it too easy for gastric secretions to move up to the esophagus.

■ If heartburn bothers you at night, raise the head of the bed slightly. (Example: Put the head of your bed up on 6-inch blocks, or buy a wedge especially made for putting between the mattress and box spring.)

■ Lose weight if you are overweight.

■ Avoid wearing tight-fitting garments around the abdomen. (Example: girdle)

■ Eat small meals. Limit alcohol.

■ Limit foods and drinks that contain air. (Examples: baked goods, waffles, whipped cream, carbonated beverages)

■ Don't drink through straws or bottles with narrow mouths.

■ Don't eat or drink for 2–3 hours before bedtime.

■ If other treatments fail:

• Take antacids. They coat your stomach and neutralize acids. For example, take 1 to 2 tablespoons of a nonabsorbable liquid antacid such as magnesium hydroxide every 2–4 hours, or ones that come in tablet form such as Tums.

• If antacids don't bring relief, consider taking an over-the-counter acid controller. (Examples: Pepcid AC, Tagamet HB, Zantac 75 and Axid AR) These not only relieve heartburn but can prevent it. {*Note:* Read labels before taking antacids or acid controllers. If you have questions, check with your doctor.}

■ Don't take baking soda. It may neutralize stomach acid at first, but when its effects wear off the acid comes back to a greater degree, causing severe gastric-acid rebound.

■ Don't smoke. It promotes heartburn.

■ If you do take aspirin, ibuprofen, naproxen sodium, or arthritis medicines, take them with food.

{*Note:* Call your doctor if you find no relief from Self-Care Tips.}

40 Hemorrhoids

Hemorrhoids are veins under the rectum or around the anus that are dilated or swollen. They are caused by repeated pressure in the rectal or anal veins. This pressure usually results from repeated straining to pass bowel movements. Rarely, they result from benign or malignant tumors of the abdomen or rectum. The risk for getting hemorrhoids increases with:

- Constipation
- Low dietary fiber intake
- Pregnancy and delivery
- Obesity

Symptoms

Symptoms of hemorrhoids include:

- Rectal bleeding
- Rectal tenderness and/or itching
- Uncomfortable, painful bowel movements, especially with straining
- A lump that can be felt in the anus
- A mucous discharge after a bowel movement

Hemorrhoids are common, and most people have some bleeding from them once in a while. Though annoying and uncomfortable, hemorrhoids are seldom a serious health problem. Reasons to seek medical treatment for hemorrhoids include:

- The presence of a painful blood clot in the hemorrhoid
- Excessive blood loss
- Infection

- The need to rule out cancer of the rectum or colon

If symptoms of hemorrhoids are not relieved with Self-Care Tips on the next page or with time, medical treatment may be necessary. This includes:

- Cryosurgery, which freezes the affected tissue
- A chemical injection into an internal hemorrhoid to shrink it
- Electrical or laser heat or infrared light to destroy the hemorrhoids
- Surgery called hemorrhoidectomy. One type, which requires general anesthesia, cuts out the hemorrhoids. Another, called ligation, uses rubber bands that are placed tightly over the base of each hemorrhoid, causing it to wither away.

Questions to Ask

Do you have severe rectal bleeding that is continuous or associated with weakness or dizziness?

 YES **Get Emergency Care**

NO

Do you have rectal bleeding:
- **Without bowel movements?**
- **That is heavy, dark red or turns brown?**
- **That lasts longer than two weeks despite using Self-Care Tips?**

YES **See Doctor**

 NO

Flowchart continued on next page

Hemorrhoids, *Continued*

Flowchart continued

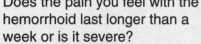

Do you have a hard lump where a hemorrhoid used to be? **YES** →  **See Doctor**

NO ↓

Does the pain you feel with the hemorrhoid last longer than a week or is it severe? **YES** →  **See Doctor**

NO ↓

 Use Self-Care

Self-Care Tips

- Take daily measures to produce soft, easily passed bowel movements such as:

  - Drink plenty of water and other fluids: at least 1¹/₂–2 quarts a day.

  - Eat foods with good sources of dietary fiber such as whole grain or bran cereals and breads, fresh vegetables, and fruits.

  - Eat prunes and/or drink prune juice.

  - If necessary add bran to your foods: about 3 to 4 tablespoons per day.

  - Exercise regularly.

  - Pass a bowel movement as soon as you feel the urge. If you wait and the urge goes away, your stool could become dry and be harder to pass.

- Lose weight if you are overweight.

- Don't strain to have a bowel movement.

- Don't hold your breath when trying to pass stool.

- Keep the anal area clean.

- Take warm baths.

- Use a sitz bath with hot water. A sitz bath device fits over the toilet. You can get one at a medical supply store or at some pharmacies.

- Use moist towelettes or wet (not dry) toilet paper after a bowel movement.

- Check with your doctor about using over-the-counter products such as:

  - Stool softeners

  - Zinc oxide preparations. (Examples: Preparation H and Hemorid)

  - Medicated wipes such as Tucks

  - Medicated suppositories

- Don't sit too much because it can restrict blood flow around the anal area.

- Don't sit too long on the toilet.

- Don't read while on the toilet.

- For itching or pain, put a cold compress on the anus for 10 minutes up to 4 times a day.

13. Abdominal Problems

41 Vomiting & Nausea

Vomiting is when you throw up what is in your stomach. Nausea is when you feel like you're going to throw up.

Causes

Common causes of nausea and vomiting are:

- Viruses in the intestines (you can get diarrhea, too)
- Morning sickness in pregnant women
- Some medications
- Spoiled food
- Eating or drinking too much

Some medical conditions cause vomiting, too. These include:

- Vertigo from an inner ear problem
- Migraine headaches
- Appendicitis
- Brain tumors
- Acute glaucoma (see page 352)
- Stomach ulcers (see page 367)
- Hepatitis – inflammation of the liver
- Meningitis – inflammation of membranes that cover the brain and spinal cord

Questions to Ask

Do you have any of these problems along with the vomiting?
- Stiff neck, fever and headache
- Black or bloody vomit
- Very bad pain in and around one eye
- Blurry eyesight
- A head injury that happened a short time ago

YES **Get Emergency Care**

NO

Dehydration is when your body loses too much water. Do you have any of these signs of dehydration?
- Feeling confused
- Very little or no urine
- Sunken eyes
- Dry skin that doesn't spring back after being pinched

YES **Get Emergency Care**

NO

Do you have all of these symptoms with the vomiting?
- Fever and shaking chills
- Pain in one or both sides of your lower back

YES **Get Emergency Care**

NO

Do you have very bad stomach pain? Does it last for more than 2 hours? Does it keep hurting even after you throw up?

YES **See Doctor**

NO

Flowchart continued on next page

Vomiting & Nausea, *Continued*

Flowchart continued

Do the whites of your eyes or does your skin look yellow? **YES** **See Doctor**

NO

Do you have any of these problems?
- Burning or stinging feeling when you pass urine
- Passing urine a lot more often than usual
- Bloody or cloudy urine
- Pain in your abdomen or over your bladder

YES **See Doctor**

NO

Do you have ear pain or a feeling of fullness in your ear? **YES** **Call Doctor**

NO

In a baby or small child, has the vomiting lasted 2 to 6 hours? For others, has the vomiting lasted more than 12 hours without getting better? **YES** **Call Doctor**

NO

Do you have a blind spot, loss of part of your visual field, or do you see sparkling lights? **YES**  **Call Doctor**

NO

Flowchart continued in next column

Are you throwing up medicine that is necessary for you to take? (Birth control pills and high blood pressure pills are examples.) **YES** **Call Doctor**

NO

 Use Self-Care

Self-Care Tips

For Vomiting:

- Don't eat solid foods. Don't drink milk.
- Drink clear liquids (water, sport drinks, such as Gatorade, flat cola, and ginger ale, etc…). Take small sips. Drink only 1 to 2 ounces at a time. Stir any carbonated beverages to get all the bubbles out before sipping them. Suck on ice chips if nothing else will stay down. {*Note:* For children, contact your child's health care provider about using over-the-counter products such as Pedialyte and Revital Ice–rehydrating freezer pops.}
- Gradually return to regular diet, but wait about 8 hours from the last time you vomited. Eat foods as tolerated. Avoid greasy or fatty foods.
- Don't smoke, drink alcohol, or take aspirin.

For Nausea Without Vomiting:

- Drink clear liquids. Eat small amounts of dry foods, such as soda crackers (if tolerated).
- Avoid things that irritate the stomach, such as alcohol and aspirin.
- For motion sickness, use an over-the-counter anti-nausea medicine, such as Dramamine. Follow package directions.

13. Abdominal Problems

42 Backaches

Most backaches come from strained muscles or ligaments in the lower back. Other causes include back injuries such as a slipped or herniated disc, arthritis (see page 336), osteoporosis (see page 363), and urinary tract infections (see page 174).

Treatment

Most backaches caused by strained muscles and ligaments can be treated with self-care. (See "Self-Care Tips" on pages 134 and 135.) Other causes need a medical evaluation and treatment specific to the problem. For example, surgery to repair a herniated disk may be needed if other non-surgical measures don't bring relief.

The goals of treatment are to treat the cause of the backache, relieve the pain, promote healing, and avoid reinjury.

Prevention

Improper lifting causes a lot of backaches. Here are some lifting "dos and don'ts" to help you avoid straining your back.

Dos

- Wear good shoes with low heels, not sandals or high heels.

- Stand close to the thing you want to lift.

- Plant your feet squarely, shoulder width apart.

- Bend at the knees, not at the waist. Keep your knees bent as you lift.

- Pull in your stomach and rear end. Keep your back as straight as you can.

- Hold the object close to your body.

- Lift slowly. Let your legs carry the weight.

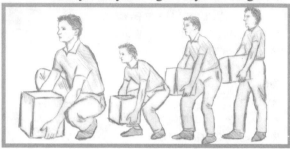

- Get help or use a dolly to move something that is too big or very heavy.

Don'ts

- Don't lift if your back hurts.

- Don't lift if you have a history of back trouble.

- Don't lift something that's too heavy.

- Don't lift heavy things over your head.

- Don't lift anything heavy if you're not steady on your feet.

- Don't bend at the waist to pick something up.

- Don't arch your back when you lift or carry.

- Don't lift too fast or with a jerk.

- Don't twist your back when you are holding something. Turn your whole body, from head to toe.

- Don't lift something heavy with one hand and something light with the other. Balance the load.

- Don't try to lift one thing while you hold something else. For example, don't try to pick up a child while you are holding a grocery bag. Put the bag down, or lift the bag and the child at the same time.

Backaches, *Continued*

Questions to Ask

Is the back pain <u>extreme</u> and felt across the upper back (not just on one side) and did it come on suddenly (within about 15 minutes) with no apparent reason such as an injury or back strain? {*Note:* These may be symptoms of a dissecting aortic aneurysm.}

YES Get Emergency Care

NO

Did the back pain start inside your chest and move to the upper back? {*Note:* You may be having a heart attack. The pain may be dull and you may not feel it in the chest at all.}

YES Get Emergency Care

NO

Was the back pain sudden with a cracking sound?

YES Get Emergency Care

NO

Did the pain come after a recent fall, injury, or violent movement to the back and are you having a hard time moving your arm or leg? Do you also have numbness or tingling in your legs, feet, toes, arms, or hands and/or loss of bladder or bowel control?

YES Get Emergency Care

NO

Flowchart continued in next column

Did the pain come on all of a sudden after being in a wheel-chair or a long stay in bed, or are you over 60 years old?

YES See Doctor

NO

Is the pain severe (but not a result from a fall or injury to the back), and has it lasted for more than 5–7 days or is there also a sense of weakness, numbness or tingling in the feet or toes?

YES  See Doctor

NO

Does the pain travel down the leg(s) below the knee?

YES  See Doctor

NO

Does it hurt more when you move, cough, sneeze, lift, or strain? Or, have you lost control of your bladder or bowel movements?

YES See Doctor

NO

Are any of the following also present?
- Pain, burning or itching when you urinate
- Increased urge to urinate or urinating often
- Foul-smelling urine or blood in the urine
- Abdominal pain

YES See Doctor

NO

Flowchart continued on next page

14. Muscle & Bone Problems

Backaches, *Continued*

Flowchart continued

Is the pain felt on one side of the small of your back, just above your waist, and do you feel sick and have a fever of 101°F or higher?

YES →  See Doctor

NO ↓

Do you also have any of the following?
- Joint stiffness and pain
- Redness, heat, or swelling in affected joints
- Cracking or grating sounds with joint movement

YES → See Doctor

NO ↓

 Use Self-Care

Self-Care Tips

Relieve the Pain

- Take an over-the-counter medicine for pain. Acetaminophen will help with pain, but not with swelling. {*Note:* See "Pain relievers" in "Your Home Pharmacy" on pages 22 and 23.}

- Don't "overdo it" after taking a painkiller. You can hurt your back more, and then it will take longer to heal.

Activity

Continue your regular activities as much as you can. Rest the back if you must, but don't rest in bed more than 2–3 days, even if your back hurts a lot. Your back muscles can get weak if you don't use them or if you stay in bed more than 3 days. Bed rest should only be used for persons with severe limitations (due mostly to leg pain). Other tips:

- Get comfortable when you are lying, standing, and sitting. For example, when you lie on your back, keep your upper back flat, but your hips and knees bent. Keep your feet flat on the bed. Tip your hips down and up until you find the best spot.

- Put a pillow under your knees or lie on your side with your knees bent. This will take pressure off your lower back.

- When you get up from bed, move slowly, roll on your side, and swing your legs to the floor. Push off the bed with your arms.

Cold Treatment

Cold helps with bruises and swelling. For the first 48 hours after back symptoms start, apply a cold pack (or bag of ice) to the painful area. Lie on your back with your knees bent, and put the cold pack under your lower back. Do this for 5–10 minutes at a time, several times a day.

Backaches, *Continued*

Heat Treatment

Heat makes blood flow, which helps healing. But don't use heat on a back strain until 48 or more hours after back symptoms start. Use cold treatment first (see "Cold Treatment" on page 134). If used sooner, heat can make the pain and swelling worse. Use a moist heating pad, a hot-water bottle, hot compresses, a hot tub, hot baths, or hot showers. Use heat for 10 minutes at a time. Do this several times a day. Be careful not to burn yourself.

Massage

Massage won't cure a backache, but it can loosen tight muscles.

Braces or Corsets

Braces and corsets support your back and keep you from moving it too much. They do what strong back muscles do, but they won't make your back stronger.

Spinal Manipulation

This treatment, usually done by a chiropractor, uses the hands to apply force to "adjust" the spine. This can be helpful for some people in the first month of low back symptoms.

Check with your doctor about spinal manipulations. You may need a referral from your doctor to see a professional who does this form of treatment.

More Tips

- Try some mild stretching exercises (in the morning and afternoon) to make your stomach and back muscles stronger. Ask your doctor for his or her advice on exercising.
- Don't sit in one place longer than you need to. It strains your lower back.
- Sleep on a firm mattress.
- Never sleep on your stomach. Sleep on your back or side, with your knees bent.
- If your back pain is chronic or doesn't get better on its own, see your doctor. He or she can evaluate your needs. Your doctor may refer you to a chiropractor, physical therapist, or physiatrist (a physical therapy doctor).

Sciatica

Sciatica is inflammation of the sciatic nerve, which starts in the lower spine and goes down the back of the legs. Pressure on the nerve (from tight muscles, herniated disk, etc.) causes a sharp pain that can be felt in the buttock and may extend to the thigh, knee, or foot. To prevent sciatica:

- Don't strain the muscles in your lower back. (See the "Dos" and "Don'ts" under "Prevention" on page 132.)
- Do exercises to strengthen your stomach muscles. These exercises help make your back stronger.

Treatment for mild sciatica is rest, heat and over-the-counter medicine for pain. Physical therapy may be helpful. In some cases, surgery to repair a herniated disk may be needed.

43 Broken Bones

There are different kinds of broken bones.

- Simple or closed fractures:
  The broken bone is not visible through the skin nor is there a skin wound near the fracture site. An example of this is a greenstick fracture. It is called this because the X-ray resembles the pattern of a very young splintered green twig.

- Compound or open fracture:
  A bone may separate partially or completely and a skin wound is also present. The bone can protrude through the skin or the skin has been cut due to the injury.

Bones in children are more pliable and may resist breakage more than bones in adults. In most cases, children's bones are still growing, especially the long bones of their arms and legs. Damage to the ends of these bones should be looked at carefully because of the risk of stunting the bone's growth.

Bones in some senior citizens become dangerously thin with age and break easily. Also, many women after menopause and some elderly men suffer from osteoporosis, a condition which weakens the bones. (See "Osteoporosis" on page 363.)

Sometimes, broken bones may cause future deformities and limited movement if not properly cared for. Broken bones can also be very painful.

Prevention

- Make sure you and your child wear the right protective gear for each activity. Items to wear might include a helmet, shoulder, knee and wrist pads, and a mouth guard.

- Check that everyone in the car is wearing a seat belt. Don't start the engine until everyone has buckled up.

Questions to Ask

Does the person have an injury to the head, neck, and/or back? **YES**

NO

(*Note:* See "Head Injuries" on page 313 and "Neck/Spine Injuries" on page 319.)

Does the victim have severe bleeding and/or an open fracture? **YES**

NO

(*Note:* See "First Aid for Major Bleeding" on page 97.)

Does the person have any of these problems?
- A broken bone in the pelvis or thigh
- Cold, blue skin under the fracture
- Numbness below the fracture
- Sweating, dizziness, thirst, or an ashen skin color
- Any deformity at the fracture site

YES

(*Note:* See "Immobilize the injured area" under Self-Care Tips on page 137.)

NO

Flowchart continued on next page

Broken Bones, *Continued*

Flowchart continued

Is the pain so severe that the person is unable to bear weight on the injured limb and/or is there a lot of bruising around the injury?

YES → **See Doctor**

NO ↓

Use Self-Care

{*Note:* See "Immobilize the injured area" under Self-Care Tips on this page.}

{*Note:* If you have answered NO to all of the above questions you probably do not have a broken bone. If you are not sure whether or not a bone has been broken, consult your doctor.}

Self-Care Tips

{*Note:* The Self-Care Tips below list things you can do when a bone has been broken before getting medical care.}

▪ Immobilize the injured area. Make a splint:

- Use rolled-up newspapers and magazines, an umbrella, a stick, a cane, or rolled-up blankets. Place this type of item around the injury and gently hold it in place with a necktie, strip of cloth, or belt. Splint a joint above and below the fracture.

- Or, lightly tape or tie an injured leg to the uninjured one, putting padding between the legs, if possible. Or, tape an injured arm to the chest, if the elbow is bent, or to the side if the elbow is straight, placing padding between the body and the arm.

- Check the pulse in the limb with the splint. If you cannot find it, the splint is too tight and must be loosened at once.

- Check for swelling, numbness, tingling, or a blue tinge to the skin. Any of these signs indicates the splint is too tight and must be loosened right away to prevent permanent injury.

- For a broken arm, make a sling out of a triangular piece of cloth. Place the forearm in it and tie the ends around the neck so the arm is resting at a 90-degree angle.

- Keep the person quiet to avoid moving the injured area.

▪ Apply a cold compress to the injured area to help reduce swelling and inflammation.

▪ Take an over-the-counter medicine to reduce pain and swelling. Acetaminophen will help the pain, but not the swelling. Don't take aspirin if there is bleeding. {*Note:* See "Pain relievers" in "Your Home Pharmacy" on pages 22 and 23.}

14. Muscle & Bone Problems

44 Dislocations

A dislocation is a separation of the end of a bone and the joint it meets. Bones that touch in the joints sometime separate when they are overstressed.

Injuries related to dislocations include damage to the membrane lining the joint as well as tears to nearby muscles and ligaments.

Causes

- Injuries from contact sports or falls
- Rheumatoid arthritis
- Inborn joint defects
- Joints weakened by previous injury
- Suddenly jerking a toddler's hand or arm
- Force applied in the wrong direction that snaps the ball of the upper arm bone out of the shoulder socket

The shoulders are especially prone to dislocation injuries. The elbow is a common site in toddlers. Fingers, hips, ankles, elbows, jaws, and even the spine can be dislocated as well. A dislocated vertebrae in the spine often damages the spinal cord and can paralyze body parts lower than the injury site.

Signs and Symptoms

A dislocated joint is:

- Misshapen
- Very painful
- Swollen
- Discolored

Sometimes it is hard to tell a dislocation from a broken bone. It is best to seek medical attention if you suspect a dislocation. It is unwise to try to put a dislocated bone back into its socket.

When treated professionally, you can usually expect the dislocated joint to function within 24 to 48 hours. Activity may need to be limited for the next 4 to 6 weeks, though, to give the injury enough time to heal.

Prevention

- Protect a previously injured joint by wrapping it with an elastic bandage or tape.
- Wear protective pads (shoulder, wrist, knee, etc.) when taking part in contact sports or in other activities in which you may fall or otherwise get injured.

Questions to Ask

Is there an injury to the neck or spine? **YES** → Get Emergency Care

NO ↓

{*Note:* See "Neck/Spine Injuries" on page 319.}

Is there severe bleeding around the injury? **YES** → Get Emergency Care

NO ↓

{*Note:* See "First Aid for Major Bleeding" under Self-Care Tips on page 97.}

Flowchart continued on next page

Dislocations, *Continued*

Flowchart continued

Are there any of these problems?
- An area that is deformed
- A limb that is pale, cold or numb
- A limb that is very painful and/or swollen or one that can't bear weight

YES → 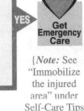 **Get Emergency Care**

{*Note:* See "Immobilize the injured area" under Self-Care Tips on page 137.}

NO ↓

 Use Self-Care

{*Note:* If you have answered NO to all of the above questions you probably do not have a dislocation. If you are not sure, consult your doctor.}

Self-Care Tips

{*Note:* All dislocations need medical attention. Seek help as soon as possible after the injury. The Self-Care Tips below list things you can do for a dislocation before and after you get medical care.}

- Dislocations, like other joint injuries, are often best treated by **R.I.C.E.** (rest, ice, compression and elevation) during the first 24–48 hours after the injury.

R Rest. Rest the injured area as much as possible.

I Ice. Ice the injured area as soon as possible. Immediately putting ice on the injury helps to speed recovery because it not only relieves pain but also slows blood flow, reducing internal bleeding and swelling.

- Put ice cubes or crushed ice in a heavy plastic bag with a little water. You can also use a bag of frozen vegetables. Wrap the ice pack in a towel before placing it on the injured area.

- Apply the ice pack to the injured area for 10–20 minutes. Reapply it every two hours and for the next 48 hours during the times you are not sleeping.

C Compression. Apply a snug elastic bandage to the injured joint. Numbness, tingling, or increased pain means the bandage is too tight. Remove the bandage every 3–4 hours and leave off for 15–20 minutes each time you do so.

E Elevation. Raise the injured body part above the level of the person's heart. Place it on a pillow, folded blanket, or stack of newspapers.

- Take an over-the-counter medicine to reduce inflammation and pain. Acetaminophen eases soreness but does not help with inflammation. {*Note:* See "Pain relievers" in "Your Home Pharmacy" on pages 22 and 23.}

14. Muscle & Bone Problems

45 Shoulder & Neck Pain

Pain in the shoulder and neck is common. Driving a golf ball, cleaning windows, or reaching for a jar can strain and injure shoulder muscles and tendons, especially in people who are out of condition. Fortunately, this discomfort rarely suggests a serious condition. Causes of shoulder and neck pain include:

- Poor posture and/or unnatural sleeping positions. Sleeping on a soft mattress can give you a stiff neck the next morning.

- Tension and stress. When you feel tense, the muscles around your neck can go into spasms.

- Tendinitis, inflammation of a tendon, the cord-like tissue that connects muscles to bone. Left untreated, tendinitis can turn into "frozen shoulder," a stiff, painful condition that may limit your ability to use your shoulder. "Wry" neck is a similar condition.

- Bursitis, an inflammation of the sac (bursa) that encases the shoulder joint. Bursitis can be caused by injury, infection, overuse, arthritis, or gout.

- Osteoarthritis. Unlike rheumatoid arthritis, osteoarthritis develops from normal wear-and-tear of the joints as we age or from repeated injuries. Aging can cause the joints to wear out, producing bony spurs that can press on nerves and cause pain.

- Accidents and falls. Collarbones can break during falls or auto accidents.

- Motor vehicle accidents. You can develop a whiplash injury when your vehicle is hit from behind.

- Pinched nerve. Arthritis or an injury to your neck can pinch a nerve in your neck. Pain from a pinched nerve usually runs down the arm on one side only.

Sometimes shoulder and neck pain signal serious medical problems, especially with other symptoms such as stiff neck, sudden and severe headache, dizziness, chest pain or pressure, and/or loss of consciousness.

Prevention

- Stretching and strengthening routines, especially before exercising, helps prevent tendinitis. So can using the right equipment and following the proper technique.

- Avoid injuries to the shoulder by wearing seat belts in cars and trucks and using protective gear during sporting events.

- Avoid vigorous exercise unless you are fit. If you are out of condition, start to strengthen your muscles gradually and slowly increase exercise intensity.

- Don't sleep on your stomach. You are likely to twist your neck in this position.

- Sleep on a firm mattress. Use a feather, polyester, or special neck (cervical) pillow. Use a thinner pillow or none at all if you have pain when you wake up.

{*Note:* See also "To Prevent Muscle Tension When You Work on a VDT" on page 59.}

Shoulder & Neck Pain, *Continued*

Keep the muscles in your shoulders strong and flexible to prevent injury. These exercises can help:

- Stretch the back of your shoulder by reaching with one arm under your chin and across the opposite shoulder. Gently push the arm toward your collarbone with the other hand. Hold for 15 seconds. Repeat 5 times, then switch sides.

- Raise one arm and bend it behind your head to touch the opposite shoulder. Use the other hand to gently pull the elbow toward the opposite shoulder. Hold for 15 seconds. Repeat 5 times, then switch sides.

- Holding light weights, lift your arms out horizontally and slightly forward. Keeping your thumbs toward the floor, slowly lower your arms halfway, then return to shoulder level. Repeat 10 times.

- Sit straight in a chair. Flex your neck slowly forward and try to touch your chin to your chest. Hold for 10 seconds and go back to the starting position. Repeat 5 times.

- Sit straight in a chair. Look straight ahead. Slowly tilt your head to the right, trying to touch your right ear to your right shoulder. Do not raise your shoulder to meet your ear. Hold for 10 seconds and straighten your head. Repeat five times on this side and then on your left side.

Questions to Ask

Did you have a serious injury that caused shoulder and/or neck pain that is not going away and/or is getting worse?

YES → Get Emergency Care

NO ↓

Flowchart continued in next column

Are heart attack signs present with the shoulder and neck pain?
- Chest pressure or pain
- Feelings of chest tightness, squeezing, or heaviness that last more than a few minutes, or go away and come back
- Chest discomfort with: Shortness of breath or trouble breathing; nausea and/or vomiting; sweating; uneven pulse or heartbeat or sense of doom

YES → Get Emergency Care

NO ↓

Do you have a stiff neck along with a severe headache, fever, nausea, and vomiting?

YES → Get Emergency Care

NO ↓

Do you have any of the following?
- Severe or persistent pain, swelling, spasms, or a deformity in your shoulder
- A shoulder that is painful and stiff and is very hard to move at all
- Stabbing pain, numbness, or tingling
- Pain, tenderness, and limited motion in the shoulder, arm, or hand

YES → See Doctor

NO ↓

Flowchart continued on next page

Shoulder & Neck Pain, *Continued*

Flowchart continued

Does the shoulder pain interfere with your sleep? Or is the shoulder stiff only in the morning?

YES → **Call Doctor**

NO

Use Self-Care

Self-Care Tips

Treating Tendinitis

■ Take an over-the-counter medicine to reduce the pain and inflammation. Acetaminophen eases muscle soreness but does not help with inflammation. {*Note:* See "Pain relievers" in "Your Home Pharmacy" on pages 22 and 23.}

R.I.C.E. Rest, ice, compression and elevation, is the accepted treatment for tendinitis. While the pain could linger for weeks, with the proper and immediate treatment it usually disappears in a few days. {*Note:* See **R.I.C.E.** on page 139.}

■ Apply heat once the swelling is gone. This helps to speed up healing, relieve pain, relax muscles, and reduce joint stiffness.

• Use a heating pad set on low (adults only). Or use a hot-water bottle, heat pack, or hot, damp towel wrapped around the injured area for moist heat. {*Note:* Damp heat should be no warmer than 105°F.}

• Apply heat to the injured area for 20–30 minutes, 2–3 times a day.

■ Try liniments and balms. These also relieve the discomfort of sore muscles. They provide a cooling or warming sensation. Although these ointments only mask the pain of sore muscles and do nothing to promote healing, massaging them into the shoulder increases blood flow to help relax the muscles.

Treating Bursitis

Arthritis or prolonged use of a joint can cause the pain and discomfort of bursitis. To control flare-ups of bursitis:

■ Apply ice packs to the sore shoulder.

■ Take a hot shower, apply a hot compress or heating pad set on low (adults only) to the affected shoulder, or rub the area with a deep-heating liniment.

Treating Neck Pain from Whiplash Injury

(See "If You Suspect a Whiplash Injury" on page 321.)

Dealing with Arthritis and Osteoporosis

See the section on arthritis on page 336 and the section on osteoporosis on page 363 for information on these conditions.

14. Muscle & Bone Problems

46 Sports Injuries

"Break a leg" means good luck only in the theater. Take care to avoid injury when exercising.

Prevention

Common sense can prevent many sports injuries. Some typical injuries and ways to prevent them are listed below. The top six are:

Knee Injury

Knees are very prone to injury.

- Avoid locking your knees.
- Do not bend knees past 90° when doing half knee bends or squats.
- Avoid twisting knees by keeping feet flat as much as possible (during stretches).
- Use the softest surface available when you exercise.
- Wear proper shoes with soft, flexible soles.
- When jumping, land with your knees bent.

Muscle soreness

Muscle soreness is a symptom of having worked out too hard or too long.

- Do warm-up exercises, such as those that stretch the muscles, before your activity, not only for vigorous activities such as running but even for less vigorous ones such as golf.
- Don't overdo it. "No pain, no gain" is not true.

- After vigorous activities, go through a cool-down period. Do the activity at a slower pace for 5 minutes. For example, after a run, walk or walk/jog for 5 minutes.

Blisters

Blisters are due to poor-fitting shoes or socks.

- Wear shoes and socks that fit well. The widest area of your foot should match the widest area of the shoe. You should also be able to wiggle your toes with the shoe on, in both a sitting and standing position. The inner seams of the shoe should not rub against areas of your feet.
- Wear preventive taping, if necessary.

Side Stitch

Side stitch is a sharp pain felt underneath the rib cage.

- Don't eat or drink 2 hours prior to exercise.
- Do proper breathing by raising abdominal muscles as you breathe in.
- Don't "work through pain." Stop the activity, then walk slowly.

Shinsplints

Shinsplints are mild-to-severe aches in front of the lower leg.

- Strengthen muscles in this region.
- Keep calves well stretched.
- When using an indoor track or a crowded road, don't always run in the same direction.

14. Muscle & Bone Problems

143

Sports Injuries, *Continued*

Achilles Tendon Pain

Achilles tendon pain is caused by a stretch, tear, or irritation to the tendon that connects the calf muscles to the back of the heel.

- Do warm-up stretching exercises before the activity. Stretch the Achilles tendon area and hold that position. Don't bounce.

- Wear proper-fitting shoes that provide shock absorption and stability.

- Avoid running shoes with a heel counter that is too high.

- Avoid running on hard surfaces like asphalt and concrete.

- Run on flat surfaces instead of uphill. Running uphill aggravates the stress put on the Achilles tendon.

Serious Sport Injuries

Less common, but more severe injuries can occur during sports, especially contact sports like football. These include:

- Broken bones (see page 136)

- Joint dislocations (see page 138)

- Strains and sprains (see page 146)

- Head injuries (see page 313)

- Neck/spine injuries (see page 319)

- Abdominal injuries, such as injuries to the spleen or liver

Take measures to prevent serious injuries during contact sports.

- Wear the right protective gear and clothing for the sport. Items to wear include a helmet, shoulder, knee and wrist pads, a mouth guard, etc.

- Train in the sport so you learn how to avoid injury. "Weekend athletes" are prone to injury.

- Follow the rules that apply to the sport.

Questions to Ask

Are any of these signs present?
- A bone sticks out or bones in the injured part make a grating sound.
- The injured body part looks crooked or the wrong shape.
- A loss of feeling in the injured body part
- Inability to put weight on the injured body part
- Severe pain or difficulty moving the heel

YES Get Emergency Care

{*Note:* See "Immobilize the injured area" under Self-Care Tips on page 137.}

NO

Flowchart continued on next page

14. Muscle & Bone Problems

Sports Injuries, *Continued*

Flowchart continued

Are there any of these problems?
- The skin around the injury turns blue and/or feels cold and numb.
- There is bad pain and swelling or the pain is getting worse.
- It hurts to press along the bone.

YES → See Doctor

NO → Use Self-Care

Self-Care Tips

■ Stop what you're doing and use R.I.C.E. – rest, ice, compression, and elevation. Do this at the first sign of serious discomfort or pain. (See R.I.C.E. on page 139.)

■ Take an over-the-counter medicine to reduce inflammation and pain. {*Note:* See "Pain relievers" in "Your Home Pharmacy" on pages 22 and 23.}

■ Do M.S.A. techniques once the injured area begins to heal. M.S.A. stands for movement, strength, and alternate activities.

M Movement – Work at establishing a full range of motion as soon as possible after an injury. This will help maintain flexibility during healing and prevent the scar tissue formed by the injury from limiting future performance.

S Strength – Gradually strengthen the injured area once the inflammation is controlled and a range of motion is re-established.

A Alternate Activities – Do regular exercise using activities that do not strain the injured part. This should be started a few days after the injury, even though the injured part is still healing.

14. Muscle & Bone Problems

145

47 Sprains & Strains

A sprain happens when you overstretch or tear a ligament (fibrous tissue that connects bones), a tendon (tissue that attaches a muscle to a bone), or a muscle. A strain occurs when you overstretch or overexert a muscle or tendon. Sprains and strains hurt and swell up. The amount of pain and swelling depends on the extent of damage.

Common causes for sprains and strains are falls, twisting a limb, sports injuries, and overexertion.

Prevention

Common sense can prevent many sprains and strains. General safety measures to prevent slips and falls:

- Clear ice from porches and walkways in winter weather.

- Wear shoes and boots with nonskid soles.

- Put sturdy handrails on both sides of stairways.

- Use rubber mats or adhesive-backed strips in bathtubs and shower stalls. A support bar is a good idea, too.

- Make sure light switches are located near all room entrances inside of the house and to entrances outside.

- Use a night light between the bedroom and bathroom or in the hallway at night.

- Don't leave shoes, toys, tools, and other things where people can trip over them.

- Use nonskid floor wax.

- Secure carpet to the floor. Make sure rugs have nonskid backing.

- Be careful whenever you use a ladder. Make sure it is steady. The ladder should be tall enough that you don't have to stand on the top 3 steps.

To Prevent Sprains and Strains from Sports Injuries:

- Ease into any exercise program. Start off with things that are easy for you. Build up gradually.

- Warm-up your muscles with slow easy stretches before you exercise. You should do this for all sports. Don't bounce.

- Don't overdo it. If muscles or joints start to hurt, ease up.

- Cool-down after hard exercises. Do the activity at a slower pace for 5 minutes. For example, after a run, walk or stroll for 5 minutes so your pulse comes down gradually.

- Wear shoes that fit you and the exercise you do.

Also, see the "Dos" and "Don'ts" of proper lifting in the section "Backaches," on page 132.

Treatment for sprains and strains will depend on the extent of damage done to the muscle, ligament, tendon, etc. Self-care measures may be all that are needed for mild injuries. Severe sprains may require medical treatment. Some sprains require a cast. Others may need surgery if the tissue affected is torn.

Sprains & Strains, *Continued*

Questions to Ask

Did the strain or sprain occur with great force from a vehicle accident or a fall from a high place?

YES → **Get Emergency Care**

NO ↓

Are any of these signs present?
- A bone sticks out or bones in the injured part make a grating sound.
- The injured body part looks crooked or the wrong shape.
- A loss of feeling in the injured body part
- Inability to move or put weight on the injured body part

YES → **Get Emergency Care**

{*Note:* See "Immobilize the injured area" under Self-Care Tips on page 137.}

NO ↓

Does the skin around the injury turn blue and/or feel cold and numb?

YES → **See Doctor**

NO ↓

Are any of these problems present?
- There is bad pain and swelling or the pain is getting worse.
- It hurts to press along the bone.

YES → **See Doctor**

NO ↓

 Use Self-Care

Self-Care Tips

■ Stop what you're doing. Then use **R.I.C.E.** (See **R.I.C.E.** on page 139).

■ Take an over-the-counter medicine for pain and inflammation. {*Note:* See "Pain relievers" in "Your Home Pharmacy" on pages 22 and 23.}

Also note, for specific areas of the body:

■ Remove rings right away if you sprain your finger or hand. (If you don't, and your fingers swell up, someone may have to cut the rings off.)

■ If you have a badly sprained ankle, use crutches. They help keep weight off the ankle, so it can heal.

Call your doctor if the sprain or strain does not improve after doing the Self-Care Tips for 4 days.

14. Muscle & Bone Problems

48 Anemia

Anemia means that either your red blood cells or the amount of hemoglobin in your red blood cells is low. Hemoglobin is a protein that carries oxygen in your red blood cells. Symptoms of anemia are tiredness, weakness, and paleness. Paleness could be pale skin. It could also be paleness around the gums, nailbeds, or the linings of the lower eyelids.

Iron-deficiency anemia is the most common form of anemia. In the United States, 20 percent of all women of childbearing age have iron-deficiency anemia (compared to 2 percent of adult men). The primary cause is blood lost during menstruation. But eating too few iron-rich foods or not absorbing enough iron can make the problem worse. Pregnancy, breast-feeding a baby, and blood loss from the gastrointestinal tract (either due to ulcers or cancer) can also deplete iron stores. Older persons who have poor diets, especially when they live alone, often have iron-deficiency anemia.

Folic-acid deficiency anemia is another type of anemia. It occurs when folic-acid levels are low. Not enough folic acid in the diet and/or poor absorption leads to this type. The need for this vitamin more than doubles during pregnancy. Folic acid may prevent certain birth defects such as spina bifida if taken before conception and in the early months of pregnancy.

Other less common forms of anemia include pernicious anemia (inability of the body to properly absorb vitamin B_{12}), sickle cell anemia (see page 370), and thalassemia anemia (an inherited disorder).

Alcohol, certain medicines, and some chronic diseases can also cause anemia.

Questions to Ask

Do you have blood in your stools or urine or have black, tarlike stools, with these problems?
- Lightheadedness
- Weakness
- Shortness of breath
- Severe abdominal pain

YES → Get Emergency Care

NO ↓

Are you dizzy when you stand up or when you exert yourself? **YES** → See Doctor

NO ↓

Do you have ringing in your ears? **YES** → See Doctor

NO ↓

For Women:
- Do you have vaginal bleeding between periods?
- Has menstrual bleeding been heavy for several months?
- Do you normally bleed 7 days or more every month?
- Do you suspect that you are pregnant?

YES → Call Doctor

NO ↓

Flowchart continued on next page

Anemia, *Continued*

Flowchart continued

Do symptoms of anemia (paleness, tiredness, listlessness and weakness) persist despite using Self-Care Tips (listed below) for at least 2 weeks?

YES Call Doctor

NO Use Self-Care

Self-Care Tips

Tips for Getting and Absorbing Iron

- Eat foods that are good sources of iron. Concentrate on green, leafy vegetables, lean, red meat, beef liver, poultry, fish, wheat germ, oysters, dried fruit, and iron-fortified cereals. {*Note:* Red meat not only supplies a good amount of iron, it also increases absorption of iron from other food sources.}

- Eat foods high in vitamin C, such as citrus fruits, tomatoes, and strawberries. Vitamin C helps your body absorb iron from food.

- Don't drink a lot of tea—it contains tannins, substances that can inhibit iron absorption. (Herbal tea is okay, though.)

- Take an iron supplement. But check with your doctor first. {*Note:* Recent research is suggesting that high levels of iron in the blood may increase the risk for heart attacks.}

- Avoid antacids, phosphates (which are found in soft drinks, beer, ice cream, etc.), and the food additive EDTA. These block iron absorption.

Tips for Getting and Absorbing Folic Acid

- Eat good food sources of folic acid every day. Some good sources are asparagus, brussels sprouts, spinach, romaine lettuce, collard greens, and broccoli. Other good sources are black-eyed peas, cantaloupe, orange juice, oatmeal, whole-grain cereals, wheat germ, and liver and other organ meats.

- Eat fresh, raw fruits and vegetables often. Don't overcook food. Heat destroys folic acid.

- Take the daily vitamin supplement your doctor suggests or prescribes.

- Don't smoke.

- Don't drink alcohol. It interferes with absorption of folic acid.

Tips for Getting B_{12}

- Eat animal sources of food–lean meat, fish, poultry, and nonfat or low-fat dairy products. Some cereals also have vitamin B_{12} added to them. {*Note:* The usual cause of a B_{12} deficiency is not a lack of it in the diet but the inability to absorb it from food. The cause for this needs to be identified and treated. Some persons may need to get monthly B_{12} shots.}

- Strict vegetarians (vegans) who eat no animal sources of food should get vitamin B_{12} from a supplement or foods fortified with the vitamin.

15. Other Health Problems

149

49 Chest Pain

Chest pain can come from a lot of things. These include:

- A heart attack
- Angina (see page 334)
- Lung problems. (Examples: pneumonia (see page 369), bronchitis (see page 81), a blood clot in the lung, a collapsed lung or an injured rib)

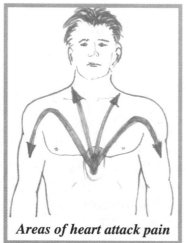

Areas of heart attack pain

- A hiatal hernia
- Heartburn (see page 126)
- Shingles (see page 109)
- A pulled muscle
- Mitral valve prolapse. A common disorder, especially in women, in which the mitral valve of the heart fails to close properly. In most people, this is not a serious problem.
- Anxiety (see page 180)
- Swallowing too much air

How do you know when you need medical help for chest pain? It's not always easy to tell. If you're not sure why your chest hurts, it's best to check it out. Getting help for a heart attack or lung injury could save your life.

Questions to Ask

Are any of these problems present?
- Chest pressure or pain (may spread to the arm, neck, or jaw)
- Feelings of chest tightness, squeezing, or heaviness that last more than a few minutes, or go away and come back
- Chest discomfort with: Shortness of breath or trouble breathing; nausea and/or vomiting; sweating; uneven pulse or heartbeat; or sense of doom

YES → Get Emergency Care

NO ↓

Did a serious injury cause the chest pain? Does it hurt all the time and/or is it getting worse?

YES → Get Emergency Care

NO ↓

Does the chest pain occur in a person who has had a recent operation or illness that has kept them in bed?

YES → Get Emergency Care

NO ↓

Does the chest pain occur in a person with a history of heart problems or in a person with angina, and not respond to prescribed medicine?

YES → Get Emergency Care

NO ↓

Flowchart continued on next page

Chest Pain, *Continued*

Flowchart continued

Is there trouble breathing along with the chest pain? Does it get worse when taking deep breaths or when you touch your chest or ribs? **YES** See Doctor

NO

Are one or more of the following present?
- Fever
- Coughing up mucus of any color (green, yellow, gray, etc.)

YES See Doctor

NO

Do you have any of these problems with the chest pain?
- Palpitations
- Lightheadedness
- Dizziness, feeling faint
- Fatigue
- Anxiety
- A heart murmur heard by a health care provider

YES See Doctor

NO

Does the chest pain come with belching and/or a burning feeling just above the stomach? Does it come and go before, during, or after eating? Does it worsen when bending or lying down?

YES See Doctor

NO

Flowchart continued in next column

Do all of these conditions describe the chest pain?
- It's only on one side of the chest.
- It's unaffected by breathing.
- A burning feeling and a skin rash are at the same place as the chest pain.

YES Call Doctor

NO

Use Self-Care

Self-Care Tips

For Chest Pain that Results from a Pulled Muscle or Minor Injury to the Rib Cage:

- Do not strain the muscle or ribs while pain is felt.

- Rest.

- Take an over-the-counter medicine for pain. {*Note:* See "Pain relievers" in "Your Home Pharmacy" on pages 22 and 23.}

- Do call your doctor, though, if the pain lasts longer than two days.

15. Other Health Problems

Chest Pain, *Continued*

For Chest Pain Associated with a Hiatal Hernia:

- Lose weight if you are overweight.

- Eat 5–6 small meals a day, instead of 3 large ones.

- Avoid tobacco, alcohol, coffee, spicy foods, peppermint, chocolate, citrus juices, and carbonated beverages.

- Do not eat food or drink milk 2 hours before going to bed.

- Don't bend over or lie down after eating.

- Do not wear tight clothes, tight belts, or girdles.

- Raise the head of your bed about 6 inches (40-degree angle) when you sleep.

For Chest Pain that Results from Anxiety and Hyperventilation:

- Talk about your anxiety with family, friends, and clergy. If this is not enough, you may need the help of a counselor or psychiatrist.

- When you hyperventilate, cover your mouth and nose with a paper bag. Breathe into the paper bag slowly and rebreathe the air. Do this in and out at least 10 times. Remove the bag and breathe normally a few minutes. Repeat breathing in and out of the paper bag as needed.

- Don't take too much aspirin or other drugs that have salicylates.

For Chest Pain Associated with Mitral Valve Prolapse (MVP):

- Eat healthy foods. Avoid caffeine.

- After checking with your doctor, exercise regularly to improve cardiovascular fitness.

- Deal with and control stress and avoid anxiety-producing situations, if possible.

- Don't smoke.

15. Other Health Problems

Fatigue

Fatigue is feeling tired, drained of energy and exhausted. Fatigue makes it hard for you to do normal daily activities. Feelings of inadequacy, low motivation and little desire for sex can also be symptoms of fatigue. There are many causes of fatigue.

Causes

Possible physical causes that need medical care include:

- Chronic fatigue syndrome. The fatigue lasts for 6 months or more (see page 341)
- Lupus (the systemic type)
- Multiple sclerosis (see page 361)
- Low thyroid (see page 372)
- Leukemia
- Heart disease
- HIV/AIDS (see page 356)
- Anemia (see page 148)
- Alcohol or drug abuse (see page 188)
- Migraine headaches (see page 158)

Other physical causes include:

- PMS (see page 243)
- Lack of sleep
- Crash dieting and eating poorly, which results in vitamin and mineral deficiencies
- Side effects from allergies or chemical sensitivities
- Living or working in hot, humid conditions
- Prolonged effects of the flu or a bad cold

Possible emotional causes:

- Burnout
- Boredom
- Change (facing a major life crisis or decision like divorce or retirement)
- Depression and/or anxiety (see "Depression" on page 186 and "Anxiety" on page 180)

Treatment

The first thing to do is find the cause(s) of the fatigue so you know what to treat. For example, iron supplements can help with the fatigue that results from iron-deficiency anemia. It is important to keep track of any other symptoms that take place with the fatigue, so both physical and emotional causes can be identified and dealt with.

Questions to Ask

Do any of these problems occur with the fatigue?
- Chest pressure or pain (may spread to the arm, neck, or jaw)
- Chest discomfort with: Shortness of breath or trouble breathing; sweating; uneven pulse or heartbeat; nausea or vomiting; or sense of doom
- Loss of balance or weakness, especially in one part or one side of the body
- Thoughts of suicide

YES → Get Emergency Care

NO

Flowchart continued on next page

15. Other Health Problems

Fatigue, *Continued*

Flowchart continued

Do you have any of these problems with the fatigue?
- Loss of weight or appetite
- Yellow skin and/or eyes (jaundice)
- Blurry or double vision
- Throwing up a lot
- Feeling anxious, and not being able to calm down

YES See Doctor

NO

Do you have 2 or more of these problems with fatigue?
- Swollen lymph glands
- Sore throat
- Headache
- Painful swelling in the neck, armpit, or groin
- Fever
- Night sweats
- Excessive thirst and/or urination

YES See Doctor

NO

Flowchart continued in next column

Do you have or have you had any of these problems?
- Arthritis or rheumatism for more than 3 months
- Fingers that get pale, numb, or uncomfortable in the cold
- Mouth sores for more than 2 weeks
- Low blood counts from anemia, low white-cell count, or low platelet count
- A rash on your cheeks for more than 1 month
- Skin rash after being in the sun
- Pain for more than 2 days when taking deep breaths
- Fainting episode
- Seizure, convulsion, or fit

YES See Doctor

NO

Did you start to feel fatigued after taking medicine?

YES 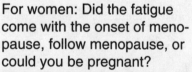 Call Doctor

NO

For women: Did the fatigue come with the onset of menopause, follow menopause, or could you be pregnant?

YES Call Doctor

NO

Flowchart continued on next page

Fatigue, *Continued*

Flowchart continued

Has the fatigue lasted for more than two weeks and kept you from doing your usual activities for no apparent reason?

YES — Call Doctor

NO

Use Self-Care

Self-Care Tips

Depending on the reasons for your fatigue, the following things may help restore your energy levels:

- **Eat better** – Eating too much and "crash dieting" are both hard on your body. Don't skip breakfast. Stay away from high-fat and/or rich, sugary snacks. Eat whole-grain breads and cereals, and raw fruits and vegetables every day. It may help to eat 5–6 light meals a day, instead of 3 large ones.

- **Get more exercise** – Exercise can give you more energy, especially if you sit all day at work. Exercise can calm you, too. Try taking a walk in the open air if you feel tired. It can help.

- **Cool off** – Working or playing in hot weather can drag you down. Living or working in a warm place without fresh air is bad too. Rest in a cool, dry place as often as you can. Drink plenty of water. Open a window when you can.

- **Rest and relax** – A good night's sleep can make you feel much better. But you can relax during the day too. Take breaks during your work day Practice deep breathing or meditation.

- **Change your routine** - Try to do something new and interesting every day. If you already do too much, make time for some peace and quiet.

- **Lighten your work load** - Assign tasks to others when you can, both at work and at home. Ask for help when you need it from family and friends. Hire help if necessary.

- **Do something for yourself** - Plan time to do things that meet only your needs, not just those of others.

- **Avoid too much caffeine and alcohol, and don't use illegal drugs** - These can trigger fatigue.

15. Other Health Problems

Fever

A body temperature of 98.6°F is average. Many healthy people walk around with a temperature a degree or so above or below average. Normal body temperature can range from 97°F to 100°F. Body temperature goes up and down during the day too. Your temperature is usually lowest in the morning and higher in the evening.

You can take your temperature by mouth, rectum (the opening where you pass solid waste), or under the arm using a mercury or digital thermometer. Thermometers you put in your ear are easy to use but cost a lot more than mercury and digital thermometers. A rectal reading is one degree higher than one by mouth or ear.

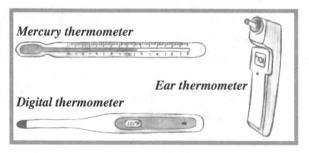

Mercury thermometer

Ear thermometer

Digital thermometer

Taking your temperature by mouth after you drink a hot liquid like soup or tea can make you think you have a fever when you don't. Other factors that can temporarily change your temperature include:

- Wearing too many clothes (if you're over-dressed enough to raise your body temperature)

- Exercise

- Hot, humid weather

- Hormones (The hormones in a woman's body make her temperature go up at certain times of the month.)

If you've ruled out other factors and your temperature is higher than 99°F, you might have a fever. If your temperature is higher than 100°F, you probably have a fever.

Adults probably don't have to do anything to treat a fever if they feel okay. But be sure to treat a fever if you don't feel good, or if it goes over 104°F (102°F in the elderly). When you treat a fever you are treating a symptom. It is important to find and treat the cause of the fever.

Questions to Ask

Do any of these problems come with the fever?
- Seizure
- Listlessness
- Abnormal breathing
- Stiff neck
- Excessive irritability
- Confusion

YES Get Emergency Care

NO

Are any of these problems also present with the fever?
- Ear pain
- Persistent sore throat
- Vomiting
- Diarrhea
- Urinary pain, burning, or frequency

YES See Doctor

NO

Flowchart continued on next page

Fever, *Continued*

Flowchart continued

Does the fever occur in a child less than 2 months old? **YES** See Doctor

NO

In an adult, is the fever over 104°F (102°F in an elderly person), or has it lasted more than 4 days despite efforts to reduce the fever? **YES** See Doctor

NO

Has the person recently had surgery or does the person have a chronic illness, such as heart disease, lung disease, kidney disease, cancer, or diabetes? **YES** Call Doctor

NO

Does the fever occur in a baby younger than 6 months old? **YES** Call Doctor

NO

Has the fever done any of the following?
• Gone away for more than 24 hours and then come back
• Come soon after a visit to a foreign country
• Come after having a DTP or MMR shot <u>and</u> is present with dizziness
YES Call Doctor

NO

Flowchart continued in next column

In a child, is the fever over 101°F (or 102°F rectally) and has it not gone down In 48 hours despite efforts to reduce the fever? **YES** Call Doctor

NO

 Use Self-Care

Self-Care Tips

- Drink fruit juice, water, and soft drinks.
- Take a sponge bath with warm (about 70°F) water. (Sponging with alcohol has no advantage and often makes people feel ill because of alcohol's pungent odor.)
- Take the appropriate dose of an over-the-counter medicine to reduce fever. {*Note:* See "Pain relievers" in "Your Home Pharmacy" on pages 22 and 23.}
- Rest in bed.
- Don't wear too many clothes or use too many blankets.
- Don't do heavy exercise.

15. Other Health Problems

157

52 Headaches

There are different kinds of headaches. The most common types are:

Tension or Muscular Headaches

You feel a dull ache in your forehead, above your ears, or at the back of your head. You get a tension headache when the muscles in your face, neck, or head get tight. This can happen when you:

- Don't get enough sleep
- Feel "stressed out"
- Read
- Do boring work
- Stay in one position for a long time, such as working at a computer

Migraine Headaches

These happen when blood vessels in your head open too wide or close too tight. Women get migraines more than men. People in the same family often get them. These are symptoms of a migraine headache:

- One side of your head hurts more than the other.
- You feel sick to your stomach or throw up.
- You see spots.
- Light hurts your eyes.
- Your ears ring.

Sinus Headaches

Your sinuses are behind your cheeks, around your eyes, and in your nose. You get a sinus headache when your sinuses are under pressure. Anybody can get a sinus headache. People with allergies like hay fever often get them.

A sinus headache makes your forehead, cheekbones, and nose hurt. It hurts more if you bend over or touch your face. You can get a sinus headache from:

- A cold
- Allergies
- Dirty or polluted air
- Other breathing problems
- Airplane travel

Headaches can also result from:

- A sensitivity to certain foods and drinks
- Alcohol
- Cigarette smoke
- Exposure to chemicals and/or pollution
- Poison
- Side effects from some medications

A headache can be a symptom of many health conditions, too. Some of these are:

- Allergies
- Arthritis in the jaw joint
- Depression (see page 186)
- Fever (see page 156)
- High blood pressure (see page 354)
- Low blood sugar
- Infections
- Pinched nerve in the neck

Headaches, *Continued*

- Shingles (see on page 109)
- Dental problems (see "Dental Problems & Injuries" on pages 276–281)

Less often, a headache can be a symptom of a serious health problem that needs immediate medical attention. Examples are:

- Acute glaucoma (see page 352)
- Stroke (see page 371)
- Tumor, blood clot, or ruptured blood vessel (aneurysm) in the brain

Prevention

- Try to anticipate when pain will strike. Keep a headache journal that records when, where, and why headaches seem to occur.
- Note early symptoms and try to abort a headache in its earliest stages. Take pain medicine such as acetaminophen right away.
- Exercise regularly. This seems to keep some kinds of headaches at bay.
- Avoid foods and beverages known to trigger headaches in sensitive people. Try to figure out which foods and beverages affect you. Problem items may include:
  - Alcoholic beverages, especially red wine
  - Aspartame (the artificial sweetener in NutraSweet)
  - Bananas (if more than $\frac{1}{2}$ banana a day)
  - Caffeine from coffee, tea, cola soft drinks, chocolate, or some medications
  - Citrus fruits (if more than $\frac{1}{2}$ cup a day)
  - Cured meats such as frankfurters

- Food additives such as monosodium glutamate (MSG)
- Hard cheeses such as aged cheddar or provolone
- Nuts and peanut butter
- Onions
- Sour cream
- Soy sauce
- Vinegar

Questions to Ask

Is the headache associated with any of the following?
- A serious head injury
- A blow to the head that causes severe pain, enlarged pupils, vomiting, confusion, or lethargy
- Loss of consciousness

YES Get Emergency Care

{Note: See "Head Injuries" on page 313.}

NO

Is the headache associated with any of the following?
- Severe pain in and around one eye
- Blurred vision
- Double vision
- Slurring of speech
- Mental confusion
- Personality change
- A problem in moving arms or legs
- Unusual sleepiness

YES Get Emergency Care

NO

Flowchart continued on next page

15. Other Health Problems

Headaches, *Continued*

Flowchart continued

Has the headache been occurring for more than 2 to 3 days and does it keep increasing in frequency and intensity? **YES** **Get Emergency Care**

NO

Does the headache come with all of the following?
• Fever
• Drowsiness
• Nausea
• Vomiting
• Stiff neck
YES **Get Emergency Care**

NO

Has the headache come on suddenly and does it hurt more than others you have had? **YES** **See Doctor**

NO

Has the headache occurred at the same time of day, week, or month? **YES** **Call Doctor**

NO

Have you noticed the headache only after taking newly prescribed or over-the-counter medicines? **YES** **Call Doctor**

NO

Use Self-Care

Self-Care Tips

For On-the-Spot Headache Relief:

■ Take an over-the-counter medicine for pain. Take it right away. (Pain relievers work best when the headache starts.) {*Note:* See "Pain relievers" in Your Home Pharmacy" on pages 22 and 23.}

■ Rest in a quiet, dark room with your eyes closed.

■ Massage the base of your head with your thumbs. Start under your ears and work back towards the center of your head. Also, gently massage both temples, your shoulders, neck and jaw.

■ Take a warm bath or shower.

■ Place a cold or warm washcloth over the area that aches. Use the one that feels better. Or, put an ice pack on the back or top of the head if this brings relief.

■ Relax. Try thinking of a calm, happy place. Breathe slowly and deeply.

53 Hyperventilation

Hyperventilation means breathing too deeply and faster than normal. Hyperventilating can be scary for any child or adult. When you hyperventilate, your heart pounds and it feels like you can't get enough air. Your arms, legs, and mouth tingle and may feel numb because you give off too much carbon dioxide in the exhaled air. This makes the carbon dioxide level in your blood and brain tissue fall. Other symptoms and signs include visual changes, a feeling of impending doom, and sometimes loss of consciousness.

The symptoms usually last 20 to 30 minutes, but it may seem like hours to anyone having them. Though scary, hyperventilation is not usually dangerous.

Causes of Hyperventilation

- Anxiety (the most common cause)
- Severe stomach pains
- Heart or lung disease
- Extensive physical injuries
- Panic attacks
- Disorders of the central nervous system

Prevention

Probably the best way to prevent hyperventilation is to avoid situations and activities that cause anxiety. To help yourself or your child avoid hyperventilating:

- Learn meditation and practice it every day. Meditation is a form of mental relaxation. It relieves stress as you focus on a single word or visual image.

- Practice relaxing your muscles.
  - Lie down in a quiet room.
  - Close your eyes and take deep breaths.
  - Start with your feet. Tense the muscles in one foot, hold for 10 seconds, and relax them. Repeat with the other foot.
  - Then, tense and relax the muscles in your legs. Then repeat with the muscles in your back, stomach, hands, arms, shoulders, neck, and face.

- Talk to friends, family, or even a counselor to help relieve anxiety.

- Keep a journal to help you focus on your problems and find solutions you can live with.

- Exercise on a regular basis. People in good physical shape are less likely to buckle under stress.

- Reduce caffeine. Drink less coffee, tea, and colas. Eat less chocolate.

Questions to Ask

Are you also having chest pain and/or pain that spreads to the arm, neck, back, or jaw? **YES** → Get Emergency Care

NO

Do you also have asthma, emphysema, or a serious lung or heart problem? **YES** → Get Emergency Care

 NO

Flowchart continued on next page

15. Other Health Problems

Hyperventilation, *Continued*

Flowchart continued

Do you hyperventilate often and/or have you had 4 or more panic attacks in 4 weeks' time?

YES  **See Doctor**

NO **Use Self-Care**

Self-Care Tips

Breathing into a paper bag increases the amount of carbon dioxide in the blood and relieves the symptoms. Follow these steps:

- Loosely cover your nose and mouth with a small paper bag.

- Breathe slowly into the bag and rebreathe the air in the bag about 10 times.

- Set the bag aside and breathe normally for a couple of minutes.

- Repeat steps 2 and 3 until the symptoms lessen or go away.

- Try to breathe slowly. Focus on taking one breath every 5 seconds.

(*Note:* If you continue to hyperventilate after using Self-Care Tips, call your doctor.)

54 Insomnia

Do you ever find yourself wide awake long after you go to bed at night? Well, you're not alone. An estimated 40 million Americans have insomnia. They either have trouble falling asleep at night, wake up in the middle of the night, or wake up too early and can't get back to sleep. And when they're not asleep, insomniacs worry about whether or not they'll be able to sleep. They are also irritable and feel fatigued during the day.

Once in a while, a sleepless night is nothing to lose sleep over. But if insomnia bothers you for three weeks or longer, it can be a real medical problem. Some medical problems that lead to insomnia include:

- Overactive thyroid gland
- Heart or lung conditions that cause shortness of breath when lying down
- Depression and anxiety disorders
- Allergies and early-morning wheezing
- Any illness, injury, or surgery that causes pain and/or discomfort, which interrupts sleep (Example: arthritis)
- Sexual problems (Example: impotence)
- Hot flashes that interrupt sleep
- Any disorder (urinary, gastrointestinal, or neurological) that makes it necessary to urinate or have a bowel movement during the night
- Side effects of certain medications (Examples: decongestants, cortisone medications)

Other things that lead to insomnia:

- Emotional stress
- Too much noise when falling asleep. This includes a snoring partner.
- The use of stimulants, such as caffeine from coffee, tea, colas, and stay-awake pills such as NoDoz
- Lack of physical exercise
- Lack of a sex partner

Questions to Ask

Do you have trouble falling or staying asleep due to any of the following?
- Pain or discomfort due to illness or injury
- The need to wake up to use the bathroom (even after using Self-Care Tips)

YES → Call Doctor

NO

Has your sleep been disturbed since you began taking medication of any kind?

YES → Call Doctor

NO

Do you still have trouble sleeping after 3 weeks, with or without Self-Care Tips (see page 164)?

YES → Call Doctor

NO

 Use Self-Care

See Self-Care Tips on next page

15. Other Health Problems

Insomnia, *Continued*

Self-Care Tips

Many old-fashioned remedies for sleeplessness work, and work well. Next time you find yourself unable to sleep, try these time-tested cures.

- Avoid caffeine in all forms after lunchtime. (Coffee, tea, chocolate, colas, and some other soft drinks contain this stimulant, as do certain over-the-counter and prescription medications. Check the labels for content.)

- Avoid long naps during the day. (Naps decrease the quality of nighttime sleep.)

- Avoid more than 1 or 2 servings of alcoholic beverages at dinnertime and during the rest of the evening. Even though alcohol is a sedative, it can disrupt sleep. Always check with your doctor about using alcohol if you are taking medications.

- Have food items rich in the amino acid L-tryptophan, such as milk, turkey, or tuna fish, before you go to bed. Eating foods with carbohydrates, such as cereal, breads and fruits may help as well. (Do not, however, take L-tryptophan supplements.)

- Take a long, warm bath before bedtime. (This soothes and unwinds tense muscles, leaving you relaxed enough to fall asleep.)

- Read a book or do some repetitive, calm activity. Avoid distractions that may hold your attention and keep you awake, such as watching a suspense movie.

- If insomnia is due to waking up to use the bathroom, avoid drinking liquids for 2–3 hours before going to sleep.

- Make your bedroom as comfortable as possible. Create a quiet, dark atmosphere. Use clean, fresh sheets and pillows, and keep the room temperature comfortable (neither too warm nor too cool.)

- Ban worry from the bedroom. Don't allow yourself to rehash the mistakes of the day as you toss and turn. You're off duty now. The idea is to associate your bed with sleep.

- Develop a regular bedtime routine. Locking or checking doors and windows, brushing your teeth, and reading before you turn in every night primes you for sleep.

- Count those sheep! Counting slowly is a soothing, hypnotic activity. By picturing repetitive, monotonous images, you may bore yourself to sleep.

- Try listening to recordings made especially to help promote sleep. Check local bookstores.

- Don't take over-the-counter sleeping pills or friends' or relatives' sleeping pills. Only take sleep medicine with your doctor's permission.

- Talk to your doctor before using melatonin, a product marketed to promote sleep.

55 Repetitive Motion Injuries

Repetitive motion injuries (RMIs), also called repetitive strain injuries (RSIs), can occur when you perform the same activity over and over for a long period of time either at work, at home, during sports, and/or with hobbies. The types of movements involved include repeated:

- Drilling or hammering
- Lifting
- Pushing or pulling
- Squeezing
- Twisting
- Wrist, finger, and hand movements

The injuries that result from RMIs are most often:

- Tendinitis – Constant wear and tear on wrists, elbows, and shoulders may create tiny tears in the tendons that cause swelling, inflammation, and pain. Tendinitis tends to hurt more at night than during the day. Treatment for tendinitis varies with the cause and how severe it is. Tennis elbow is one example of this RMI.

- Eyestrain – Results, for example, from working with video display terminals (VDTs). (See "Eyestrain from Computers" on page 59.)

- Backaches – Often due to poor posture or improper lifting. (See "Backaches" on page 132.)

- Carpal tunnel syndrome (CTS) – Develops when tissues swell inside the carpal tunnel, a narrow tunnel in the wrist. Soft tissue in this tunnel enlarges, pinching the nerves that pass through it. Women are more likely to suffer from CTS than men because their carpal tunnel is usually smaller. Pregnancy can also increase a woman's risk for CTS, though the pain usually disappears after the baby is born. CTS is easier to treat and less likely to cause future problems if it is diagnosed early. (See "For Preventing Wrist and Hand Injuries" in this section on page 166.) Once diagnosed, CTS can be treated with:

  - Physical therapy
  - Wearing a splint at night
  - Taking anti-inflammatory medicines such as aspirin, ibuprofen, or naproxen sodium
  - Changing the workplace setup to reduce pressure in the wrist

Sometimes surgery is necessary if these measures aren't enough.

Repetitive motion injuries are on the increase. Disability claims for these injuries have more than doubled in the last 10 years. In many cases, computers are the culprits. A writer or busy secretary, for example, often strikes the keys about 200,000 times a day; that's like your fingers taking a 10-mile walk. And chairs without lumbar support can cause back pain. Misplaced monitors can bring on eyestrain and stiff necks. No wonder many keyboard operators experience tendinitis and CTS.

Repetitive Motion Injuries, *Continued*

Questions to Ask

Do you have one or both of these problems?
- Severe or persistent pain, swelling, or spasm
- Tenderness or stiffness and limited motion in the affected area such as the shoulder, arm, or wrist

 YES  See Doctor

NO

Does pain in your hand, shoulder, or wherever wake you from sleep?

YES Call Doctor

NO

Have you had one or both of these problems?
- Pain, numbness, and tingling in your hand for more than 2 weeks
- Inability to make a fist for a couple of weeks

YES Call Doctor

NO

Do you frequently drop objects, and does your thumb feel weak?

YES Call Doctor

NO

 Use Self-Care

Self-Care/Prevention Tips

For Preventing Wrist and Hand Injuries:

Whenever your hands and wrists perform the same activity time and again, you increase your risk for CTS and tendinitis. Change how you do a task and you may avoid some of these injuries.

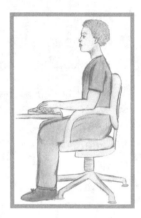

- Keep your wrists straight when typing. Make sure your fingers are lower than your wrists and don't rest the heels of your hands on the keyboard. Buy a wrist rest for your keyboard to keep your wrists higher than the keyboard. Drop and tip your keyboard or try one of the new ergonomic keyboards.

- Do not hold an object in the same position for a long time. Even simple tasks such as hammering a nail can cause injury when performed over a period of time.

- Give your hands a break by resting them for a few minutes each hour.

- Lift objects with your whole hand or, better yet, with both hands. Gripping or lifting with the thumb and index finger puts stress on your wrist.

Repetitive Motion Injuries, *Continued*

- If your line of work causes pain in your hands and wrists, see if you can share different jobs with someone else. Or alternate the stressful tasks with other work.

- Exercise your hands and wrists as often as possible.

  - Stretch your hands. Place them in front, spread your fingers as far apart as possible and hold for 5 seconds. Relax. Repeat 5 times with each hand.

  - Turn your wrists in a circle, palms up and then palms down. Relax your fingers and keep your elbows still. Repeat 5 times.

  - Drop your hands downwards. Shake your hands up and down, then sideways, until the tension is gone.

For Carpal Tunnel Syndrome:

- Lose weight. CTS is linked to obesity; the excess tissue can press on the carpal tunnel.

- Take an over-the-counter medicine to reduce the pain and inflammation. {*Note:* See "Pain relievers" in "Your Home Pharmacy" on pages 22 and 23.}

- Use a wrist splint. Many drug and medical supply stores carry splints that keep the wrist angled slightly back with the thumb parallel to the forearm. This position helps to keep the carpal tunnel open.

For Preventing Tendinitis:

- Use proper posture, proper equipment, and proper technique when doing repetitive tasks.

- Take stretch breaks several times a day.

- Do stretching and strengthening exercises to keep your shoulder, neck, and arm muscles strong and flexible.

See also: "Treating Tendinitis" on page 142; "To Prevent Eyestrain" on page 59; "Dos and Don'ts" (of Lifting) under "Prevention" in "Backaches" on page 132 and "Self-Care Tips for Backaches" on pages 134 and 135.

15. Other Health Problems

56 Snoring

Snoring is the sound heard when the airway is blocked during sleep. It can result from a number of things: obesity, enlarged tonsils and adenoids, deformities in the nasal passages, etc. Smoking, heavy drinking, overeating, especially before bedtime, and nasal allergies can lead to snoring by swelling the nasal passages and blocking the free flow of air. Also, persons who sleep on their backs are more likely to snore because the tongue falls back toward the throat and partly closes the airway. Nine out of 10 snorers are men, and most of them are age 40 or over.

Snoring can be merely a nuisance or it can be a signal of a serious health problem, sleep apnea. Sleep apnea is a condition where breathing is stopped for a time period of at least 10 seconds, but usually 20–30 seconds or even up to 1 or 2 minutes during sleep. It is more common in men than in women and typically affects men who are middle-aged and older. It can result from:

- An obstructed airway. This is more common as people age, especially those who are obese or who have smoked for many years.

- A central nervous system disorder such as a stroke, a brain tumor, or even a viral brain infection

- A chronic respiratory disease

Sleep apnea may require surgery.

Questions To Ask

Do you notice the following signs of sleep apnea during your daytime hours?
- Sleepiness or chronic day-time drowsiness
- Poor memory
- Lack of concentration
- Irritability
- Falling asleep while driving or working
- Loss of sex drive
- Headaches

YES **See Doctor**

NO

Has someone else noticed that breathing has stopped for 10 seconds or longer (sleep apnea) in the midst of snoring?

YES **See Doctor**

NO

Has snoring persisted despite using the Self-Care Tips on the next page?

YES **Call Doctor**

NO

 Use Self-Care

See Self-Care Tips on next page

Snoring, *Continued*

Self-Care Tips

■ Sleep on your side. Prop an extra pillow behind your back so you won't roll over. Try sleeping on a narrow sofa for a few nights to get accustomed to staying on your side.

■ Sew a large marble or tennis ball into a pocket on the back of your pajamas. The discomfort it causes may prompt you to sleep on your side.

■ If you must sleep on your back, raise the head of the bed by putting bricks or blocks between the mattress and box springs. Or buy a wedge especially made to be placed between the mattress and box spring to elevate the head section. Elevating the head prevents the tongue from falling against the back of the throat.

■ If you are heavy, lose weight. Excess fatty tissue in the throat can cause snoring.

■ Don't drink alcohol or eat a heavy meal within 3 hours before bedtime. For some reason, both seem to foster snoring.

■ If necessary, take an antihistamine or decongestant before retiring to relieve nasal congestion (which can also contribute to snoring). {*Note:* Older men should check with their doctor before taking decongestants. Decongestants that have ephedrine can give older men urinary problems.}

■ Get rid of allergens in the bedroom such as dust, down-filled (feathered) pillows and bed linen (this may also relieve nasal congestion).

■ Try over-the-counter "nasal strips." These keep the nostrils open and lift them up, keeping nasal passages unobstructed.

57 Urinary Incontinence

If you have urinary incontinence, you suffer from a loss of bladder control or your bladder fails to retain urine properly. As a result, you can't keep from passing urine, even though you may try to hold it in. Urinary incontinence is not a normal part of aging, but often affects older persons because the sphincter muscles that open the bladder into the urethra become less efficient with aging.

Although you might feel embarrassed if you have urinary incontinence, you should nevertheless let your doctor know about it. It could be a symptom of a disorder that could lead to more trouble if not treated.

Causes

In most cases, the problem is curable and treatable.

Two categories of urinary incontinence are acute incontinence and persistent incontinence.

The acute form is generally a symptom of a new illness or condition (e.g., bladder infection, inflammation of the prostate, urethra or vagina, and constipation).

Side effects of some medications, such as water pills, tranquilizers, and antihistamines can also result in acute urinary incontinence.

Acute urinary incontinence comes on suddenly. It is often easily reversed when the condition that caused it is treated.

Persistent incontinence comes on gradually over time. It lingers or remains, even after other conditions or illnesses have been treated. There are many types of persistent incontinence. The 3 types that account for 80 percent of cases are:

- **Stress Incontinence** – Urine leaks out when there is a sudden rise in pressure in the abdomen (belly). The amount ranges from small leaks to large spills. This usually happens with coughing, sneezing, laughing, lifting, jumping, running, or with straining to have a bowel movement. Stress incontinence is more common in women than in men.

- **Urge Incontinence** – This inability to control the bladder when the urge to urinate occurs comes on suddenly, so there is often not enough time to make it to the toilet. This type typically results in large accidents. It can be caused by a number of things, including an enlarged prostate gland, a spinal cord injury, multiple sclerosis, or Parkinson's disease.

- **Mixed Incontinence** – This type has elements of both stress and urge incontinence.

Other types of persistent incontinence are:

- **Overflow Incontinence** – Constant dribbling of urine occurs because the bladder overfills. This may be due to an enlarged prostate, diabetes, or multiple sclerosis.

- **Functional Incontinence** – With this, a person has trouble getting to the bathroom fast enough, even though he or she has bladder control. This can happen in a person who is physically challenged.

Urinary Incontinence, *Continued*

- **Total Incontinence** – In this rare type, with complete loss of bladder control, urine leakage can be continual.

Treatment

Care and treatment for urinary incontinence will depend on the type and cause(s). The first step is to find out if there is an underlying problem and to correct it. Treatment can also include pelvic floor exercises, called Kegel exercises, and other self-care measures (see Self-Care Tips in this section on pages 172–173). Medication, collagen injections (for a certain type of stress incontinence), or surgery to correct the specific problem may be needed.

Your primary doctor may evaluate and treat your incontinence or send you to a urologist, a doctor who specializes in treating problems of the bladder and urinary tract.

Questions to Ask

Have you lost control of your bladder after an injury to your spine or back?

YES → Get Emergency Care

NO ↓

Do you have these problems?
- Fever and shaking chills
- Back pain (sometimes severe) in one or both sides of the lower back or just at your midline
- Nausea and vomiting

YES → Get Emergency Care

NO ↓

Flowchart continued in next column

Does your loss of bladder control come with any of these symptoms?
- Loss of consciousness
- Inability to speak or slurred speech
- Loss of sight, double or blurred vision
- Sudden, severe headaches
- Paralysis, weakness, or loss of sensation in an arm or leg and/or the face on the same side of the body
- Change in personality, behavior, and/or emotions
- Confusion and dizziness

YES → 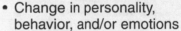 Get Emergency Care

NO ↓

Is the loss of bladder control more than temporary after surgery or an abdominal injury?

YES → See Doctor

NO ↓

Do you have any of these problems?
- Burning
- Frequent urination
- Blood in the urine or cloudy urine
- Abdominal or low back pain

YES → 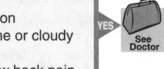 See Doctor

NO ↓

Flowchart continued on next page

Urinary Incontinence, *Continued*

Flowchart continued

With the loss of bladder control, do you have diabetes or any of these symptoms of diabetes?
- Extreme thirst
- Unusual hunger
- Excessive loss or gain in weight
- Blurred vision
- Easy fatigue, drowsiness
- Slow healing of cuts and/or infections

YES → See Doctor

NO ↓

If you are a man, do you have any of these problems?
- Dribbling urine and/or feeling the need to urinate again after you have finished urinating
- Voiding small amounts of urine often during the day
- The need to urinate while sleeping
- An intense and sudden need to urinate often
- A slow, weak, or interrupted stream of urine

YES → See Doctor

NO ↓

Do you leak urine when you cough, sneeze, laugh, jump, run, or lift heavy objects?

YES → Call Doctor

NO ↓

Flowchart continued in next column

Did you lose some bladder control only after taking a new medicine or after taking a higher dose of a medicine you were already taking?

YES → Call Doctor

NO ↓

 Use Self-Care

Self-Care Tips

- Avoid or limit drinks, foods, and medicines that have caffeine (e.g., coffee, tea, colas, chocolate, and No-Doz).

- Limit carbonated drinks, alcohol, citrus juices, greasy and spicy foods, and items that have artificial sweeteners. These can irritate the bladder.

- Drink 1–2 quarts of water throughout the day.

- Go to the bathroom often, even if you don't feel the urge. When you urinate, empty your bladder as much as you can. Relax for a minute or two and then try to go again. Keep a diary of when you have episodes of incontinence. If you find that you have accidents every 3 hours, for example, empty your bladder every $2\frac{1}{2}$ hours. Use an alarm clock or wristwatch with an alarm to remind you.

- Wear clothes you can remove quickly and easily when you use the bathroom. Examples are elastic-waist bottoms and items with velcro closures or snaps instead of buttons and zippers. Also, look for belts that are easy to undo, or don't wear belts at all.

Urinary Incontinence, *Continued*

- Wear absorbent pads or briefs.

- Ask your doctor if you would benefit from using self-catheters. A self-catheter is a clear, straw-like device, usually made of flexible plastic, that you insert into the opening of the urethra; it helps you empty your bladder completely. Your doctor will need to show you how to use one. You need a prescription for self-catheters.

- Empty your bladder before you leave the house, take a nap, and go to bed.

- Keep the pathway to your bathroom free of clutter and well lit. Make sure the bathroom door is left open until you use it.

- Use an elevated toilet seat and grab bars if these will make it easier for you to get on and off the toilet.

- Keep a bedpan, plastic urinal (for men), or portable commode chair near your bed. You can get these at medical supply stores and drugstores.

Kegel Exercises

To strengthen your pelvic floor muscles, do Kegel exercises . They can help treat or cure stress incontinence. Even elderly women who have leaked urine for years can benefit greatly from these exercises. Here's how to do them:

- First, identify where your pelvic floor muscles are. One way to do this is to start to urinate, then hold back and try to stop. If you can slow the stream of urine, even a little, you are using the right muscles. You should feel muscles squeezing around your urethra and anus.

- Next, relax your body, close your eyes and just imagine that you are going to urinate and then hold back from doing so. You should feel the muscles squeeze like you did in the step before this one.

- Squeeze the muscles for 3 seconds and then relax them for 3 seconds. When you squeeze and relax, count slowly. Start out doing this 3 times a day. Gradually work up to 3 sets of 10 contractions, holding each one for 10 seconds at a time. You can do them in lying, sitting, and/or standing positions.

- Women can also use pelvic weights prescribed by their doctor. A woman inserts a weighted cone into the vagina and squeezes the correct muscles to keep the weight from falling out.

- When you do these exercises:
  - Do not tense the muscles in your belly or buttocks.
  - Do not hold your breath, clench your fists or teeth, or make a face.
  - If you are not sure you're doing the exercise right, consult your doctor.

- Squeeze your pelvic floor muscles right before and during whatever it is (coughing, sneezing, jumping, etc.) that causes you to lose urine. Relax the muscles once the activity is over.

- It may take several months to benefit from pelvic floor exercises and you have to keep doing them daily to maintain their benefit.

58 Urinary Tract Infections (UTIs)

Your urinary tract is made up of these parts:
- Kidneys
- Ureters (tubes that connect the kidneys to the bladder)
- Bladder
- Urethra (the tube through which urine is passed)

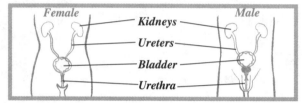

Female   *Male*

Kidneys

Ureters

Bladder

Urethra

Causes

UTI's result when bacteria infect any part of the urinary tract. The bladder is the most common site.

The risk for getting a UTI is greater for:
- Sexually active women – bacteria from intercourse can move from the urethra to the bladder
- Women who use a diaphragm
- Men and women who have had UTI's in the past
- Anyone with a condition that doesn't allow urine to pass freely. Kidney stones, an enlarged prostate, and multiple sclerosis are some examples.

Symptoms

- A strong need to go to the bathroom
- Going to the bathroom more often than usual
- A sharp pain or burning in the urethra when you pass urine
- Blood in the urine
- Feeling like your bladder is still full after you pass urine
- Soreness in your belly, back, or sides
- Chills, fever, sick stomach, throwing up

{*Note:* You can have a UTI without symptoms.}

Treatment

An antibiotic to treat the specific infection and pain relievers (if necessary) are the usual course of treatment.

Prevention

Here are some things you can do to keep from getting UTIs:
- If you're a woman, wipe from front to back after using the toilet. This keeps bacteria away from the opening of the urethra.
- Drink plenty of liquids. Drink fruit juices, especially cranberry juice.
- Empty your bladder as soon as you feel the urge. Don't give bacteria a chance to grow.
- Drink a glass of water before you have sex. Go to the bathroom as soon as you can after sex.
- If you use a lubricant when you have sex, use a water-soluble lubricant like K-Y Jelly.
- Wear cotton underpants. Bacteria like a warm, wet place. Cotton helps keep you cool and dry because it lets air flow through.
- Don't take bubble baths if you have had UTIs before. Take showers instead of baths.
- Don't wear tight-fitting undergarments, jeans and/or slacks.
- If you use a diaphragm, clean it after each use. And, have your doctor check your diaphragm periodically to make sure it still fits properly.

Urinary Tract Infections (UTIs), *Continued*

Questions to Ask

Do you have all of these symptoms?
- Fever and shaking chills
- Pain in one or both sides of your lower back
- Vomiting and nausea

YES → **Get Emergency Care**

NO ↓

Do you have these problems?
- Burning or stinging feeling when you pass urine
- Passing urine a lot more often than usual
- Bloody or cloudy urine
- Pain in your abdomen or over your bladder
- Feeling like you're going to throw up

YES → **See Doctor**

NO ↓

Do you have any of these problems?
- Constant urge to urinate.
- You feel like your bladder is still full after you urinate.
- Your urine smells bad.
- It hurts to have sex.

YES →  **See Doctor**

NO ↓

Do you get UTIs a lot?

YES → 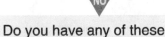 **Call Doctor**

NO ↓

Flowchart continued in next column

Have you had symptoms for more than 3 days, without getting better? Did medication the doctor prescribed give you side effects, such as a skin rash, or make you sick?

YES → **Call Doctor**

NO ↓

 Use Self-Care

Self-Care Tips

- Avoid alcohol, spicy foods, and coffee.
- Drink at least 8 glasses of water a day. Cranberry juice is good, too.
- Get plenty of rest.
- Check for fever twice a day. Take your temperature in the morning and then in the evening.
- Take an over-the-counter medicine for pain. {*Note:* See "Pain relievers" in "Your Home Pharmacy" on pages 22 and 23.} Or, take an over-the-counter medicine made for the pain that comes with a bladder infection. (Example: Uristat) {*Note:* Uristat helps with symptoms but doesn't get rid of the infection. If you take Uristat, you should still see your doctor.}
- Go to the bathroom as soon as you feel the need. Empty your bladder completely every time you pass urine. If you have a condition that keeps you from doing this, such as that which occurs in some persons with multiple sclerosis, ask your doctor about using intermittent self-catheters.
- Empty your bladder as soon as you can after sex.

{*Note:* See your doctor if you don't feel better in 3 days.}

15. Other Health Problems

59 Alcoholism

Alcoholism is used here to describe alcohol abuse and/or dependence. Alcohol abuse is the repeated use of alcohol that results in daily living problems. Examples include:

- Failing to fulfill work, school, or home duties
- Getting arrested for drunk driving, disorderly conduct, etc.
- Having relationship problems such as arguments or physical fights

Alcohol dependence is alcohol addiction. It means not being able to stop using alcohol without some degree of distress. The distress can be from:

- Cravings for alcohol
- The need for more and more alcohol to get the desired effect
- Withdrawal symptoms when blood alcohol levels decline

Causes

A tendency to become alcoholic is increased if family members are alcoholic. Men and women are about 4 times more likely to become alcoholic if one of their parents was, and 10 times more likely if both parents were. Environmental factors also play a role. For example, the more a person drinks, the greater the risk. Also, being able to consume a lot of alcohol (having a high tolerance) is a risk factor, not a safeguard, for alcoholism.

Alcohol abuse and/or dependence can develop in several ways:

- Drinking in excess on an almost daily basis
- Drinking a lot at certain times, such as every weekend

- Drinking a lot in binges, with or without long periods of not drinking
- Drinking infrequently, but with loss of control over drinking and/or behavior problems while drinking

Alcoholism is a disease which affects the alcoholic's physical health, emotional well-being and behavior.

Physical Effects of Alcohol

- Can impair mental/physical reflexes. The chart below describes the typical effects as blood alcohol content (BAC) increases.

Alcohol in Blood (percent)	Typical Effects (varies per individual)
0.05	Loosening of judgment, thought, and restraint. Release of tension; carefree sensation.
0.08	Tensions and inhibitions of everyday life lessened.
0.10*	Voluntary motor action affected; hand and arm movements, walk, and speech clumsy.
0.20	Severe impairment. Staggering; loud, incoherent speech. Emotionally unstable. One hundred times greater risk of traffic accident.
0.30	Deeper areas of brain affected, causing confusion and stuporous.
0.40	When asleep, difficult to arouse. Incapable of voluntary action. Equivalent to surgical anesthesia.
0.50	Coma. Anesthesia of center controlling breathing and heartbeat. Death.

* For most states, blood alcohol content (BAC) of 0.10 is the indicator for driving while intoxicated.

Alcoholism, *Continued*

- Can increase the risk of diseases such as cancer of the brain, tongue, mouth, esophagus, larynx, liver, and bladder; cirrhosis of the liver and hepatitis; gastritis and brain damage when used heavily. It can also cause heart and blood pressure problems.
- Can lead to malnutrition
- Is known to cause birth defects

Emotional and Behavioral Effects of Alcohol

- May cause someone to do things they might not do otherwise, such as driving at dangerous speeds or other daredevil acts
- May result in anger, violent behavior, or depression which can intensify as more alcohol is consumed. Can result in suicide.
- May result in memory loss, the inability to concentrate, and problems in other intellectual functions
- Can make family life chaotic. The divorce rate is 7 times higher among alcoholics. Also, children of alcoholics often have emotional problems lasting into adulthood.
- Often results in decreased work attendance and performance as well as problems in dealing with employees and coworkers

Treatment

Treating alcoholism as an illness is important. Recovery requires lifelong changes. Types of treatment are:
- Self-help groups such as:
  - Alcoholics Anonymous (AA)
  - Rational Recovery (RR)
  - Women for Sobriety (WFS)
  - Men for Sobriety (MFS)

  (See "Places to Get Information & Help" under "Alcohol/Drug Abuse" on pages 374 and 375.)

- Alcohol treatment programs. Many types exist:
  - Outpatient treatment is held in hospitals, clinics, or other alcohol rehabilitation centers. It focuses on education and is often set up in a group format. Substance abuse counselors, psychologists, social workers, etc., staff this type of treatment, which generally lasts from 6–10 weeks.
  - Day treatment programs in which the person checks into a facility all day, but goes home at night. Individual and group therapy as well as education are provided. This type of treatment is suitable for persons with more severe problems than can be helped by outpatient programs. It is less costly than inpatient treatment.
  - Inpatient treatment is usually a 14–28-day stay in a hospital or other residential treatment facility. The alcoholic may need to go through detoxification. The focus of treatment is to rehabilitate the person to not use alcohol. This is done through education and individual and group therapy.
  - "Aftercare" eases the person back into the "real world" through individual counseling, group therapy, and support group meetings such as AA, after inpatient or outpatient treatment is finished. This can last one year. The person continues with individual and group therapy and support group meetings such as AA.
  - Psychotherapy, which can be individual, family, and/or group therapy
- Medications. One called Naltrexone, blocks the craving for alcohol and the pleasure of getting high. Another one, called Antabuse, causes physical reactions such as vomiting when drinking alcohol. Antabuse is rarely used.

16. Mental Health Conditions

177

Alcoholism, *Continued*

Questions to Ask:

{Note: "Counselor" in this section may also refer to self-help support groups such as Alcoholics Anonymous (AA).}

Have you had memory lapses or blackouts due to drinking? **YES**  **See Doctor OR See Counselor**

NO

Do you continue to drink even though you have health problems caused by alcohol? **YES** 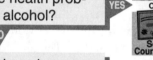 **See Doctor OR See Counselor**

NO

Do you get withdrawal symptoms such as headaches, chills, shakes, and a strong craving for alcohol, and, as a result, drink more to get rid of these symptoms? **YES** 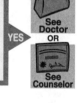 **See Doctor OR See Counselor**

NO

Do you take part in high-risk behaviors such as: unsafe sex in a nonmonogamous relationship or driving a boat or car or working with hazardous machinery when under the influence of alcohol? **YES**  **See Doctor OR See Counselor**

NO

Flowchart continued in next column

Has drinking caused trouble at home, at work, and/or with relationships with others? **YES**  **See Doctor OR See Counselor**

NO

Do you have to drink alcohol for any of the following reasons?
- To get through the day or unwind at the end of the day
- To cope with stressful life events
- To escape from ongoing problems

YES  **See Doctor OR See Counselor**

NO

Do you answer yes to 2 or more of the following questions?
- Have you ever tried to cut down on your drinking?
- Have you ever been annoyed by anybody criticizing your drinking?
- Have you ever felt guilty about your drinking?
- Have you ever had an eye-opener (drink) in the morning?

YES  **See Doctor OR See Counselor**

NO

 Use Self-Care

See Self-Care Tips on next page

Alcoholism, *Continued*

Self-Care Tips

Tips to Reduce the Risks Associated with Drinking:

- Know your limit and stick to it or don't drink any alcohol.

Know Your Limit[1]

Body Weight	# of Drinks[2] During a 2-Hour Period									
100 lbs.	1	2	3	4	5	6	7	8	9	10
120	1	2	3	4	5	6	7	8	9	10
140	1	2	3	4	5	6	7	8	9	10
160	1	2	3	4	5	6	7	8	9	10
180	1	2	3	4	5	6	7	8	9	10
200	1	2	3	4	5	6	7	8	9	10
220	1	2	3	4	5	6	7	8	9	10
240	1	2	3	4	5	6	7	8	9	10

Be Careful Driving BAC* to .05	Driving May Be Impaired BAC .05-.09[3]	Do Not Drive BAC .10 and up

[1] This chart provides averages only. Individuals may vary, and factors such as food in the stomach, medication, and fatigue can affect your tolerance.

[2] One drink is $1\frac{1}{4}$ oz. of 80-proof liquor, 12 oz. of beer, or 4 oz. of wine.

[3] The BAC percentages for impairment and intoxication vary from state to state.

* BAC = blood alcohol content

Developed by Techniques for Alcohol Management. Used with permission.

If you're in doubt about your ability to drive, play it safe. Don't drive!

- Drink slowly. You are apt to drink less.

- Pour less alcohol and more mixer in each drink.

- Alternate an alcoholic beverage with a non-alcoholic one.

- Eat when you drink. Food helps to slow alcohol absorption.

- Talk to persons who will listen to your feelings and concerns without putting you down. You will be less likely to turn to alcohol to "drown your sorrows."

- Find ways to calm yourself other than with alcohol. Examples include hobbies, relaxation exercises, physical activities, music, movies, etc.

- Realize that you are a role model for your children. They learn what they see. When you drink, do so responsibly.

- Don't mix drinking with driving, drugs, or operating machines. Doing so can be fatal.

- Don't rely on coffee or fresh air to make you sober. Even though you see these things done on TV, they won't make a person sober.

- Don't have any alcohol if you are pregnant.

- Contact your Employee Assistance Program (EAP) at work for information and other suggestions.

60 Anxiety

Anxiety is a feeling of dread, fear or distress over a real or imagined threat to your mental or physical well-being.

Symptoms

Symptoms of anxiety are both physical and psychological. They include:

- Rapid pulse and/or breathing rate
- Racing or pounding heart
- Dry mouth
- Sweating
- Trembling
- Shortness of breath
- Faintness
- Numbness/tingling of the hands, feet, or other body part
- Feeling a "lump in the throat"
- Stomach problems
- Insomnia

A certain amount of anxiety is normal. It can prompt you to study for a test. It can alert you to seek safety when you are in physical danger. Anxiety is not normal, though, when there is no apparent reason for it or when it overwhelms you and interferes with your day-to-day life.

Causes

Anxiety can be a symptom of medical conditions such as:

- A heart attack
- An overactive thyroid gland (hyperthyroidism)
- Low blood sugar (hypoglycemia)
- An excess of hormones made by the glands located above the kidneys called the adrenal glands (Cushing's syndrome)
- A side effect of some medications
- A withdrawal reaction from nicotine, alcohol, drugs or medicines such as sleeping pills

Anxiety can also be a symptom of a number of illnesses known as anxiety disorders. These include:

- Phobias (see page 203)
- Panic attacks and panic disorder (see page 200)
- Obsessive-Compulsive Disorder – An anxiety disorder where the sufferer has persistent, involuntary thoughts or images (obsessions) and engages in ritualistic acts such as washing their hands according to certain self-imposed rules (compulsions).
- Post-Traumatic Stress Disorder – A condition where a person reexperiences a traumatic past event like a wartime situation, hostage taking or rape. Symptoms include nightmares, flashbacks of the event, excessive alertness and emotional numbness to people and activities.

Anxiety, *Continued*

Treatment

When anxiety is mild and/or does not interfere with daily living, it can be dealt with using self-help. (See Self-Care Tips in this section on page 183.)

Treatment for anxiety includes:

- Treating any medical condition which causes the anxiety

- Medication. Examples include antianxiety medicines such as Xanax, and antidepressants such as Tofranil and Prozac. Another medicine, Tenormin, which is usually used for high blood pressure, has been shown to help persons with the anxiety that comes with stage fright.

- Psychological counseling

- Changing jobs or other life situations

- Self-help groups such as Agoraphobics in Motion (AIM). (See "Places to Get Information & Help" under "Anxiety/Phobias" on page 375.)

Anxiety disorders are some of the most common conditions people suffer with. They often respond to treatment.

Questions to Ask

Are any of these symptoms of a heart attack present with the anxiety?
- Chest pressure or pain (may spread to the arm, neck, or jaw)
- Chest discomfort with any of these problems: Shortness of breath or trouble breathing; nausea or vomiting; sweating; uneven heartbeat or pulse; or sense of doom

 YES **Get Emergency Care**

NO

Are these symptoms present with the anxiety?
- Excessive hair growth
- Round face and puffy eyes
- Skin changes – reddening, thinning, and stretch marks
- High blood pressure

YES **See Doctor**

 NO

Do you have these symptoms with the anxiety?
- Rapid heartbeat
- Hyperactivity
- Weight loss
- Muscle weakness, tremors
- Bulging eyes
- Feeling hot or warm all the time

YES 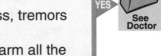 **See Doctor**

 NO

Flowchart continued on next page

Anxiety, *Continued*

Flowchart continued

If you have been through or seen a traumatic event, do you suffer from any of these problems?
- Nightmares, night terrors, and/or flashbacks of the event
- Lack of concentration, poor memory, sleep problems
- Feelings of guilt for surviving the event
- Startled easily by loud noises or anything that reminds you of the event
- Lack of interest in the activities and people you once enjoyed

YES → 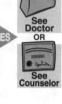 See Doctor OR See Counselor

NO ↓

Do you have anxiety only under the following conditions?
- When you don't eat or when you do too much physically, especially if you are diabetic
- During the 2 weeks before your menstrual period if you are a woman

YES → Call Doctor

NO ↓

Does the anxiety come only after 1 or both of the following?
- Taking an over-the-counter (OTC) or prescription medicine
- Withdrawing from medication, nicotine, alcohol, or drugs

YES → Call Doctor

NO ↓

Flowchart continued in next column

Have you had any of these problems?
- Panic attacks followed for 1 month by fears of getting another one
- Worry about what would happen with another panic attack, or
- A change in what you do related to panic attacks such as avoiding places, not being able to leave the house or be left alone

YES → Call Doctor OR Call Counselor

NO ↓

Do any of the following keep you from doing your daily activities?
- Checking something over and over again, such as seeing if you've locked the door even though it is locked
- Repeated, unwanted thoughts such as worrying you could harm someone
- Repeated, senseless acts such as washing your hands over and over again

YES → Call Doctor OR Call Counselor

NO ↓

Flowchart continued on next page

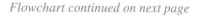

16. Mental Health Conditions

Anxiety, *Continued*

Flowchart continued

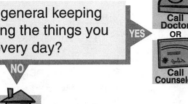

Is anxiety in general keeping you from doing the things you need to do every day?

YES → Call Doctor OR Call Counselor

NO → Use Self-Care

Self-Care Tips

- Look for the cause of the stress that results in anxiety and deal with it through the use of stress management techniques. (See "Self-Care Tips" under "Stress" on pages 212 and 213.)

- Lessen your exposure to things that cause you distress.

- Talk about your fears and anxieties with someone you trust such as a friend, spouse, teacher, etc.

- Eat healthy and at regular times. Don't skip meals.

- If you are prone to low blood sugar episodes, eat 5–6 small meals per day instead of 3 larger ones. Avoid sweets on a regular basis, but carry a quick source of sugar with you at all times, such as a small can of orange juice. This will give you a quick source of sugar in the event that you do get a low blood sugar reaction.

- Exercise regularly.

- Limit or avoid caffeine intake after noon. Caffeine can worsen anxiety and lead to poor sleeping patterns. If you must drink coffee, switch to decaffeinated. Also use decaffeinated teas, colas, and other sodas. Limit your intake of chocolate.

- Avoid nicotine and alcohol.

- Avoid medicines that have a stimulating effect, which can cause anxietylike symptoms. Examples are over-the-counter diet pills and pills to keep you awake.

- Do some form of relaxation exercise daily. Examples include biofeedback, deep muscle relaxation, meditation, and deep breathing exercises.

- Don't "bite off more than you can chew." Plan your schedule for what you can handle both physically and mentally.

- Rehearse for events that are coming up about which you have felt anxious in the past or think will cause anxiety. Imagine yourself feeling calm and in control during the event several times before it really occurs.

- Be prepared to deal with symptoms of anxiety if you think they will happen. For example, if you have hyperventilated in the past, carry a paper bag with you. If you do hyperventilate, cover your mouth and nose with the paper bag. Breathe into the paper bag slowly and re-breathe the air. Do this in and out at least 10 times. Remove the bag and breathe normally a few minutes. Repeat breathing in and out of the paper bag as needed.

- Help others. The positive feelings from this can help you overcome or forget about your anxiety.

16. Mental Health Conditions

183

61 Codependency

"Codependency" is used to describe the condition where a person becomes the "caretaker" of an addicted or troubled individual. The individual can be addicted to alcohol, drugs, or gambling. Or, he or she can be troubled by a physical or emotional illness. Codependents can be this individual's spouse, lover, child, parent, sibling, coworker, or friend.

Below are typical roles that codependents play:

- Enabler – allows the person to continue his or her self-destructive or troubled behavior, or denies that the person has a problem

- Rescuer – makes excuses for the person's behavior, or saves the person from unpleasant situations, i.e. putting an alcoholic to bed after he/she passes out

- Caretaker – takes care of all household and financial chores which hold the family together

- Joiner – rationalizes that the person's behavior is normal by simply allowing it to take place or by taking part in the same behavior as the addicted or troubled individual

- Hero – becomes the "super person" to preserve the family image

- Complainer – blames the person and makes him or her the scapegoat for all problems

- Adjuster – withdraws from the family and acts like he/she doesn't care

Most codependents do not realize they have a codependency problem. They focus more energy on another's actions and needs than on their own. They think they are actually helping the troubled person, but they are not.

Questions to Ask

Do you do 3 or more of the following?
- Think more about another person's behavior and problems than about your own life
- Feel anxious about the addicted or troubled persons behavior and constantly check on them to try to catch them in their bad behavior
- Worry that if you stop trying to control the other person, that he or she will fall apart
- Blame yourself for this person's problems
- Cover up or "rescue" this person when they are caught in a lie or other embarrassing situation related to their addiction or other problem
- Deny that this person has a "real" problem with drugs, alcohol, etc., and become angry and/or defensive when others suggest there is an addiction or other substance abuse problem

YES
See Counselor

NO
Use Self-Care

See Self-Care Tips on next page

Codependency, *Continued*

{*Note:* You may not be truly codependent, but you should become aware of how your behavior may be enabling an addicted or troubled individual.}

Self-Care Tips

Most codependents are not in touch with their codependency and may need help to see it. The following self-help tips are general suggestions. For many people, these are not easy to do without the help of a counselor.

■ Read books on codependency. You can find these in the library and bookstores. You may find you identify with what you read and gain understanding.

■ Focus on these three C's:

- You did not **cause** the other person's problem.

- You can't **control** the other person.

- You can't **cure** the problem.

■ Don't lie, make excuses, or cover up for the abuser's drinking, drug, or other problem. Admit to yourself that this way of living is not normal and that the abuser or troubled person has a real problem and needs professional help.

■ Refuse to come to the person's aid. Every time you bail the abuser out of trouble, you reinforce their helplessness and your hopelessness.

■ If you or your children are being physically, verbally, or sexually abused, do not allow it to continue. There are shelters for victims of domestic violence. (See "Places to Get Information & Help" under "Domestic Violence" on page 375.)

■ Know that there are many support groups which help codependents. Examples are self-help groups for family and friends of substance abusers such as Al-Anon, Alateen, and Children of Alcoholics Foundation (COAF). (See "Places to Get Information & Help" under "Alcohol/Drug Abuse" on pages 374 and 375.) Other self-help and support groups are offered through community health education programs.

■ Continue with your normal family routines. For example, include the drinker when he/she is sober.

■ Focus on your own feelings, desires, and needs. Negative thoughts may be brewing just below the surface. It's important to vent them in healthy ways. Begin to do what is good for your own well-being.

■ Allow children to express their feelings openly. Show them how by expressing your own feelings.

■ Set limits on what you will and won't do. Be firm and stick to these limits. It's natural to want to take care of those you love, but in this case, it doesn't help.

■ Engage in new experiences and interests. Find diversion from your loved one's problem.

■ Take responsibility for yourself and others in the family to live a better life whether your loved one recovers or not.

16. Mental Health Conditions

185

62 Depression

Depression is marked by sadness, hopelessness, helplessness, pessimism, and a loss of interest in life. Symptoms of depression include long-lasting crying spells, fatigue, loss of interest or pleasure in ordinary activities including sex, changes in eating and sleeping patterns, lack of concentration, and thoughts of suicide or death.

Causes

A lot of things can lead to depression:

- Life changes such as the birth of a baby, divorce, retirement, loss of a job, or death of a loved one. (See "Grief/Bereavement" on page 198.)

- Worrying about financial problems

- Chronic or acute medical conditions

- Abuse of alcohol, drugs, and some medications

- Lack of natural, unfiltered sunlight between late fall and spring in some sensitive people. This is called Seasonal Affective Disorder (SAD). It only strikes people that are prone to this disorder.

- A side effect of medicines such as some to treat high blood pressure

- Holiday "blues"

Depression can, however, be a disease in and of itself.

Treatment

Whatever the cause, depression can be treated. Treatment includes medication such as antidepressants, psychotherapy, and other therapies specific to the cause of the depression, such as exposure to bright light (similar to sunlight) for depression that results from SAD.

Questions to Ask

Have you just tried to commit suicide or are you planning ways to commit suicide? YES → **Get Emergency Care**

NO

Has there been a lot less interest or pleasure in almost all activities most of the day, nearly every day for at least 2 weeks? Or, have you been in a depressed mood most of the day nearly every day and have you had any of the following for at least 2 weeks?
- Feeling slowed down or restless and unable to sit still
- Feeling worthless or guilty
- Changes in appetite or weight loss or gain
- Thoughts of death or suicide
- Problems concentrating, thinking, remembering, or making decisions
- Trouble sleeping or sleeping too much
- Loss of energy or feeling tired all the time
- Headaches
- Aches and pains
- Digestive problems
- Sexual problems
- Feelings of pessimism or hopelessness
- Worried or anxious feeling

YES →  **See Doctor** OR **See Counselor**

 NO

Flowchart continued on next page

Depression, *Continued*

Flowchart continued

Has depression interfered with daily activities for more than 2 weeks? Have you withdrawn from normal activities during this time? **YES** 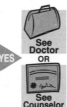 See Doctor OR See Counselor

NO

Has the depression occurred as the result of any of the following?
• A medical problem
• Taking over-the-counter or prescription medicine
• Abusing alcohol or drugs **YES** Call Doctor

NO

Does the depression come with dark, cloudy weather or winter months and does it lift when spring comes? **YES** Call Doctor

NO

Are you feeling depressed now and do any of the following apply?
• You have been depressed before and not gotten treatment.
• You have been treated for depression in the past and it has returned.
• You have taken medication for depression in the past. **YES**  Call Doctor OR Call Counselor

NO

Flowchart continued in next column

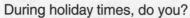

During holiday times, do you?
• Withdraw from family and friends?
• Dwell on past holidays to the point that it interferes with your present life? **YES** 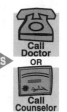 Call Doctor OR Call Counselor

NO

 Use Self-Care

Self-Care Tips

To Overcome Mild, Situational Depression:

■ Be with positive people. They'll lift your morale.

■ Do something to help someone else. This will focus your attention away from yourself.

■ Get some physical exercise every day. Walk, jog, bike, play tennis, etc.

■ Do something different. Walk or drive to a new place. Try a new restaurant.

■ Take a vacation doing something you enjoy.

■ Tackle a new project or do something that lets you express yourself, such as writing or painting.

■ Relax. Listen to soft music, take a warm bath or shower. Do relaxation exercises.

■ Talk to someone who will let you express the tensions and frustrations you are feeling.

■ Avoid drugs and alcohol. These can cause or worsen depression.

{*Note:* For information on depression see "Places to Get Information & Help" under "Depression" on page 375.}

63 Drug Dependence & Abuse

Drug dependence and abuse both involve the misuse of one or more drugs. These can be prescription medicines and/or illicit drugs.

Drug dependence is addiction. A person keeps using a drug even though doing so results in problems that affect the person's mind, physical health, and/or behaviors. Features of drug dependence include:

- Cravings for the drug
- Need for increased amounts of the drug to get the desired effect
- Withdrawal symptoms

Drug abuse is the repeated use of a drug that results in distress and daily living problems. Examples are:

- Failure to fulfill work, school, or home obligations
- Legal problems such as getting arrested for disorderly conduct
- Physical harm that results from things such as a car accident
- Relationship problems such as arguments or physical fights

A person can abuse a drug without becoming addicted to it. Addicts, however, usually have distress and the daily problems that result from drug abuse.

See chart below for facts on different drugs.

Drug Facts

Type of Drug—Common Names	Possible Effects	Dangers of Use/Abuse
Cocaine—Blow, crack, crank, "C," coke, nose candy, rock, white girl	Increased alertness and energy, euphoria (followed by depression), increased pulse rate and blood pressure, decreased appetite, insomnia, irritability, paranoia	Severe depression, convulsions, heart attack, lung damage, hallucinations, coma, brain damage, risk of infection (hepatitis, AIDS) from using contaminated needles, death
Depressants—Alcohol (see "Alcoholism" on page 176), barbiturates, sedatives, tranquilizers, downers, ludes, reds, yellow jackets	Drowsiness, slurred speech, drunkenness, memory loss, sudden mood shifts, depression, lack of coordination	Shallow breathing, dilated pupils, clammy skin, weak and rapid pulse, coma, possible death

Chart continued on next page

16. Mental Health Conditions

Drug Dependence & Abuse, *Continued*

Drug Facts

Type of Drug— Common Names	Possible Effects	Dangers of Use/Abuse
Hallucinogens— Acid, LSD, PCP (angel dust), mescaline, designer drugs: DMT, MDA, STP, MMDA, MDMA, ecstasy, peyote	Alter mood and perception of time and space, delusions, hallucinations. Can "see sounds" and "hear colors." Rapid mood swings. Feelings of loss of control, helplessness, panic. Elevation in body temperature, heartbeat, and breathing. Blurred vision, tremors, lack of coordination	Brain damage, behavior can be unpredictable, unstable (violent with PCP). Can have flashbacks and re-experience symptoms of past hallucinogen use even though not taking the drug at the present time. Psychosis (unconsciousness, seizure, coma possible with PCP)
Inhalants— Solvents such as gasoline, kerosene, lighter fluid, nail polish remover; aerosols such as hair sprays, vegetable cooking sprays; anesthetics such as ether, chloroform, nitrous oxide (laughing gas), spray paints, especially gold and silver. {*Note:* These substances are known as inhalants when the vapors from them are used for the purpose of getting high.}	Slow heart rate, breathing and brain activity. Headaches, dizziness, nausea, lack of coordination, slurred speech, blurred vision. Euphoria, increased energy, bloodshot eyes, nosebleed	Suffocation, heart failure, unconsciousness, seizures, brain damage, possible death
Marijuana— Pot, grass, reefer, herb, jay, joint, smoke, weed and AMP (marijuana mixed with formaldehyde)	Euphoria, relaxes inhibitions, increases appetite, dry mouth	Feelings of panic, impaired short term memory, decreased ability to concentrate, fatigue, paranoia, possible psychosis

Chart continued on next page

16. Mental Health Conditions

Drug Dependence & Abuse, *Continued*

Drug Facts

Type of Drug— Common Names	Possible Effects	Dangers of Use/Abuse
Narcotics— Heroin (dope, horse, smack, brown sugar, schoolboy), codeine (also in prescription medicine such as Tylenol with codeine, Robitussin AC), opium (Dovers powder, paregoric), morphine, methadone, Darvon, Percodan, Demerol	Slowed breathing, heart rate and brain activity. Increase in the body's tolerance to pain. Constipation, euphoria, relaxation, sense of peace. Impaired memory and/or attention span, slurred speech	Lethargy, weight loss. Risk of infection (hepatitis, AIDS) from using contaminated needles. Impaired judgement in social and/or work functioning. Convulsions, coma, possible death
Stimulants— Speed, uppers, crank, amphetamines	Increased alertness, blood pressure, pulse rate. Elevates mood	Fatigue, confusion, agitation, severe anxiety, appetite, and/or weight loss. Hallucinations, convulsions, possible death

Treatment

Using drugs can cause physical and emotional problems. Drug use and abuse affects the users and their families, friends, and coworkers. It is also costly, not only to the drug abusers and their families, but to their employers as well. If you are drug-dependent or abusing drugs, get help. You can get help through:

- Your doctor
- Your Employee Assistance Program (EAP) at work
- A drug treatment clinic
- A mental health center or provider
- Self-help groups such as Narcotics Anonymous (NA). (See "Places to Get Information & Help" under "Alcohol/Drug Abuse" on pages 374 and 375.)

The treatment for drug dependence and abuse varies, and depends on the drug(s) being used and the person's needs. Types of treatment include:

- Emergency medical care. This may be needed for drug overdoses or for violent or out-of-control behaviors.

- Medical treatment for physical problems due to the use of a drug(s) and/or for proper care and supervision from drug withdrawal. Medical treatment can be given in outpatient or inpatient settings. The goal for treatment is to get to the point where all mood-altering chemicals are not used.

Drug Dependence & Abuse, *Continued*

Medical treatment involves the use of a number of things. These include:

- An initial and ongoing evaluation of the person's physical, mental, and social condition

- Diagnostic and lab tests

- "Detoxifying" the person of the abused substance. In many cases, the only thing needed for "detox" is time. In others, such as heroin addiction, another drug (in this case, methadone) is given to replace the heroin so as to minimize withdrawal effects. The amount of methadone is slowly reduced until the person no longer needs it. Some persons may need to be on methadone for a long time.

- Counseling. This can be individual, family, and/or group therapy. Counseling helps the drug addict or abuser identify the needs for drug use and helps the person set up life-coping skills. Counseling can be provided on an outpatient basis or in inpatient settings.

- Medical nutrition therapy from a registered dietitian if the drug abuse has resulted in nutrient deficiencies.

- Support groups such as Narcotics Anonymous (NA), Cocaine Anonymous (CA) and Alcoholics Anonymous (AA). (See "Places to Get Information & Help" under "Alcohol/Drug Abuse" on pages 374 and 375.)

Questions to Ask

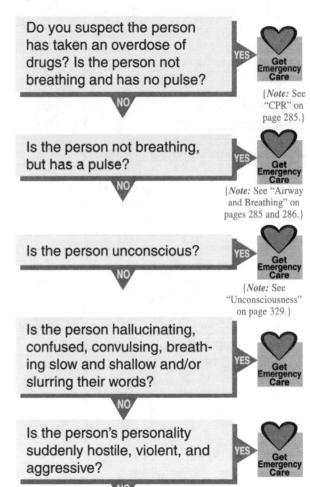

Do you suspect the person has taken an overdose of drugs? Is the person not breathing and has no pulse? — YES — Get Emergency Care

{*Note:* See "CPR" on page 285.}

Is the person not breathing, but has a pulse? — YES — Get Emergency Care

{*Note:* See "Airway and Breathing" on pages 285 and 286.}

Is the person unconscious? — YES — Get Emergency Care

{*Note:* See "Unconsciousness" on page 329.}

Is the person hallucinating, confused, convulsing, breathing slow and shallow and/or slurring their words? — YES — Get Emergency Care

Is the person's personality suddenly hostile, violent, and aggressive? — YES — Get Emergency Care

{*Note:* Use caution. Protect yourself. Do not turn your back to the victim or move suddenly in front of him or her. If you can, see that the victim does not harm you or himself/herself. Remember, the victim is under the influence of a drug. Call the police to assist you if you cannot handle the situation.}

Flowchart continued on next page

16. Mental Health Conditions

Drug Dependence & Abuse, *Continued*

Flowchart continued

Have 3 or more of the following applied to you in the last 12 months due to drug use?

• You need more of a drug to get intoxicated or reach a desired effect.

• You get withdrawal symptoms if you stop taking or take less of the drug. Examples of withdrawal symptoms include:
- Shaking   - Irritability
- Sleeplessness - Depression
- Headaches - Paranoia
- Hallucinations - Anxiety

• You have to take the drug or one similar to it to relieve or avoid withdrawal symptoms.

• You take the drug in larger amounts often or over a longer period of time than you intended.

• You have not been able to cut down or control your use of a drug even though you want to.

• You spend a lot of time doing things necessary to get the drug, use the drug, or re-cover from its effects.

• You give up important social, work or leisure activities or do them less often so you can use the drug.

• You continue to take the drug even though you know it results in physical or psycho-logical problems or makes these problems worse.

YES See Counselor

NO

Flowchart continued in next column

Have you or someone else accidentally taken more than the prescribed dose of a prescription or over-the-counter medicine?

YES Call Doctor

NO

{*Note:* If physician is not available, call Poison Control Center. Follow instructions given.}

Has 1 or more of the following taken place in the last 12 months due to drug use?

• Failure to fulfill your major duties at work, school, or home

• Taking part in situations that could cause physical harm while under the influence of a drug, such as driving or operating a machine

• Legal problems, such as getting arrested for drunk driving or disorderly conduct

• Relationship problems due to the effects of the drug such as physical fights or arguments with others

YES Call Counselor

NO

Use Self-Care

See Self-Care Tips on next page

16. Mental Health Conditions

Drug Dependence & Abuse, *Continued*

Self-Care Tips

To Prevent Dependence on Prescription Medication:

- Use the medication only as prescribed.

- Discuss the effects of taking more than one medicine and/or taking medicine with alcohol with your physician and pharmacist. Have your prescriptions filled at the same pharmacy. The pharmacist can check for harmful interactions with all the medicines you take.

- Don't increase the dosage or take it more often than your physician tells you to. Consult your physician first.

- Don't use medicine prescribed for someone else.

- Ask your physician about the risks of addiction when he or she prescribes medicines, especially sleeping pills, tranquilizers, and strong pain relievers. Find out how long you will need to take the medicine. Ask if there are ways to treat your problem without medicine.

- Find out how to gradually reduce the usage of a medicine to avoid harmful side effects.

Ways to Lower the Chances of Letting Drugs Affect Your Life or Someone Else's Life:

- Learn as much as you can about the harmful effects of drugs.

- Contact your Employee Assistance Program (EAP) person at work for information and suggestions.

- Change your lifestyle. Try to stay out of situations where drugs are available.

- If your friends insist that you take drugs in order to socialize with them, make it clear that you are serious about stopping.

- Attend self-help group meetings for drug users. Examples include Narcotics Anonymous (NA) and Cocaine Anonymous (CA). (See "Places to Get Information & Help" under "Alcohol/Drug Abuse" on pages 374 and 375.)

- Talk to persons who will listen to your feelings and concerns without judging you. You will be less likely to turn to drugs to "drown your sorrows."

- Listen to calm music.

- Do deep breathing exercises.

- Do things that you know and do well in order to feel confident. For example, learn and practice martial arts, sew, paint, take part in volunteer work.

- Get regular vigorous exercise such as swimming, jogging, or walking.

- Learn something new. Take a night school course or community education class that you are interested in.

- Realize that you are a role model for your children. They learn what they see. When you take prescription drugs, do so responsibly.

- Don't mix drugs with alcohol, driving, or operating machines. These combinations can be fatal.

16. Mental Health Conditions

64 Eating Disorders (Anorexia Nervosa & Bulimia)

Anorexia nervosa and bulimia are two kinds of eating disorders. Anorexia nervosa is a form of self-starvation. Bulimia is eating large amounts of foods (binging) and then forcing oneself to throw up or using laxatives and water pills to get rid of what was overeaten (purging). These eating disorders are both a form of self-abuse.

Symptoms

Anorexia nervosa and bulimia seem like opposite conditions, but they share these common traits:

- Fear of overeating and gaining weight
- Depression
- Low self-esteem, poor body image
- Self-destructive outlook, self-punishment for some imaginary wrong
- Disturbed family relationships
- Increased rate of illness due to low weight, frequent weight gain/loss and/or poor nutrition
- Abnormal preoccupation with food and feeling out of control

Anorexia Nervosa Sufferers:

- Are mostly female, and/or preteen, teenage or college age
- Tend to place too much emphasis on body image and perfection
- May feel the need to be perfect to gain parental attention.
- Have marked physical effects – loss of head hair, slowed heart rate, low blood pressure, absence of menstrual periods

- Tend to experience more extreme depression than bulimics
- Develop osteoporosis in later life due to lack of calcium and decreased production of estrogen if menstruation stops. Excessive exercise can contribute to this as well.
- May have severe damage to heart and vital organs due to an excessive loss of weight and to a mineral imbalance from vomiting and/or poor nutrition

Approximately 1% of American females have anorexia.

Bulimia Sufferers:

- Can be overweight, underweight, or normal weight
- Are mostly female and older teen or young adult
- Binge eat and then vomit (purge) and/or take laxatives or water pills (diuretics) to "undo" the binge
- Have severe health problems that come from the binge-purge cycle of eating. These include stomach lining damage, irregular heartbeat, kidney damage from low potassium levels, and damage to tooth enamel from vomiting.
- Repress anger because they can't express emotions in an assertive way. They fear upsetting important people in their lives.

Eating Disorders (Anorexia Nervosa & Bulimia), *Continued*

Approximately 2% of college students and 1% of U.S. women overall have bulimia. Bulimia can follow anorexia and vice versa.

There is no one cause for these eating disorders. There are many factors. They include:

- A possible genetic link
- Metabolic and biochemical problems or abnormalities
- Pressure from society to be thin
- Personal or family pressures
- Fear of entering puberty or becoming sexually active

Treatment

Treatment for anorexia and/or bulimia includes:

- Medical diagnosis and care – the earlier, the better
- Psychotherapy – individual, family, and/or group
- Behavior therapy
- Medication – antidepressant medicine is sometimes used.
- Medical nutrition therapy
- Support group participation
- Outpatient treatment programs
- Hospitalization – if your weight loss makes you 25% or more below normal weight and/or has affected vital functions

Treatment can vary in length as well as method. It can take from a few months to several years.

Questions to Ask

Have you lost a significant amount of weight by dieting and exercising on purpose (not due to any known illness) and do you have any of these problems?
- An intense fear of gaining weight or of getting fat
- You see yourself as fat even though you are at normal weight or are underweight.
- You continue to diet and exercise excessively even though you have reached your weight goal.

YES → See Doctor

 NO

Are you aware that your eating pattern is not normal and are you afraid that you will not be able to stop binge eating? Are you depressed after binging on food?

YES → See Doctor

 NO

Flowchart continued on next page

16. Mental Health Conditions

Eating Disorders (Anorexia Nervosa & Bulimia), *Continued*

Flowchart continued

Do you have a combination of these problems along with abnormal eating habits?
- Irregular heartbeat
- Slow pulse, low blood pressure
- Rapid tooth decay
- Low body temperature, cold hands and feet
- Thin hair (or hair loss) on the head, babylike hair on the body (lanugo)
- Dry skin, fingernails that split, peel, or crack
- Problems with digestion, bloating, constipation
- Three or more missed periods (in a row), delayed onset of menstruation, infertility
- Periods of depression and lethargy, euphoria and/or hyperactivity
- Tiredness, weakness, muscle cramps, tremors
- Lack of concentration

YES See Doctor

NO

Do you do one or both of the following?
- Hoard food
- Leave the table right after meals to "go to the bathroom" to induce vomiting and/or spend long periods of time in the bathroom from taking laxatives and/or water pills

YES See Doctor

NO

Flowchart continued in next column

Do you have recurrent episodes when you eat a large amount of food at a very fast pace <u>and</u> do at least 3 of the following?
- Eat high-calorie, easily eaten foods during a binge
- Binge eat with no one watching
- Stop the binge eating when you get stomach pain, go to sleep, interact socially, or induce vomiting
- Attempt to lose weight over and over with severe diets, self-induced vomiting, and/or laxatives or water pills
- Have weight changes of more than 10 pounds due to binging and fasting

YES See Doctor

NO

If you have answered NO to all of the above questions you are probably not suffering from anorexia nervosa and/or bulimia. If you are not sure, though, see a counselor for a professional assessment.

{*Note:* Eating disorders are too complex and physically harmful to be treated with self-care alone. Experts agree that experienced professionals should treat people who have eating disorders. See "Places to Get Information & Help" under "Eating Disorders" on page 375.}

See Prevention Tips on next page

Eating Disorders (Anorexia Nervosa & Bulimia), *Continued*

Prevention

The following tips may help prevent an eating disorder:

■ Accept yourself and your body. You don't need to be or look like anyone else. Spend time with people who accept you as you are, not people who focus on "thinness."

■ Eat nutritious foods. Focus on complex carbohydrates (whole grains, beans, etc.), fresh fruits and vegetables, low-fat dairy foods, and low-fat meats.

■ Eat at regular times during the day. Don't skip meals. If you do, you are more likely to binge when you eat.

■ Avoid white flour, sugar, and "junk" foods high in calories, such as cakes, cookies or pastry, which have fat and sugar. Bulimics tend to binge on junk food. The more they eat, the more they want.

■ Get regular moderate exercise. If you find that you are exercising excessively, make an effort to get involved in nonexercise activities with friends and family.

■ Find success in things that you do. Your work, hobbies, and volunteer activities will promote self-esteem.

■ Learn as much as you can about eating disorders from books and organizations that deal with them.

■ Parents who want to help daughters avoid eating disorders should promote a balance between their daughters' competing needs for both independence and family involvement.

16. Mental Health Conditions

197

65 Grief/Bereavement

Grief is a deep sadness or sorrow that results from a loss. The loss can be from something big or small. It can be from something positive or negative.

Causes

Examples of things that cause grief include changes in:

- A job (new or lost job, a promotion or demotion, or retirement)
- Relationships (getting separated or divorced or having a child leave home)
- Health (illness or injury)
- Life matters (death of a family member or friend, loss of property or moving to a new place)

Bereavement is a process of grieving most often linked with the death of a loved one. There are many factors that shape our response to a loss such as death. These factors include:

- Age
- Health
- How sudden the loss was
- Cultural background
- Religious beliefs
- Financial security
- Social network
- History of other losses or traumatic events

Each of these factors can add to or reduce the pain of grieving. Trying to deny grief or avoid it only seems to create more serious problems later on. To come through the process in a healthy way, it is best to understand what coping with loss is all about.

Stages of Grief

Before a griever can feel "whole" or healed, they generally go through four stages:

1. Shock. The person feels dazed or numb.

2. Denial and Searching. The person:
   - Is in a state of disbelief
   - Asks questions such as "Why did this happen?" Or "Why didn't I prevent this?"
   - Looks for ways to keep their loved one or loss with them
   - Thinks he or she sees or hears the deceased person
   - Just begins to feel the reality of the event

3. Suffering and Disorganization. The person:
   - Has feelings such as guilt, depression, anxiety, loneliness, fear, hostility
   - May place blame on everyone and everything, including themselves
   - May get physical symptoms such as headaches, stomachaches, constant fatigue, shortness of breath
   - Withdraws from routine and social contacts

4. Recovery and Acceptance. The person:
   - Begins to look at the future instead of focusing on the past
   - Adjusts to the reality of the loss
   - Develops new relationships
   - Develops a positive attitude

The normal period of grieving the loss of a loved one lasts from 1 to 3 years, but could take longer.

Grief/Bereavement, *Continued*

Questions to Ask

Have you just tried to commit suicide or are you planning ways to commit suicide? **YES**
Get Emergency Care

NO

Are you thinking about committing suicide? **YES**
See Doctor OR See Counselor

NO

Are you abusing medication and/or alcohol to make yourself feel better? Do you need these to cope or "numb" your pain? **YES**
See Doctor OR See Counselor

NO

Do you have one or more of these problems due to grief?
- Extreme stress on your marriage and/or your children
- Not able to cope day-to-day
- Ongoing problems such as insomnia, excessive crying, depression, feelings of guilt, eating too much or too little food

YES
See Doctor OR See Counselor

NO

Flowchart continued in next column

Have you refused to sort through the deceased's belongings after a significant time? **YES**
See Counselor

NO

Use Self-Care

Self-Care Tips

- Eat regular meals.

- Get regular physical exercise such as walking.

- Allow friends and family to assist you. Tell them how you really feel. Don't hold your feelings inside. Visit them, especially during the holidays, if you would otherwise be alone. Traveling during the holidays may also be helpful. It is also important to reminisce. Being reminded of the past can be essential to the process of coming to grips with a loss.

- Try not to make major life changes such as moving during the first year of grieving.

- Join a support group for the bereaved if someone close to you has died. People and places to contact include your EAP representative, churches or synagogues, funeral homes, and hospice centers.

- Contact social agencies such as the American Association for Retired Persons (AARP) and local mental health centers. (See "Places to Get Information & Help" under "Grief" on page 376 and under "Senior Citizen Health" on page 377.)

16. Mental Health Conditions

Panic Attacks

A panic attack is a brief period of acute anxiety that comes on all of a sudden. It occurs when there is no real danger. It comes without warning. A panic attack lasts only a few minutes, but seems to last for hours.

Symptoms

Four or more of the following symptoms come with a panic attack:

- Shortness of breath or smothering sensations
- Sweating
- Choking feeling
- Racing heart rate or palpitations
- Chest pain or discomfort
- Feeling dizzy, faint, or light-headed
- Trembling or shaking
- Nausea or abdominal distress
- Hot flashes or chills
- Numbness, tingling in the hands or feet
- Feelings of unreality or being detached from oneself
- Fear of going crazy or losing control
- Fear of dying

A person having a panic attack may rush to an emergency room because they think they really are having a heart attack or feel like they are going to die.

Persons who have repeated panic attacks begin to avoid situations they associate with past attacks. For example, if the panic attack took place in a grocery store and the person had to leave the store to get home to feel safe, the person avoids future trips to the grocery store. This can lead to a phobia called agoraphobia. (See "Phobias" on page 203.)

A person who has 4 or more panic attacks in any 4 week period could have panic disorder. The disorder can also be present if the person has less than 4 panic attacks in 4 weeks, but is afraid of having another panic attack.

Panic attack symptoms can be symptoms of many medical conditions. These include heart attack and low blood sugar. The symptoms can also be a side effect of drug abuse or some medications. It is important, then, to rule out any other medical reasons for panic attack symptoms to know what the real problem is. Most persons who have panic disorder consult with their doctor 10 or more times before their condition is accurately diagnosed.

Treatment

Treatment for panic disorder includes:

- Medication. Certain antidepressants and anti-anxiety medicines are used.
- Therapy. One type helps the person "reshape" the way they think to avoid panic attacks. Another type uses relaxation methods and a gradual exposure to situations they have avoided due to fear of another panic attack.
- Support groups. These provide understanding and positive feedback to the sufferer.

16. Mental Health Conditions

Panic Attacks, *Continued*

Questions to Ask

Do all of these apply to you?
- You have been to your doctor more than once with symptoms like those of a heart attack such as chest pain, irregular heartbeat, and shortness of breath.
- You've been told that your heart and physical health are fine from a thorough examination and proper testing.
- You continue to have panic attack symptoms.

YES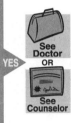
See Doctor OR See Counselor

NO

Do you have recurrent panic attacks that come when you don't expect them and have 1 or more of these problems?
- Continued concern about having more attacks
- Worry about what will happen as the result of a panic attack such as having a heart attack, losing control, or "going crazy"
- A noted change in things you normally do because of past panic attacks

YES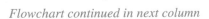
See Counselor

NO

Flowchart continued in next column

Do you avoid certain situations or places because they make you feel anxious and you think they will put you in danger?

YES
See Counselor

NO

Do you use alcohol or drugs to help you deal with situations that provoke the thought of another panic attack?

YES
Soo Counselor

NO

Use Self-Care

Self-Care Tips

These can help you or someone else.

{*Note:* Many of these tips are used in the context of therapy first before the person can do them on their own.}

Ways to Deal with Panic that has Limited Symptoms and Duration:

- Talk over the source of your anxiety with family, friends, and clergy. If this is not enough, you may need the help of a professional counselor.

- Face the fear. Accept it. Don't fight it. (This may need external help.)

- Remind yourself you are in no real danger.

- Try to imagine that you are "floating" on water.

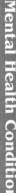
16. Mental Health Conditions

Panic Attacks, *Continued*

■ Let time pass. Try to think ahead to what tasks you need to do when the panic will be gone.

■ Keep things with you that will provide comfort and a sense of control in case another panic attack occurs. Examples:

- Keep a paper bag handy if you think you might hyperventilate (overbreathe). Breathe into the paper bag slowly and rebreathe the air. Do this in and out at least 10 times. Remove the bag and breathe normally a few minutes. Repeat breathing in and out of the paper bag as needed.

- Keep the name and phone number of a person to call in case of an emergency.

■ Do one or more mental "stress rehearsals." Imagine yourself feeling calm and handling the situation well.

■ Minimize your exposure to things that cause you distress.

■ Prepare for stressful situations. For example, if you need to give a group talk or presentation:

- Have materials you will need ready ahead of time. Make sure you have the equipment, such as slides and a slide projector. Check to see that they are in working order.

- Write an outline and key points on note cards, if necessary.

- Anticipate problems that could occur and prepare to address them ahead of time.

- Rehearse what you will do and say.

■ Learn and practice relaxation techniques such as:

- Deep breathing exercises

- Tensing and relaxing muscles

- Yoga

- Self-hypnosis

■ Limit caffeine.

{*Note:* see "Places to Get Information & Help" under "Anxiety/Phobias" on page 375.}

Phobias

A phobia is an irrational fear of a specific situation, activity, or object. The phobia compels the sufferer to avoid whatever is feared because with it comes a number of troubling symptoms such as:

- Anxiety
- Rapid heartbeat
- Sweating
- Hot or cold flashes
- Choking, smothering feelings
- Shaking
- Dizziness, faintness
- The need to flee the situation
- Panic attack, sometimes. (See "Panic Attacks" on page 200.)

Children may express their anxiety by:

- Crying
- Clinging
- Tantrums
- Freezing in place

Types of Phobias

- **Specific Phobias.** These are sometimes called simple phobias. The irrational fear is of specific objects such as snakes, dogs, closed spaces, or heights. (See box in next column for some common phobias.)

Fear of:	Known as
Heights	Acrophobia
Spiders	Arachnophobia
Thunder	Asterophobia
Lightning	Ceraunophobia
Enclosed spaces	Claustrophobia
Dirt, Germs	Mysophobia
Snakes	Ophidiophobia
Darkness	Nyctophobia
Fire	Pyrophobia
Foreigners, Strangers	Xenophobia
Animals	Zoophobia

Most of the time, simple phobias develop during childhood and often go away with time. Those that continue into adulthood rarely go away without treatment.

- **Social Phobias.** The irrational fear is of being embarrassed or humiliated in public. Examples of situations leading to this include:
  - Public speaking (this is the most common social phobia)
  - Stage fright
  - Eating in public
  - Talking to coworkers
  - Asking someone out on a date

- **Agoraphobia.** The irrational fear is of being alone in public places in which the person:
  - Feels trapped with no way to escape (or thinks it would be difficult to escape)
  - Would be very embarrassed or helpless when phobic symptoms occur
  - Fears being totally unable to take care of himself or herself if help was not around

Phobias, *Continued*

Agoraphobia can occur with or without panic disorder. (See "Panic Attacks" on page 200.) It most often comes after having panic attacks because the sufferer avoids the places where panic attacks occurred. He or she fears that something about the location caused the panic attack. The fear of having another panic attack can result in avoiding going out in public. In severe cases, persons with agoraphobia don't leave their home at all.

Treatment

Treatment for phobias depends on the type of phobia and how much the fear keeps a person from normal life activities. Methods of treatment include:

■ Behavior therapy – one type is called exposure therapy. This type exposes the person to the feared situation or object in one of two ways:

Gradual exposure. This is called "systematic desensitization." A therapist works with the person in gradual steps. First the person learns relaxation methods to deal with the physical responses to his or her phobia. Second, the person imagines the source of the phobia. Next, the person looks at pictures of the feared object or ones that depict the feared situation. Finally, the person is gradually exposed to the situation or feared object.

Direct exposure. This is known as "flooding." The person is exposed to the feared object or situation all at once (in the presence of a therapist). The person stays in that situation until his or her anxiety is markedly less than its previous level. Sessions doing this are repeated until the person can handle the phobic situation alone.

■ Group therapy and/or self-help support group therapy such as Agoraphobics in Motion (A.I.M.).

■ Medication. Types include certain antidepressants, antianxiety medicines, tranquilizers and ones known as beta blockers. These medicines block or reduce the panic symptoms that come with phobic situations. In so doing, they help a person confront the feared situation when they might have been too afraid to do so otherwise.

Medications are especially helpful for persons who have agoraphobia with panic disorder. Certain beta blockers can be useful for persons who suffer from stage fright.

Questions to Ask

Do you have all of these problems?
• Panic disorder (see page 200)
• Anxiety about being in places or situations from which escape might be difficult or embarrassing or in which you could not get help if you had a panic attack
• You avoid places outside of the home alone, such as ones that involve:
- Being in a crowd
- Standing in a line
- Being on a bridge
- Traveling in a car, bus or train

YES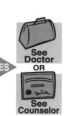
See Doctor OR
See Counselor

NO

Flowchart continued on next page

16. Mental Health Conditions

Phobias, *Continued*

Did you answer yes to parts 2 and 3 of the first question, but you don't have panic disorder or get panic attacks? **YES** → See Counselor

↓ **NO**

Are there certain objects or situations which cause you to feel intense fear or terror to the point that you lose control of yourself? **YES** → See Counselor

↓ **NO**

Do you avoid certain situations, objects, persons, or places to the point that doing so is interfering with tasks you want to get done? **YES** → See Counselor

↓ **NO**

 Use Self-Care

Self-Care Tips

The following tips are ways to deal with phobias that do not disrupt your daily life. They may also be employed with or after professional treatment.

- List your irrational fears. Writing them down helps you to identify them. Try to figure out why you have the fears, what you think they mean, what they might symbolize, and what you can do to deal with them. Doing these things can give you some control over your fears.

- Learn and practice relaxation techniques. These allow you to feel more comfortable and show that you can control the physical symptoms which result from your phobia. They also help you remain in the situation long enough to realize that you are not in any danger. Two important relaxation techniques to use are:

  - Controlled Breathing. When you panic, you overbreathe or hyperventilate, which makes you dizzy. This causes your heart to race and makes you feel weak and tremble. Take a few deep breaths and hold each one to the count of 3, then exhale slowly to the count of 3. This will help restore normal breathing, slow your pulse, and remedy your dizziness and shakiness.

  - Tension Control. When you panic, you tense your muscles, making them feel hard and uncomfortable. Relax each muscle group (arms, legs, neck, shoulders) until you feel the tension subside. Practice this technique until you can relax your muscles simply by thinking about relaxing them.

- If you have a fear of speaking in public, enroll in a public speaking course such as Dale Carnegie.

- If you are afraid of flying, take a course designed to help people conquer this fear.

- Also, see "Self-Care Tips: Ways to Deal with Panic that has Limited Symptoms and Duration" on pages 201 and 202.

- See a counselor if Self-Care Tips do not help you deal with your phobia on your own. (See also, "Places to Get Information & Help" under "Anxiety/Phobias" on page 375.)

68 Sexual Concerns

A lot of people have concerns about their sex life. Common concerns and problems that affect one or both sex partners include:

- Little or no desire for sexual relations

- Different levels of desire for sex between partners

- Disgust or distress with having sex or even thinking about it

- Failure to become aroused before sex and/or the inability to stay aroused until the sex act is completed

- Impotence in males. This means not being able to sustain an adequate erection.

- Premature ejaculation in the male. Ejaculation comes too early. Some experts define "too early" as 2–4 minutes. The concern, though, is not the exact amount of time, but that ejaculation comes with a minimum amount of stimulation sooner than the person wants it to come.

- Delay in or absence of orgasm in either the female or male

- Pain during intercourse

- Painful, sustained erection

There are a lot of reasons these things take place:

- Psychological factors. Examples are:
  - Sexual trauma from things such as rape, incest, past sexual embarrassments or failures
  - Worry or anxiety about sexual performance

  - Guilt or inner conflicts about sex such as when a person's sexual needs, wishes, or thoughts go against family, religious, or cultural teachings
  - Depression
  - Relationship problems and/or lack of communication of wants and needs between sex partners

- Physical conditions that affect a person's sexual response. Examples include disorders that involve:
  - The heart and blood vessels. Less blood can flow to the genitals. Even the arteries and veins in the penis can be involved.
  - The nervous system, with a condition like multiple sclerosis
  - The body's glands such as with diabetes and/or any condition that alters the making or release of sex hormones
  - The use of any substance that alters the sexual response. These include some medications, drugs, alcohol and/or smoking. For example, some antidepressants may lead to impotence or failure to achieve orgasm.
  - Surgery. For example, prostate surgery can result in impotence.
  - Injuries such as ones that cause damage to nerves used in the sexual response or that result in scar tissue that interferes with sensations felt during sex

Sexual Concerns, *Continued*

Treatment

A medical evaluation is the first step. It can determine if physical conditions, medications, etc., are the cause of the problem(s). A physical exam and certain tests can be done. These include:

- Hormonal studies

- Ones that check for neurological problems

- Ones that measure the flow of blood and the conditions of the veins and arteries in the penis

- Blood and urine tests to detect diabetes, urinary tract infections, etc.

- X-rays and/or ultrasound, if needed, which can help detect endometriosis, vaginal scar tissue, ovarian tumors, etc., in women.

When a physical condition is found that causes the sexual concern or problem, treating it can get rid of or help with the problem. For example, several treatments exist for impotence. These include:

- A special vacuum that is placed over the penis to remove air. This causes an erection.

- Self-injections of a prescription medicine

- Penile implant surgery

If no physical condition is found to be at fault, measures to deal with psychological causes can help. These include therapies of many kinds:

- Individual counseling

- Counseling with both partners

- Sex therapy

- Behavior therapy

Questions to Ask:

Does it hurt to have sex and are any of these problems present?
- The urge to go to the bathroom very badly or passing urine a lot more often than usual
- Burning or stinging feeling when passing urine
- The feeling that the bladder is still full after voiding
- Bad-smelling urine
- Bloody or cloudy urine
- Pain in the abdomen or over the bladder
- Stomachaches or feeling like throwing up

YES  **See Doctor**

NO

Do you have signs of "Anxiety" (see page 180) and/or "Depression" (see page 186)?

YES 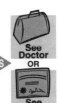 **See Doctor OR** **See Counselor**

NO

Do any of the following cause a great deal of distress?
- Little or no desire for sex
- Disgust with having sex or even thinking about it
- Failure to get aroused before sex and/or the inability to stay aroused until the sex act is completed
- Delay or absence of orgasm

YES **See Counselor**

NO

Flowchart continued on next page

16. Mental Health Conditions

Sexual Concerns, *Continued*

Flowchart continued

For Men Only:

Does impotence occur with any of the following?
- Prostate surgery
- Medication for:
  - High blood pressure
  - Allergies (antihistamines)
  - Depression
  - Anxiety
  - Muscle relaxation
  - Any other prescriptions or over-the-counter medicine
- Drugs such as cocaine
- Excessive use of alcohol

YES See Doctor

NO

Does impotence occur with one or more of these problems?
- An urge to urinate right away or the need to urinate often, especially at night
- Not being able to empty the bladder completely
- A feeling of hesitancy or delay or straining to urinate
- A weak or interrupted urinary stream

YES See Doctor

NO

Flowchart continued in next column

Does impotence occur with diabetes or the following signs of diabetes?
- Constant or frequent urination
- Extreme thirst
- Unusual hunger
- Weight loss or gain
- Fatigue
- Slow healing of cuts or wounds, especially on the feet
- Irritability

YES 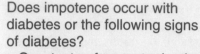 See Doctor

NO

Are any of these problems present?
- Pain in the penis during intercourse
- Sustained erection that is painful
- Sores and/or painful blisters on the genital area and/or anus
- A discharge of pus from the penis
- Pain and swelling in the scrotum

YES See Doctor

NO

Do one or both of the following cause a great deal of distress?
- Not being able to sustain an adequate erection
- Ejaculation that comes too soon

YES See Counselor

NO

Flowchart continued on next page

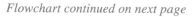

16. Mental Health Conditions

Sexual Concerns, *Continued*

Flowchart continued

For Women Only:

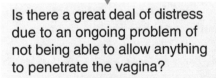

Is intercourse very painful with or without any of the following?
- Heavy, painful periods
- A yellowish-green vaginal discharge
- Chronic pain in the abdomen or a dull and constant ache on either or both sides of your pelvis
- Abnormal bleeding from the vagina
- Itching and burning around the vagina
- A large, painless, ulcerlike sore (chancre) or painful blisters in the genital area, anus, or mouth

YES → See Doctor

NO ↓

Has sex been painful and given less pleasure since having an intrauterine contraceptive device (IUD) inserted?

YES → See Doctor

NO ↓

Is there a great deal of distress due to an ongoing problem of not being able to allow anything to penetrate the vagina?

YES → See Doctor OR See Counselor

NO ↓

 Use Self-Care

Self-Care Tips

- Stay healthy:
  - Eat well.
  - Exercise regularly.
  - Get enough sleep.
  - Don't ignore signs of illnesses.
  - Follow your doctor's advice for a chronic illness, if you have one, to help prevent possible problems with sexual satisfaction.
  - Practice safe sex to prevent sexually transmitted diseases.
  - Limit alcohol. A little alcohol can act as an aphrodisiac. Too much, however, can lead to unsafe sex, violent behavior, etc.
  - Don't smoke.

The following things can help enhance the desire for sex. This is especially important for couples who both work outside the home and also have children. By the time they get into bed each night, sex seems like too much bother.

- Make a point to spend at least 15 minutes of uninterrupted time with your partner each day. If you can't meet face to face, call each other on the telephone.
- Remember to express your affection for each other every day.
- Plan to spend part of a day alone together at least once a week. Make a date to take a walk in the park, go out for dinner, or share other activities you both enjoy.
- Schedule a weekend away together every 2 months or so.

16. Mental Health Conditions

Sexual Concerns, *Continued*

- Go to bed together at the same time. Tell yourself that what you haven't accomplished by 11 p.m. can wait until the next day.

- Relax by giving each other a massage or taking a shower together.

- Keep the television set out of the bedroom. Watching TV can be sexual suicide.

Don't worry if your sexual encounters occasionally fail. Fatigue and stress are known to cause temporary impotence, a decrease in vaginal lubrication, or the inability to have an orgasm. Don't let yourselves become preoccupied with performance; just take pleasure in being together. Enjoy hugging, kissing, and caressing.

For Premature Ejaculation

- The squeeze technique. If a man feels he's about to ejaculate prematurely, he firmly pinches the penis directly below the head using the thumb and first two fingers of one hand and squeezes for 3 to 4 seconds. (This technique was developed by William H. Masters, M.D. and Virginia E. Johnson, founders of the Reproductive Biology Research Foundation).

- The start/stop method. The couple should abstain from intercourse for 2 weeks, but focus on touching. The man concentrates on the sensations in his penis as his partner touches his genitals and brings him to an erection. The man asks his partner to stop just before ejaculation. After a few minutes, his partner continues to arouse him, then stops again. This sequence is repeated twice more with ejaculation occurring the fourth time. Then each time the couple has sex, foreplay is prolonged.

For Lack of Sexual Response in Women

Couples can practice certain techniques to address sexual unresponsiveness in a woman. A few simple methods follow:

- For the first week, limit lovemaking to cuddling, kissing, and nuzzling. Don't touch the genitals or breasts.

- During the second week, the man should gently touch his partner's vaginal area during lovemaking, but stop before she reaches orgasm to increase vaginal lubrication.

- During the third week, repeat the first 2 phases, then proceed with intercourse. If the vagina isn't adequately lubricated, apply a water-soluble lubricant such as K-Y Jelly to the penis to facilitate penetration. (Penetration may also be easier if the woman is on top.)

If a tight vaginal opening still makes penetration painful or impossible, the following exercise may help:

- The woman should gently place the tip of her partner's little finger against her vagina and gently push his finger into her vagina. If this feels uncomfortable, she should stop and wait a few minutes.

- The couple should continue this exercise until the man can insert 2 fingers in his partner's vagina without causing pain or discomfort. (It may take several attempts over a period of weeks for this technique to work.)

{*Note:* The above techniques do not guarantee success. If they do not help improve your sexual concerns, consider professional help from a sex therapist.}

69 Stress

Stress is the way our bodies react to any change in the status quo (good, bad, real, or even imagined). Some physical symptoms created by stress include:

- Increased heart rate
- Rapid breathing
- Tense muscles
- Increased blood pressure

Emotional reactions include:

- Irritability
- Anger
- Losing one's temper
- Yelling
- Lack of concentration
- Being jumpy

When left unchecked, stress can lead to a variety of health problems including:

- Insomnia
- Back pain
- High blood pressure
- Heart disease
- A lowering of the body's immune system. In fact, the American Academy of Family Physicians states that about two-thirds of all visits to the family doctor are for stress-related disorders.

Questions to Ask

Do you have one or both of these problems?
- You are so distressed that you have recurrent thoughts of suicide or death.
- You have impulses or plans to commit violence.

YES → Get Emergency Care

NO ↓

Do you have any of these problems often?
- Anxiety
- Nervousness
- Crying spells
- Confusion about how to handle your problems

YES → See Doctor

NO ↓

Are you abusing alcohol and/ or drugs (illegal or prescription) to deal with stress?

YES → See Doctor

NO ↓

Flowchart continued on next page

16. Mental Health Conditions

Stress, *Continued*

Flowchart continued

Have you been a part of a traumatic event in the past (e.g., armed combat, airplane crash, rape, or assault) and do you now experience any of the following?
- Flashbacks (reliving the stressful event), painful memories, nightmares
- Feeling easily startled and/or irritable
- Feeling "emotionally numb" and detached from others and the outside world
- Having a hard time falling asleep and/or staying asleep
- Anxiety and/or depression

YES → See Counselor

NO

Do you withdraw from friends, relatives and coworkers and/or blow up at them at the slightest annoyance?

YES → See Counselor

NO

Do you suffer from a medical illness that:
- You are unable to cope with
- Leads you to neglect proper treatment

YES →  Call Doctor OR Call Counselor

NO

 Use Self-Care

Self-Care Tips

Being able to manage stress is important in living a healthy, happy, and productive life. Here are some techniques and strategies to help you deal with stress.

- Maintain a regular program of healthy eating, good health habits, and adequate sleep.

- Exercise regularly. This promotes physical fitness as well as emotional well-being.

- Balance work and play. All work and no play can make you feel stressed. Plan some time for hobbies and recreation. These activities relax your mind and are a good respite from life's worries. Plan one or more vacations during the year. Don't do work on your vacation.

- Help others. We concentrate on ourselves when we're distressed. Sometimes helping others is the perfect remedy for whatever is troubling us.

- Take a shower or bath with warm water. This will soothe and calm your nerves and relax your muscles.

- Have a good cry. Tears of sadness, joy, or grief can help cleanse the body of substances that accumulate under stress and also release a natural pain-relieving substance from the brain.

Stress, *Continued*

- Laugh a lot. When events seem too over-whelming, keep a sense of humor. Laughter makes our muscles go limp and releases tension. It's difficult to feel stress in the middle of a belly laugh. Learn to laugh as a relaxation technique.

- Find ways to learn acceptance. Sometimes a difficult problem is out of control. When this happens, accept it until changes can be made. This is better than worrying and getting nowhere.

- Talk out troubles. It sometimes helps to talk with a friend, relative, or member of the clergy. Another person can help you see a problem from a different point of view.

- Escape for a little while. When you feel you are getting nowhere with a problem, a temporary diversion can help. Go to a movie, read a book, visit a museum, or take a drive. Temporarily leaving a difficult situation can help you develop new attitudes.

- Reward yourself. Starting today, reward yourself with little things that make you feel good. Treat yourself to a bubble bath, buy the hardcover edition of a book, call an old friend long distance, add to your stamp or coin collection, buy a flower, picnic in the park during lunchtime, try a new perfume or cologne, or give yourself some "me" time.

- Do relaxation exercises daily. Good ones include visualization (imagining a soothing, restful scene), deep muscle relaxation (tensing and relaxing muscle fibers), meditation, and deep breathing.

- Budget your time. Make a "to do" list. Rank in priority your daily tasks. Avoid committing yourself to doing too much.

- View changes as positive challenges, opportunities, or blessings.

- Rehearse for stressful events. Imagine yourself feeling calm and confident in an anticipated stressful situation. You will be able to relax more easily when the situation arises.

- Modify your environment to get rid of or manage your exposure to things that cause stress.

Suicidal Thoughts

A lot of people think about suicide or say things like, "I wish I was dead" at times of great stress. For most people these thoughts are a way to express anger, frustration, and other strong emotions. They may not, in and of themselves be a sign of a problem. Suicidal thoughts could be a signal for help, though, if they:

- Don't go away or occur often

- Lead to suicidal threats, gestures, or attempts

- Are a symptom of a medical illness or mental health condition such as:

  • Depression (see page 186). Up to 70% of persons who commit suicide are known to have suffered from depression right before their deaths.

  • Bipolar disorder (manic depression) – a mood disorder characterized by mood swings from elation and/or euphoria to severe depression. Suicide can take place during either the manic or depressive episodes.

  • Schizophrenia – a group of mental disorders in which there are severe disturbances in thinking, mood, and behavior. The sufferer experiences delusions, hallucinations, disordered thinking, and/or inappropriate emotions.

  • Grief/Bereavement (see page 198). The loss of a loved one may provoke thoughts of suicide. A person may find it hard to go on living without their loved one or may want to be with him or her in death.

Suicide:

- Is more common in men than women. Men commit 4 times as many suicides as women.

- Is attempted 3 times more often by women than men. Young women attempt suicide 4 to 8 times more often than young men.

- Is committed more often by white men than by black men

- Has the highest rate in adults over age 65

- Is the third leading cause of death among 15–24 year olds behind accidents and homicide

Suicidal threats and attempts are a person's way of letting others know that he or she is in need of attention or wants someone to help them. Suicide attempts and/or threats should never be taken lightly or taken only as a "bluff." Most people who threaten and/or attempt suicide more than once usually succeed if they are not stopped.

Prevention and Treatment

Prevention and treatment include:

- Knowing the warning signs for suicide (see "Questions to Ask" on page 215)

- Taking courses that teach problem solving, coping skills, and suicide awareness in schools and in the community

- Addressing and treating the emotional and/or physical problems that lead to thoughts and attempts of suicide such as:

  • Medical treatment for physical and/or mental health conditions such as depression. This includes monitoring medicine, if used.

- Therapy such as individual and family counseling

- Keeping firearms, drugs, and other means to commit suicide away from potential victims

- Emergency care and hospitalization, if necessary, after an attempted suicide

Suicidal Thoughts, *Continued*

Questions to Ask

{*Note:* In some suicides, no warning signs are shown or noticed.}

Are any of the following present?
- Suicide attempts
- Plans being made to commit suicide
- Repeated thoughts of suicide or death

YES **Get Emergency Care**

NO

With thoughts of suicide or death, are any of these conditions present?
- Depression
- Manic depression
- Schizophrenia
- Any other mental health or medical condition

YES **See Doctor**

NO

Have thoughts of suicide come as a result of one of the following?
- Taking, stopping, or changing the dose of a prescribed medicine
- Using drugs and/or alcohol

YES **See Doctor**

NO

Flowchart continued in next column

Has there been a lot less interest or pleasure in almost all activities or a depressed mood most of the day, nearly every day for at least 2 weeks? Or, have you been in a depressed mood most of the day nearly every day and have you had any of the following for at least 2 weeks?
- Feeling slowed down or restless and unable to sit still
- Feeling worthless or guilty
- Changes in appetite or weight loss or gain
- Thoughts of death or suicide
- Problems concentrating, thinking, remembering, or making decisions
- Trouble sleeping or sleeping too much
- Loss of energy or feeling tired all the time
- Headaches
- Other aches and pains
- Digestive problems
- Sexual problems
- Feeling pessimistic or hopeless
- Being anxious or worried

YES **See Doctor**

NO

Does the person thinking about suicide have other blood relatives who committed or attempted suicide?

YES **See Counselor**

NO

Flowchart continued on next page

16. Mental Health Conditions

Suicidal Thoughts, *Continued*

Flowchart continued

Has the person recently done 1 or more of the following?
- Given away favorite things, cleaned the house, and gotten legal matters in order
- Purchased or gotten a weapon or pills that could be used for suicide
- Given repeated statements that indicate suicidal thoughts such as, "I want to be dead", "I don't want to live anymore," or "How does a person leave their body to science?"
- Made suicidal gestures such as standing on the edge of a bridge, cutting their wrists with a dull instrument, or driving recklessly on purpose

YES → See Counselor

NO ↓

Flowchart continued in next column

Have suicidal thoughts come as a result of an upset in life such as?
- A separation
- A divorce
- The death of a loved one or other loss such as the loss of a job
- A rejection
- Being ridiculed

YES →  See Counselor

NO ↓

 Use Self-Care

Self-Care Tips

If you are having thoughts of suicide:

■ Let someone know. Talk to a trusted family member, friend, or teacher. If it is hard for you to talk directly to someone, write your thoughts down and let someone else read them.

■ Call your local crisis intervention or suicide prevention hotline. Look in your local phone book or call directory assistance or the operator for the number. Follow up with a visit to your doctor or local mental health center, if instructed to do so.

{*Note:* For information on suicide see "Places to Get Information & Help" under "Suicide " on page 377.}

16. Mental Health Conditions

71 Enlarged Prostate

The prostate is a male sex gland. It makes a fluid that forms part of semen, the fluid that is released during orgasm. The prostate is about the size of a walnut. It is located below the bladder and in front of the rectum. The prostate surrounds the upper part of the urethra, the tube that empties urine from the bladder.

If they live long enough, most men will eventually get an enlarged prostate gland. Doctors call it benign prostatic hyperplasia (BPH).

Symptoms

An enlarged prostate is usually not cancerous or life- threatening. It may cause some problems such as:

- Increased urgency to urinate
- Frequent urination, especially during the night
- Delay in onset of urine flow
- Diminished or slow stream of urine flow
- Incomplete emptying of the bladder

These symptoms indicate that the prostate gland has enlarged enough to partially obstruct the flow of urine. Sometimes, BPH causes a urinary tract infection. Over time, a few men might have bladder or kidney problems or both.

Your doctor can diagnose BPH through a number of things. These include:

- A physical exam which includes asking questions about your current symptoms and past medical problems, an examination of your prostate gland, checking your urine for signs of infection, and a blood test to see if the prostate has affected your kidneys

- Tests that measure urine flow, the amount of urine left in your bladder after you urinate, and the pressure in your bladder as you urinate
- Other tests such as X-rays, cystoscopy (the doctor looks directly at the prostate and bladder), and an ultrasound (sound wave pictures of the prostate, kidneys or bladder). Many men do not need these tests. They are costly and are not very helpful for most men with BPH.

{*Note:* Men 40 years of age and older should have a digital rectal exam every year to screen for an enlarged prostate. (See "Common Health Tests & How Often to Have Them" on page 17.) Other tests that a doctor might order are a prostate–specific antigen (PSA) blood test, and a transcretal ultrasound (TRUS). Men should discuss the need for these tests with their doctor.}

Treatment

Treatment for BPH varies depending on symptoms. Treatment options include:

- Watchful waiting. This is getting no treatment, but having regular exams to see if your BPH is causing problems or getting worse.
- Medications. Examples are ones that help relax the smooth muscle of the bladder neck and prostate, such as Hytrin and one which causes the prostate to shrink, such as Proscar.
- Surgery. There are many types. Check with your doctor for the type best suited for your needs. Ask about new procedures being done, too. Surgical options include:
  - Transurethral resection of the prostate (TURP). This type relieves symptoms by increasing the diameter of the urethra as it passes through the prostate. It is a proven way to treat BPH effectively.

17. Men's Health Problems

Enlarged Prostate, *Continued*

- Transurethral incision of the prostate (TUIP). This reduces the prostate's pressure on the urethra, making it easier to urinate. TUIP may be used instead of TURP when the prostate is not enlarged as much.

- Open prostatectomy. This may be used if the prostate is very large. An incision is made in the lower abdomen to remove the prostate.

Prostate surgery can result in problems such as impotence and/or incontinence. It is important to discuss the benefits and the risks of these operations with your doctor. Most men who undergo surgery have no major problems.

Questions to Ask

Do you have 1 or more of these problems?
- A feeling that you have to urinate right away or the need to urinate often, especially at night
- A feeling that you can't empty your bladder completely
- A feeling of hesitancy, delay, or straining to urinate
- A weak or interrupted urinary stream

YES See Doctor

NO

 Use Self-Care

Self-Care Tips

■ Remain sexually active.

■ Take hot baths.

■ Avoid dampness and cold temperatures.

■ Do not let the bladder get too full. Urinate as soon as the urge arises. Relax when you urinate.

■ When you take long car trips, make frequent stops to urinate. Keep a container in the car that you can urinate in when you can't get to a bathroom in time.

■ Limit coffee, alcohol, and foods that are spicy.

■ Drink 8 or more glasses of water every day, but don't drink liquids before going to bed.

■ Reduce stress.

■ Don't smoke.

■ Avoid taking over-the-counter antihistamines or cold medicines that contain ephendrine.

Jock Itch

Jock itch is usually caused by a fungus infection. It can also result from a bacterial infection or be a reaction to chemicals in clothing, irritating garments, or medicines that you take.

Jock itch gets its name because an athletic supporter worn, then stored in a locker, and then worn again without being laundered, provides the ideal environment in which the fungi thrive. (Under similar conditions, women's clothing can develop this problem, too.) Jock itch is more likely to occur after taking antibiotics.

Symptoms

Symptoms of jock itch (in the groin and thigh area) are:

- Redness of the skin of the groin and/or scrotum
- Itching
- Scaly patches of skin

Questions to Ask

Do symptoms of jock itch persist longer than 2 weeks despite self-treatment remedies?

YES → Call Doctor

NO ↓

Use Self-Care

Self-Care Tips

To Prevent Jock Itch:

- Don't wear tight, close-fitting clothing. Wear loose-fitting underwear, such as boxer shorts, instead of briefs.
- Change underwear frequently, especially after tasks that leave you hot and sweaty.
- Bathe or shower right away after a workout. Dry the groin area well.
- Apply talc or other powder to the groin area. This will help keep this area dry. If you sweat a lot or are very overweight use a drying powder with miconazole nitrate.
- Don't store damp clothing in a locker or gym bag.
- Wash workout clothes after each wearing.
- Sleep in the nude or in a nightshirt.
- Avoid antibacterial (deodorant) soaps.

To Treat Jock Itch:

- Use over-the-counter antifungal cream, powder, or lotion. Examples are ones with clotrimazole (such as Lotrimin), miconazole (such as Micatin), and tolnaftate (such as Tinactin). Follow package directions.

73 Testicular Cancer & Self-Exam

Cancer of the testicles, the primary male sex glands, accounts for only about 1 percent of all cancers in men. It is, though, the most common type of cancer in males aged 20 to 35, but can occur in other age groups. It strikes about 5,000 males a year. Often, only one testicle is affected. The cause of testicular cancer is not known. Risk factors, though, have been given. These are:

- Undescended testicles (that are not corrected) in infants and young children. (Parents should see that their infant boys are checked at birth for undescended testicles.)

- A family history of testicular cancer

- Having an identical twin with testicular cancer

- Injury to the scrotum

Signs and Symptoms

In the early stages, testicular cancer may have no symptoms. When there are symptoms, they include:

- Small, painless lump in a testicle

- Enlarged testicle

- Feeling of heaviness in the testicle or scrotum

- Pain or discomfort in a testicle or in the scrotum

- A dull ache in the lower abdomen or the groin

- A change in the way the testicle feels

- Enlarged male breasts and nipples

- Sudden collection of fluid in the scrotum

Testicular cancer is almost always curable if it is found and treated early. Surgery is done to remove the testicle. Other things can further treat the disease:

- Chemotherapy

- Radiation therapy

- Surgical removal of lymph nodes, if necessary

Questions to Ask

Do you have severe testicular pain?

YES → Get Emergency Care

NO ↓

Can any lumps, enlargement, swelling, or change in consistency be felt in the scrotum?

YES → See Doctor

NO ↓

Is there any sense of heaviness or pain?

YES → See Doctor

NO ↓

Is there an enlargement of the breasts and nipples or a sudden feeling of puffiness in the scrotum?

YES → See Doctor

NO ↓

 Use Self-Care

See Self-Care Tips on next page

Testicular Cancer & Self-Exam, *Continued*

Self-Care Tips

Perform Testicular Self-Exam (TSE) monthly or as recommended by your doctor.

The American Academy of Family Physicians Subcommittee for Male Patients recommends the teaching of testicular self-examination between the ages of 13 and 18. The testicles are located behind the penis and contained within the scrotum. They should be about the same size and feel smooth, rubbery, and egg-shaped. The left one sometimes hangs lower than the right.

Testicular Self-Exam (TSE)

Self-examination of the testicles is best performed when the scrotum is relaxed, after a warm bath or shower. This will also allow the testicles to drop down.

How to do TSE

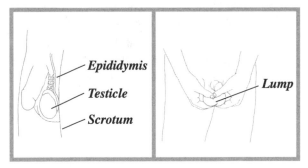

- Examine each testicle gently with both hands. The index and middle fingers should be placed underneath the testicle while the thumbs are placed on the top. Gently roll the testicle between the thumbs and fingers. One testicle may be larger than the other. This is normal.

- Find the epididymis (the soft, tube-like structure at the back of the testicle that stores and carries the sperm). Do not confuse the epididymis with an abnormal lump.

- Feel for any abnormal lumps (about the size of a pea) on the front or the side of the testicle. These lumps are usually painless.

If you do find a lump, contact your doctor right away. The lump may be due to an infection, and a doctor can decide the proper treatment. If the lump is not an infection, it is likely to be cancer. Remember that testicular cancer is highly curable, especially when detected and treated promptly. Testicular cancer almost always occurs in only one testicle. After the testicle with cancer is removed the other testicle provides full sexual functioning.

Routine testicular self-exams are important, but they cannot substitute for a doctor's examination. Your doctor should examine your testicles when you have a physical exam. You can also ask your doctor to teach you the correct way to do a TSE.

74 Breast Cancer & Self-Exam

Breast cancer is the most common form of cancer among women, accounting for 30% of cancers women get. Each year, there are approximately 185,000 new cases of breast cancer and 45,000 deaths from it. Only lung cancer causes more cancer deaths among women.

Men can also develop breast cancer, but it is very unusual. About 300 men die each year from the disease.

Breast cancer results from malignant tumors which invade and destroy normal tissue. When these tumors break away and spread to other parts of the body, it is called metastasis. Breast cancers can spread to the lymph nodes, lungs, liver, bone and brain.

Increase in age is the number one risk factor for breast cancer. The National Cancer Institute (NCI) has given the following statistics for a woman's chances of developing breast cancer:

By Age	Chances
25	1 in 19,608
30	1 in 2,525
35	1 in 622
40	1 in 217
45	1 in 93
50	1 in 50
55	1 in 33
60	1 in 24
65	1 in 17
70	1 in 14
75	1 in 11
80	1 in 10
85	1 in 9
Lifetime	1 in 8

The risk of breast cancer increases above the normal risk with these factors:

- Personal history of breast cancer increasing the risk for additional cancer in the remaining breast tissue
- Never giving birth or giving birth after age 30
- Early onset of menstruation (before age 12)
- Late menopause (after age 55)
- Family history of breast cancer for a woman whose mother, daughter, or sister has had the disease. The woman's risk increases even more if her relative's cancer developed before menopause or if it affected both breasts
- Exposure to radiation
- Diet high in fat
- Being overweight (for older women only)

Detection

Early screening for breast cancer includes:

- Mammograms – X-rays of the breast. (See "Common Health Tests & How Often to Have Them" on page 17.) Make sure you have mammograms at facilities that are accredited by the American College of Radiology (ACR). Call The National Cancer Institute Hotline at 1-800-4-CANCER to find ones in your area.
- Clinical breast exams – breast exams by a doctor or nurse
- Breast self-exam – (See "How to Examine Your Breasts" on pages 224 and 225.)

If a lump or other problem is found, the doctor can do further exams and tests to check for cancer.

Breast Cancer & Self-Exam, *Continued*

Treatment

There are a variety of treatments for breast cancer. The main treatment is surgery. Most often the cancerous area is removed. A sample of the lymph nodes in the armpit is also taken to see if the cancer has spread there.

Other treatments are radiation therapy, chemotherapy, and hormonal therapy. It is important to find out the type of cancer cell present. If the cancer is a type which spreads quickly, a more extensive surgical treatment may be chosen.

Types of Surgical Procedures:

- Lumpectomy – The lump and a border of surrounding tissue are removed.

- Partial or segmental mastectomy – The tumor and up to one-fourth of the breast tissue are removed.

- Simple or total mastectomy – The entire breast is removed.

- Modified radical mastectomy – The entire breast, the underarm lymph nodes and the lining covering the chest muscles, but not the muscles themselves, are removed.

- Radical mastectomy – The breast, lymph nodes in the armpit and the chest muscles under the breast are removed.

Ask your doctor about the benefits and risks for each surgical option and decide together which option is best for you.

Questions to Ask

Do you see or feel any lumps, thickening, or changes of any kind when you examine your breasts? For example, is there dimpling, puckering, retraction of the skin, or change in the shape or contour of the breast? **YES** See Doctor

NO

Do you have breast pain or a constant tenderness that lasts throughout the menstrual cycle? **YES**  See Doctor

NO

Do the nipples become drawn into the chest (or are they inverted totally), change shape, or become crusty from a discharge? **YES** See Doctor

NO

If you normally have lumpy breasts (already diagnosed as being benign by your doctor), do you notice any new lumps, or have any lumps changed in size, or are you concerned about having "benign" lumps? **YES** See Doctor

NO

Flowchart continued on next page

18. Women's Health Problems

Breast Cancer & Breast Self-Exam, *Continued*

Flowchart continued

Is there any nonmilky discharge when you squeeze the nipple of either breast or both breasts?

YES →  See Doctor

NO

Do you have a family history of breast cancer which leads you to be concerned even if you don't notice any problems when you examine your breasts?

YES → Call Doctor

NO

 Use Self-Care

Use Self-Care/Prevention Tips on this page and perform breast self-examination monthly.

Self-Care/Prevention Tips

- Follow a low-fat diet. Focus on fresh fruits and vegetables, whole grains, etc.

- Eat vegetables that contain a substance called sulforaphane, which may help protect against breast cancer. Examples: broccoli, cabbage, cauliflower, and brussels sprouts.

- Avoid unnecessary X-rays. Wear a lead apron when you get dental X-rays and other X-rays not of the chest.

- Breast-feed your babies. This may reduce your risk for breast cancer, especially before menopause.

- Limit your alcohol intake to 1 or 2 drinks per day at most.

How to Examine Your Breasts

It is normal to have some lumpiness or thickening in the breasts. By examining your breasts once each month, you will learn what is normal for you and notice when any changes do occur. Some women find that doing a daily or weekly self-exam works better for them. They become familiar with their breasts at all phases of their menstrual cycle. The more you can examine your breasts, the better you can learn what is normal for you. Your "job" isn't just to find lumps, but to notice if there are any changes.

Breast Self-Exam (BSE) is a Three-Step Process:

1. In the shower – With your fingers flat, gently move the pads of your fingertips over every part of each breast. Use your right hand to examine the left breast and your left 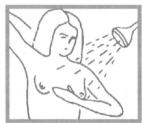 hand to examine the right breast. Check for any thickening, hard lump or knot.

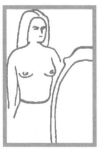 2. In front of a mirror – Holding your arms at your sides, look at your breasts. Raise your arms overhead and look for any changes in the 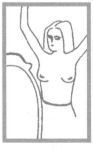 shape of either breast, or any swelling, dimpling, or changes in the nipples.

18. Women's Health Problems

Breast Cancer & Breast Self-Exam, *Continued*

3. Lying down – To examine your right breast, put 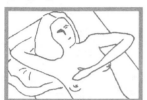 a pillow under your right shoulder. Place your right hand behind your head. Then, using the fingers of your left hand held flat, press your right breast gently in small circular motions around an imaginary clock face. Begin at the outermost top of your right breast for 12 o'clock, then move to 10 o'clock, etc., until you get back to 12 o'clock. Each breast will have a normal ridge of firm tissue.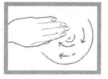

Then move in 1 inch toward the nipple. Keep circling to examine every part of your breast including the nipple. Repeat the procedure on the left breast with a pillow under the left shoulder and your left hand behind your head. Finally, squeeze the nipple of each breast gently between the thumb and index finger. Any clear or bloody discharge should be reported to your physician immediately.

18. Women's Health Problems

Cervical Cancer

Cervical cancer accounts for about 4% of all cancers found in women. Each year, about 15,000 women in the United States learn that they have this type of cancer.

Cancer of the cervix, the lower, narrow part of the uterus, can occur at any age, but is found most often in women over the age of 40.

Cells on the surface of the cervix sometimes appear abnormal but are not cancerous. It is thought that these abnormal changes are the first step in a slow series of changes that can lead to cervical cancer many years later. That is, some abnormal changes are precancerous.

Causes

Certain risk factors have been identified that increase the chance that cells in the cervix will become abnormal or cancerous. It is believed, in many cases, that cervical cancer develops when two or more of these risk factors act together:

- Having a history of the sexually transmitted human papilloma virus (HPV). There are many types of this virus. Some types put women at greater risk than others. {*Note:* Not all women who are infected with HPV develop cervical cancer, and the virus is not present in all women who have this disease.}

- Having had frequent sexual intercourse before age 18

- Having multiple sex partners. The greater the number of partners, the greater the risk.

- Having sex partners who:
  - Began having sexual intercourse at a young age

  - Have had many sexual partners
  - Were previously sexually active with a woman who had cervical cancer

- Having had a sex partner with HPV

- Smoking

- Being the daughter of a mother who took a drug known as DES during pregnancy. This drug was used from about 1940 to 1970, mostly to prevent miscarriage.

- Having a weakened immune system due to such things as:
  - Having human immunodeficiency virus (HIV)

  - Having taken drugs to prevent rejection with an organ transplant

Signs and Symptoms

Any abnormal pap test can be an early sign of cervical cancer. There are often no symptoms, though, especially in the early stages. In very late stages the symptoms include:

- Vaginal bleeding or spotting between periods

- Bleeding after intercourse

- Thick vaginal discharge that may have an odor

- Watery vaginal discharge

- Pain in the pelvic area

The final stages can result in:

- Anemia

- Appetite and weight loss

- Pain in the abdomen

- Leakage of urine and feces through the vagina

Cervical Cancer, *Continued*

Detection

Early diagnosis of cervical cancer is important. If the cancer is found early, most women can be cured. The best way to find it early is to have pap tests and pelvic exams on a regular basis. These should start when a female begins having sex or is over 18. Ask your doctor how often you should have pap tests and pelvic exams. His or her advice will be based on your age, medical history, and your risk factors for cervical cancer. Also ask your doctor about tests for sexually transmitted diseases (STDs), especially if you or your sex partner have or have had multiple sex partners.

Pap tests are the initial screening tool for cervical cancer. During this test, the doctor or nurse collects cells from the opening of the cervix and surfaces that surround it. The pap test is then checked to see:

- Whether or not the sample taken is adequate

- If the cells are normal or abnormal

- If there is an infection, inflammation, or cancer

In addition to your pap test or if an abnormal pap test is found, your doctor may use a special magnifying instrument called a colposcope. This will allow your doctor to look for any abnormal cells on the surface of the cervix. If your doctor notices a suspicious area on your cervix during this procedure, he/she may choose to take a biopsy of the area. These small pieces of cervical tissue will give your doctor an accurate diagnosis of your problem.

Treatment

Treatment will depend on the exact diagnosis. The precancerous form of cervical cancer is known as dysplasia. This can be treated with laser, conization (removal of a portion of the cervix), or cryotherapy (freezing). Surgery and/or radiation therapy may be required for cervical cancer. Chemotherapy is used in late stages. Sometimes more than one form of treatment is necessary. If the cervical cancer has not spread and a woman wants to become pregnant in the future, a conization may be done. If a woman does not want a future pregnancy, removal of the uterus may be chosen (a hysterectomy).

Questions to Ask

Do you have these problems?
- A leakage of urine and feces through the vagina
- Pain in the abdomen
- Anemia (noted by paleness, weakness, fatigue)
- Appetite and weight loss

YES 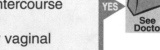 See Doctor

NO

Do you have any or these problems?
- Constant vaginal bleeding
- Spotting between periods or bleeding after intercourse
- Pelvic pain
- Thick or watery vaginal discharge

YES See Doctor

NO

Flowchart continued on next page

Cervical Cancer, *Continued*

Flowchart continued

Do you have 2 or more risk factors for cervical cancer? (See risk factors under "Causes" on page 226.) And, have you not had a pap test and pelvic exam for more than a year?

YES →  See Doctor

NO → Use Self-Care

Self-Care Tips

■ Remember to schedule and have pap tests and pelvic exams as often as your doctor suggests. Schedule these near your birthday to help you remember that they need to be done.

■ Take measures to prevent getting HPV and other sexually transmitted diseases (STDs) (see "Self-Care/Prevention Tips" on page 275)

■ Avoid douching. If you do, don't do so more than once a month.

■ Don't smoke.

■ Unless you are in a monogamous relationship in which you and your partner are free of STDs, use a latex condom every time you have sexual intercourse. Do this especially if your sex partner has a history of multiple sex partners.

Endometriosis

76

Endometriosis occurs when growth of the tissue that lines the inside of the uterus (endometrium) is found outside of the uterus in other areas of the body. It can only occur after menstruation begins in a woman. Women in their 20s, 30s, and 40s are most likely to get endometriosis.

Symptoms

The most common symptoms of endometriosis are:

- Pain before and during menstrual periods (usually worse than the pain in "normal" menstrual cramps)

- Pain during or after sexual intercourse

- Painful urination

- Lower back pain and painful bowel movements or loose stools with menstrual periods

- Pelvic soreness/tenderness

Pain, however, is not always present. Other symptoms include:

- Premenstrual vaginal spotting of blood

- Abnormally heavy or long menstrual periods

- Infertility

The exact cause of endometriosis is unknown. One theory suggests that some of the lining of the uterus during menstruation moves backwards through the fallopian tubes into the abdominal cavity where it attaches and grows. Other theories point to problems with the immune system and/or hormones. There is also some evidence that the condition may be inherited. Places where endometriosis is commonly found are:

- The outside surface of the uterus

- Fallopian tubes

- Ovaries

- The lining of the pelvic cavity

- The area between the vagina and the rectum

An accurate diagnosis of endometriosis must be made by your gynecologist. He or she may perform a laparoscopy, which is an out-patient surgical procedure. A slim telescope is inserted through a very small opening made in the navel. This allows your doctor to examine the abdominal and pelvic organs and evaluate the extent of the disease.

Treatment

The management of endometriosis is aimed at suppressing levels of the hormones estrogen and progesterone. These hormones cause endometriosis to grow. Mild to moderate endometriosis may be relieved at menopause.

Treatment for endometriosis can include surgery or medication therapy.

- Surgery:

  - Conservative surgery, such as removing areas of endometriosis using laser, cautery, or small surgical instruments to destroy the growths. These methods are used to reduce pain and to allow pregnancy to occur in some women.

  - Nonconservative surgery which removes the ovaries. The fallopian tubes and uterus can also be removed. Surgeries of this kind would likely eliminate pain, but leave a woman unable to conceive.

18. Women's Health Problems

Endometriosis, *Continued*

■ Medication therapy:

- Pain medications such as nonsteroidal anti-inflammatory drugs (NSAIDs). These include ibuprofen and naproxen sodium.

- Oral contraceptives given in a specific regimen to temporarily stop ovulation and menstruation. They are more likely to be used for very mild cases of endometriosis.

- Antiestrogens, which suppress a woman's production of estrogen. This will stop the menstrual cycle and prevent further growth of endometriosis since endometriosis needs estrogen to grow. These can have side effects such as acne, hair growth on the face, and changes in the libido.

- Progesterone, which is used to cast off the endometrial cells and thus destroy them

- Gonadotropin-releasing hormone (GnRH) agonist drugs, which will stop the production of estrogen. This causes a medically induced menopause that is temporary.

Questions to Ask

Do you have premenstrual spotting of blood and/or abnormally heavy or long menstrual periods? **YES**  Call Doctor

NO

Flowchart continued in next column

Do you have a lot of pain at any of these times?
- During sex
- When you menstruate and this has gotten worse over time
- When you urinate

YES Call Doctor

NO

Have you tried to get pregnant, but have not been able to in 12 or more months? **YES**  Call Doctor

NO

 Use Self-Care

Self-Care Tips

Self-care is very limited for endometriosis. It needs medical treatment. Things you can do to enhance medical treatment include:

■ Exercise regularly.

■ Eat a diet high in nutrients and low in fat, especially saturated fat, mostly found in coconut and palm oils, animal sources of fat, and hydrogenated vegetable fats.

■ Take an over-the-counter medicine for pain. Check with your doctor for his/her preference. {*Note:* See "Pain relievers" in "Your Home Pharmacy" on pages 22 and 23.}

■ Consider using oral contraceptives for birth control. Women who take the pill are less likely to have endometriosis.

18. Women's Health Problems

77 Fibroids

Fibroids are benign (not cancerous) tumors made mostly of muscle tissue. They are found in the wall of the uterus and sometimes on the cervix. They can range in size from as small as a pea to as large as a basketball! With larger fibroids, a woman's uterus can grow to the size of a pregnancy that is more than 20 weeks along. About 20–25% of women over 35 get fibroids. A woman is more likely to get fibroids if:

- She has not been pregnant
- She has a close relative who also had or has them
- She is African American. The risk is 3 to 5 times higher than it is for Caucasian women.

Why fibroids occur is not really known. They do, however, depend on estrogen for their growth. They may shrink or even disappear after menopause.

Signs and Symptoms

Some women with uterine fibroids do not have any symptoms or problems from them. When symptoms or problems occur, they vary due to the number, size, and locations of the fibroid(s). These include:

- Abdominal swelling, especially if they are large
- Heavy menstrual bleeding
- Bleeding between periods or after intercourse
- Pain (backache, during sex, with periods)
- Bleeding after menopause
- Anemia from excessive bleeding
- Frequent urination from pressure on the bladder
- Constipation from pressure on the rectum
- Infertility (the fallopian tubes may be blocked)
- Miscarriage (if the fibroid is inside the uterus, the placenta may not implant the way it should)

You can find out if you have fibroids when your doctor takes a medical history and does a pelvic exam. The doctor can also do other tests such as an ultrasound or a D & C to confirm their presence, location, and size. The ultrasound is the most common test for diagnosing fibroids.

Treatment

Treatment for fibroids includes:

- "Watchful waiting" if fibroids are small, harmless, and painless or not causing any problems. Your doctor will "watch" for any changes and may suggest "waiting" for menopause, since fibroids often shrink or disappear after that time. If you have problems during this "waiting" period (too much pain, too much bleeding, etc.), you may decide that you do not want to "wait" for menopause, but choose to have something done to treat your fibroids.

- Medication. One type, gonadotropin-releasing hormone (GnRH) agonists, blocks the production of estrogen by the ovaries. This shrinks fibroids in some cases but is not a cure. The fibroids return promptly when the medicine is stopped. Shrinking the fibroids might allow a minor surgery to be done instead of a major one. (See surgical methods below.) GnRH agonists are taken for a few months, but not more than 6, because their side effects mimic menopause.

- Surgery. There are two basic surgical methods:
  - Myomectomy – The fibroids are removed, but the uterus is not. There are 3 approaches.
    - Laparascopic – A laparascope is used with a laser to remove the fibroids.

Fibroids, *Continued*

- Hysteroscopic – The fibroids are cut out and the uterine lining is destroyed by laser (ablation). This makes a woman sterile (no lining, no bleeding). Laser ablation can also be done with a small electrocautery ball. This is known as "Rollerball."

- Laparotomy – Surgery in which the abdomen is opened and the fibroids are removed under direct vision. Fibroids can still be present, grow, and cause future trouble.

• Hysterectomy – Surgery that removes the uterus and the fibroids with it. Depending on the size of the fibroids, this can be done:

  - Vaginally

  - Through abdominal surgery

A hysterectomy may be recommended when the fibroid is very large or when there is severe bleeding that can't be stopped by other treatments. This leaves a woman sterile. It is the only way to get rid of fibroids for sure. A hysterectomy may also be done in the rare occasion that the fibroid becomes cancerous.

Questions to Ask

Do you have severe abdominal pain? **YES** → Get Emergency Care

NO

Flowchart continued in next column

Do you have any of these problems?
• Heavy menstrual bleeding (you saturate a pad or tampon in less than an hour)
• Bleeding between periods or after intercourse
• Bleeding after menopause
• Anemia (noted by paleness, weakness, fatigue)

YES → See Doctor

NO

Do any of these things define the pain?
• It comes during sexual intercourse.
• It comes with your menstrual periods.
• It is in the lower back, and is not caused by strain or any other condition.

YES → See Doctor

NO

Do you have to urinate often or do you feel pressure on your bladder or rectum?

YES → See Doctor

NO

 Use Self-Care

Self-Care/Prevention Tips

Maintain a healthy body weight. The more body fat you have, the more estrogen your body is likely to have, which enhances fibroid growth.
■ Exercise regularly. This may reduce your body's fat and estrogen levels.
■ Follow a low-fat diet.

78 Menopause

Menopause is when a woman's menstrual periods stop altogether. It signals the end of fertility. A woman is said to have gone through menopause when her menstrual periods have stopped for an entire year. "The change," as menopause is often called, generally occurs between the ages of 45 and 55. It can occur as early as 35 or as late as 65 years of age, though. It can also result from the surgical removal of both ovaries. The physical and emotional signs and symptoms that go with "the change" usually span 1–2 years or more (perimenopause). They vary from woman to woman. The changes themselves are a result of a number of factors. These include hormone changes such as estrogen decline, the aging process itself, and stress.

Signs and Symptoms

Physical signs and symptoms associated with menopause are:

■ Hot flashes – Sudden waves of heat that can start in the waist or chest and work their way to the neck and face and sometimes the rest of the body. They are more common in the evening and during hot weather. They can hit as often as every 90 minutes. Each one can last from 15 seconds to 30 minutes – 5 minutes is average. Seventy-five to eighty percent of women going through menopause experience hot flashes. Hot flashes bother some women more than others. Sometimes heart palpitations accompany hot flashes.

■ Irregular periods – This varies and can include:

 • Periods that get shorter and lighter for 2 or more years

 • Periods that stop for a few months and then start up again and are more widely spaced

 • Periods that bring heavy bleeding and/or the passage of many or large blood clots. This can lead to anemia.

■ Vaginal dryness – This results from hormone changes. The vaginal wall also becomes thinner. These problems can make sexual intercourse painful or uncomfortable and can lead to irritation and increased risk for infection.

■ Loss of bladder tone, which can result in stress incontinence (leaking urine when you cough, sneeze, laugh, or exercise)

■ Headaches, dizziness

■ Skin and hair changes. Skin is more likely to wrinkle. Growth of facial hair, but thinning of hair in the temple region

■ Muscles lose some strength and tone

■ Bones become more brittle, increasing the risk for osteoporosis

■ Risk for a heart attack increases when estrogen levels drop

Emotional changes associated with menopause:

■ Irritability

■ Mood changes

■ Lack of concentration, difficulty with memory

■ Tension, anxiety, depression

■ Insomnia, which may result from hot flashes that interrupt sleep

Menopause, *Continued*

Treatment

Treatment for the symptoms of menopause varies from woman to woman. If symptoms cause little or no distress, medical treatment is not needed. Self-Care Tips (see next page) may be all that is required. Hormone replacement therapy (HRT) can reduce many of the symptoms of menopause. It also offers significant protection against osteoporosis and heart disease. The risk for heart attacks, for example, is reduced by 50% with HRT. Each woman should discuss the benefits and risks of HRT with her doctor. (See "Osteoporosis" on page 363 and "Chest Pain" on page 150.)

Medication to treat depression and/or anxiety may be warranted in some women. Also, certain sedative medicines can help with hot flashes.

Questions to Ask

Do you have any of these?
- Extreme pain during intercourse
- Pain or burning when urinating
- Thick, white, or colored vaginal discharge
- Fever and/or chills

YES → 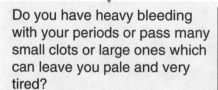 **See Doctor**

NO ↓

Do you have heavy bleeding with your periods or pass many small clots or large ones which can leave you pale and very tired?

YES → **Call Doctor**

NO ↓

Flowchart continued in next column

Have you begun menstrual periods again after going without one for 6 months?

YES →  **Call Doctor**

NO ↓

Are hot flashes severe, frequent, or persistent enough that they interfere with normal activities?

YES → **Call Doctor**

NO ↓

Do you have risk factors for osteoporosis?
- Family history of osteoporosis
- Small bone frame
- Thin
- Fair skin (Caucasian or Asian race)
- Had surgery to remove ovaries before normal menopause or menopause before 48 years of age
- Lack of calcium in diet
- Lack of weight-bearing exercise
- Alcohol abuse
- Hyperthyroidism
- Use of steroid medicine

YES → **Call Doctor**

NO ↓

Flowchart continued on next page

Menopause, *Continued*

Flowchart continued

If taking hormone replacement therapy (HRT), are you having any of the following?
• Side effects
• Return of menopausal symptoms

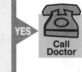
YES → **Call Doctor**

NO ↓

Use Self-Care

Self-Care Tips

To Reduce the Discomfort of Hot Flashes:

■ Wear lightweight clothes made of natural fibers.

■ Limit or avoid beverages that contain caffeine or alcohol.

■ Avoid rich and spicy foods and heavy meals.

■ Have cool drinks, especially water, when you feel a hot flash coming on and before and after exercising. Avoid hot drinks.

■ Keep cool. Open a window. Lower the thermostat when the heat is on. Use air conditioning and/or fans. Carry a small fan with you (hand or battery operated).

■ Try to relax when you get a hot flash. Getting stressed out over one only makes it worse.

■ Use relaxation techniques such as meditation, biofeedback, or yoga.

■ Ask your doctor about taking vitamin E.

■ Try having 1–2 servings per day of a food made with soy such as soy milk, soybeans, tofu, or miso.

If You Suffer from Night Sweats (Hot Flashes that Occur as You Sleep):

■ Wear loose-fitting cotton nightwear. Have changes of nightwear ready.

■ Sleep with only a top sheet, not blankets.

■ Keep the room cool.

To Deal with Vaginal Dryness and Painful Intercourse:

■ Don't use deodorant soaps or scented products in the vaginal area.

■ Use a water-soluble lubricant such as K-Y Jelly, Replens, etc. Avoid oils or petroleum-based products. They encourage infection.

■ Ask your doctor about intravaginal estrogen cream.

■ Remain sexually active. Having sex often may lessen the chance of having the vagina constrict, help keep natural lubrication, and maintain pelvic muscle tone. This includes reaching orgasm with a partner or alone.

■ Avoid using antihistamines unless truly necessary. They dry mucus membranes in the body.

To Deal with Emotional Symptoms:

■ Exercise regularly. This will also help maintain your body's hormonal balance and preserve bone strength.

■ Talk to other women who have gone through or are going through menopause. You can help each other cope.

■ Avoid stressful situations as much as possible.

■ Use relaxation techniques. Examples include yoga, meditation, listening to soft music and massages.

■ Eat nutritious foods. Check with your doctor about taking vitamin/mineral supplements.

79 Menstrual Cramps

Menstrual cramps are also called dysmenorrhea or painful periods. Most women experience them at some time during their life. They can range from very mild to severe. They may also differ from month to month or year to year. The pain felt during menstrual cramps may be accompanied by backache, fatigue, vomiting, diarrhea, and headaches. It can be made worse by premenstrual bloating (water retention).

Causes

There are two types of dysmenorrhea – primary and secondary. The primary form usually occurs in females who have just begun to menstruate. It may disappear or become less severe after a woman reaches her mid-twenties or gives birth. (Childbirth stretches the uterus.) The cause of menstrual cramps is thought to be related to hormonelike substances called prostaglandins. These are chemicals that occur naturally in the body. Certain prostaglandins cause muscles in the uterus to go into spasms.

Dysmenorrhea occurs much less often in women who do not ovulate. For this reason, oral contraceptives reduce painful periods in 70–80% of women who take them. When the pill is stopped, women usually get the same level of pain they had before they took it.

Secondary dysmenorrhea refers to menstrual cramps that are due to other disorders of the reproductive system, such as fibroids, endometriosis, ovarian cysts, and, rarely, cancer. Having an intrauterine device (IUD), especially if you've never been pregnant, can also cause menstrual cramps, except with the Progestasert IUD. It releases a small amount of progesterone into the uterus which helps with cramps and lightens menstrual flow.

Questions to Ask

Have your menstrual periods been especially painful since having an intrauterine contraceptive device (IUD) inserted? **YES** See Doctor

NO

Do you have any signs of infection such as fever and foul-smelling vaginal discharge or do you have black stools or blood in the stools? **YES** See Doctor

NO

For women who are still capable of bearing children: Do you have a heavier-than-usual blood flow or is your period late by 1 or more weeks? **YES** Call Doctor

NO

Flowchart continued on next page

Menstrual Cramps, *Continued*

Flowchart continued

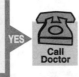

Is the pain extreme or have you had pain-free periods for years, but are now having severe cramps? **YES** → Call Doctor

NO ↓

Does cramping continue even after your period is over? **YES** → Call Doctor

NO ↓

Use Self-Care

Self-Care Tips

To Relieve Menstrual Cramps:

- Take over-the-counter ibuprofen or naproxen sodium around the clock as directed to relieve pain and inhibit the release of prostaglandins. Acetaminophen will help with pain, but not with prostaglandins. Most over-the-counter menstrual discomfort products contain acetaminophen. Read labels. {*Note:* See "Pain relievers" in "Your Home Pharmacy" on pages 22 and 23.}

- Drink a hot cup of regular tea or chamomile or mint tea.

- Hold a heating pad or hot-water bottle on your abdomen or lower back.

- Take a warm bath.

- Gently massage your abdomen.

- Do mild exercises like stretching, yoga, walking, or biking. Exercise may improve blood flow and reduce pelvic pain.

- Whenever possible, lie on your back, supporting your knees with a pillow.

- Get plenty of rest and avoid stressful situations as your period approaches.

- For birth control, consider using the pill because it blocks the production of prostaglandins, or the Progestasert IUD because its use lessens menstrual cramps.

If you still feel pain after using Self-Care Tips, call your doctor.

18. Women's Health Problems

80 Ovarian Cysts

18. Women's Health Problems

The ovaries are two almond-sized organs on either side of the uterus. They produce eggs and female hormones (estrogen, progesterone, and others). Growths called cysts can form in, on, or near the ovaries. Cysts are sacs filled with fluid or semisolid material. Ovarian cysts are commonly found in women in their reproductive years. Taking hormones does not cause cysts. Luckily, cysts are rarely cancerous.

Women more likely to get ovarian cysts are:

- Between the ages of 20 and 35

- Those who take a drug for epilepsy called Valporate. {*Note:* Do not stop taking this or any prescribed medicine without consulting your doctor.}

- Those who have endometriosis, pelvic inflammatory disease (PID), or the eating disorder bulimia

Signs and Symptoms

Most of the time, ovarian cysts are harmless and cause no symptoms. When symptoms do occur, they include:

- A feeling of fullness or swelling of the abdomen

- Weight gain

- A dull, constant ache on either or both sides of the pelvis

- Pain during intercourse

- Delayed, irregular, or painful menstrual periods

- Increased facial hair

- Sharp, severe abdominal pain, fever, and/or vomiting. This may be caused by a bleeding cyst or one that breaks or twists.

Ovarian cysts are of three basic types:

- Follicular and corpus luteum cysts. A follicular cyst is one in which the egg-making follicle of the ovary enlarges and fills with fluid. A corpus luteum cyst is a yellow mass of tissue that forms from the follicle after ovulation. These types of cysts come and go each month and are associated with normal ovarian function.

- Functional cysts. This is the most common type. These cysts are related to variations in the normal function of the ovaries. For example, they form when an egg fails to release as it should during normal ovulation. They can last 4–6 weeks. Rarely do they secrete hormones.

- Abnormal cysts, or neoplastic cysts. These result from cell growth and are mostly benign. In rare cases, they can be cancerous. Abnormal cysts require medical treatment by your doctor. Examples include:

  - Dermoid cysts. These consist of a growth filled with various types of tissue such as fatty material, hair, teeth, bits of bone and cartilage

  - Polycystic ovaries. These are caused by a buildup of multiple small cysts which cause hormonal imbalances that can result in irregular periods, body hair growth, and infertility

Ovarian Cysts, *Continued*

Detection

You can find out if you have ovarian cysts through:

- A pelvic exam. Your doctor can feel the size of your ovaries and discover abnormalities.

- An ultrasound. Sound waves create pictures of internal organs through a device placed on your abdomen or a probe inserted inside your vagina.

- A laparoscopy. A minor surgical procedure allows your doctor to see the structures inside your abdomen.

Treatment

Treatment for ovarian cysts will depend on:

- Size and type of cyst(s)

- Age and if you are in your reproductive years or have reached menopause

- Desire to have children

- Overall health status

- Severity of symptoms

Some cysts may resolve without any treatment in 1–2 months time. In others, hormone therapy with oral contraceptives may be tried to suppress cysts. If a cyst does not respond to this treatment, surgery may be needed to remove the cyst. If a cyst is found early, it may be removed leaving the ovary. Sometimes the ovary needs to be removed and surgery may include removal of the fallopian tube and uterus as well.

Questions to Ask

Do you have severe abdominal pain, fever, and vomiting? **YES** → See Doctor

NO

Do you have any of the following that are not due to other known reasons?
- Abdominal fullness or swelling
- Delayed, irregular, or painful menstrual periods
- Pain during intercourse
- Dull and constant ache on either or both sides of your pelvis

YES → Call Doctor

NO

 Use Self-Care

Self-Care/Prevention Tips

- Reduce caffeine intake.

- Have regular pelvic exams according to your doctor's recommendations.

- Take an over-the-counter medicine for pain. {*Note:* See "Pain relievers" in "Your Home Pharmacy" on pages 22 and 23.}

18. Women's Health Problems

81 Pelvic Inflammatory Disease (PID)

About one million American women have pelvic inflammatory disease (PID). It is an infection that goes up through the uterus to the fallopian tubes. One or more types of bacteria and/or other parasites are the culprits. These organisms can be carried by both women and men. They can be passed on to someone else who could then develop PID even when no symptoms are noticeable. When symptoms are present, they can vary from woman to woman. PID can be acute or chronic.

Symptoms

Symptoms of Acute PID:

- Pain in the abdomen or back (can be severe)
- Bad-smelling vaginal discharge
- Pain during intercourse
- Abdominal tenderness and/or bloating
- Difficult menstrual cramps
- High fever

Symptoms of Chronic PID:

- Pain (less severe) – often occurs halfway through the menstrual cycle or during a pelvic exam
- Skin on abdomen is sensitive
- Vaginal discharge
- Change in menstrual flow
- Nausea
- Low-grade fever

Causes

The causes of PID are:

- A sexually transmitted disease (STD) such as gonorrhea and chlamydia. The organisms that cause these STDs travel into the internal reproductive organs.

- Bacteria normally found in the intestines that get into the pelvic cavity. This most likely happens:

  - After sexual intercourse, especially having vaginal intercourse right after having anal intercourse

  - After getting an intrauterine device (IUD) put in or repositioned (low risk)

  - Because of high-risk sexual practices that increase the risk of infection, such as having multiple sex partners or having sex with a person who has many partners

  - Having had PID in the past or a recent bout with vaginitis

The symptoms of PID are a lot like those of other conditions, such as endometriosis (see page 229) and urinary tract infections (see page 174). This can make it hard to diagnose from symptoms alone. Your doctor may need to do special tests, such as an ultrasound, to find out if you have PID.

Pelvic Inflammatory Disease (PID), *Continued*

Treatment

Treatment for PID is antibiotics (sometimes more than one kind over a period of 3–4 weeks) and bed rest. If the infection is severe or if vomiting is present, intravenous (IV) antibiotics may need to be given in a hospital. Preventing further infections is important. This may include treatment for an infected sex partner so as not to get reinfected.

When PID is not treated, it can lead to blood poisoning, blood clots that break off and travel to the lungs, and bands of scar tissue in the pelvis. All of these can be life-threatening.

Permanent damage to a woman's reproductive organs and/or infertility can occur as well. Also, a woman who has had PID is at increased risk for:

- Ectopic or tubal pregnancy
- Premature labor and birth

Questions to Ask

Do you have 2 or more of the following?
- Pain in the abdomen or back (this may be severe)
- Bad-smelling vaginal discharge
- Pain during intercourse
- Abdominal tenderness and/or bloating
- Difficult menstrual cramps
- High fever

YES See Doctor

NO

Flowchart continued in next column

Do you have 2 or more of these problems?
- Pain in the abdomen or back halfway through your menstrual cycle
- Skin on your abdomen feels sensitive
- Vaginal discharge when you're not having a menstrual period
- Change in menstrual flow
- Low-grade fever

YES See Doctor

NO

Have you had an IUD inserted, especially within the last 20 days, and are you feeling discomfort from it?

YES See Doctor

NO

Have you had unprotected sex with someone who you think might have a sexually transmitted disease?

YES See Doctor

NO

 Use Self-Care

See Self-Care/Prevention Tips on next page

18. Women's Health Problems

241

Pelvic Inflammatory Disease (PID), *Continued*

Self-Care/Prevention Tips

- Wipe from front to back after a bowel movement to keep bacteria from the feces from entering the vagina.

- Change tampons and/or pads frequently when you menstruate.

- Don't have vaginal intercourse right after anal intercourse.

- Don't have sex with anyone who has not been treated for a current case of PID or STD or anyone who has partners that haven't been treated.

- Use barrier birth control methods with spermicides to reduce the risk of getting PID from an infected partner. These include the male or female condom, cervical cap, or diaphragm. Use these even if you use other contraceptives like the pill.

- If you use an IUD, have your doctor remove it if you become pregnant and then miscarry. If it is left in, your risk for PID goes up.

- Don't smoke. If you smoke, you may have a higher risk for PID.

- Don't douche. This may spread the organisms that cause infection, and in so doing, increase the risk for PID.

- Do not have sexual intercourse until the postpartum bleeding stops (after childbirth) or for 1 week after a D & C, abortion, or miscarriage. Use a condom for 2 weeks after having an IUD inserted.

- If you are at risk for PID get tested for chlamydia and gonorrhea when you get a yearly pap test. (See causes of PID on page 240).

82 Premenstrual Syndrome (PMS)

Four out of 10 menstruating women suffer from PMS (premenstrual syndrome). A syndrome is a group of signs and symptoms that indicate a disorder. There have been as many as 150 symptoms associated with PMS. The most common ones are:

- Irritability
- Anxicty
- Depression
- Headache
- Bloating
- Fatigue
- Feelings of hostility and anger
- Food cravings, especially for chocolate and sweet and salty foods

For some women, symptoms are slight and may last only a few days before menstruation. For others, they can be severe and last the whole 2 weeks before every period. Also worth noting is that other disorders women experience, such as arthritis or clinical depression, may be worse during this same premenstrual period. This is known as premenstrual magnification (PMM).

Causes

The exact cause or causes for PMS are not known. There are many theories. One points to low levels of the hormone progesterone. Others link it to nutritional or chemical deficiencies. One thing is certain, though, to be classified as PMS, symptoms must occur between ovulation and menstruation that is, anytime within 2 weeks before the menstrual period and disappear shortly after the period begins. PMS usually stops with menopause.

PMS is often confused with depression. An evaluation by your doctor can help with a correct diagnosis.

Treatment

Treatment for PMS may include:

- Medical management with medicines such as:
  - The prescribed hormone progesterone (suppositories or an oral form)
  - Water pills such as Spironolactone (Aldactone)
  - Antidepressant or antianxiety medicines
- Dietary measures such as:
  - Eating 5–6 light meals a day instead of 3 large ones. Not skipping meals.
  - Avoiding sweets
  - Limiting salt and fat
  - Avoiding caffeine and alcohol
  - Vitamin supplements.
  - Adequate intake of calcium and magnesium
- Lifestyle changes such as: regular exercise which includes 20 minutes of aerobic exercise, such as walking or aerobic dance, at least 3 times a week
- Limiting and learning to deal with stress

18. Women's Health Problems

Premenstrual Syndrome (PMS), *Continued*

Questions to Ask

Are symptoms of PMS such as anxiety, depression, and anger that leads to aggression making you feel suicidal? **YES** → Get Emergency Care

NO ↓

Do PMS symptoms make you feel out of control and unable to live your daily life? **YES** → See Doctor

NO ↓

Do you still have PMS symptoms after your period starts? **YES** → Call Doctor

NO ↓

Have you tried the Self-Care Tips and still don't feel better? **YES** → Call Doctor

NO ↓

Use Self-Care

Self-Care Tips

- Exercise 3 times a week for 20 minutes. Swimming, walking, and bicycling all relax your muscles and help you lose water weight.

- Eat 5–6 small meals a day instead of 3 large ones. Choose: whole grains, fruits, and vegetables; good food sources of calcium, such as skim milk, nonfat yogurt, collard greens, kale, calcium-fortified cereals and juices; and sources of magnesium, such as spinach, other green, leafy vegetables, and whole grain cereals.

- Limit salt, fat, and sugar. Doing so may help keep your breasts from getting sore.

- If you need to satisfy a food craving, do so in moderation. For example, if you crave chocolate, have a small chocolate bar or add chocolate syrup to skim milk. If you crave salt, eat a small bag of pretzels.

- Stay away from caffeine, alcohol, and cigarettes for 2 weeks before your period is due.

- The vitamins and minerals listed here seem to help some women. Ask your doctor if you should take any of them in supplement form and in what amounts.

  - Vitamin E
  - Vitamin B6
  - Calcium
  - Magnesium
  - L-tyrosine, an amino acid

- Take naps if you need to.

- Learn to relax. Try deep breathing, meditation, yoga, or taking a hot bath.

- Try to avoid stress when you have PMS.

83 Toxic Shock Syndrome

Toxic shock syndrome (TSS) is a potentially fatal disease that is caused by certain bacteria. It is a form of blood poisoning which results when poisons (toxins) are released by the suspect bacteria. It can result from wounds or infection in the throat, lungs, skin, or bone. Most often, though, it affects women of childbearing age, especially women who use superabsorbent tampons. These may trap the bacteria and provide a breeding ground for them, especially when the tampons are left in place for a long period of time. Also, the superabsorbent fibers in some tampons may cause microscopic tears in the vagina that allow the transmission of the bacteria's toxin. Though not common, TSS can also occur in persons following surgery including women who have had a cesarean section.

Symptoms

Symptoms come on fast and are often severe. They include:

- High, sudden fever
- Muscle aches
- Vomiting
- Diarrhea
- Sunburnlike rash, including peeling skin on hands and feet
- Rapid pulse
- Extreme fatigue and weakness
- Sore throat
- Dizziness
- Fainting
- Drop in blood pressure

Questions to Ask

Are symptoms (see "Symptoms" listed in left column) of toxic shock syndrome present? These could occur during your menstrual period or any other time of month.

YES — Get Emergency Care

NO — Use Self-Care

Self-Care/Prevention Tips

- Never use tampons if you've experienced TSS in the past.
- Use sanitary napkins instead of tampons whenever possible.
- Alternate tampons with sanitary pads or mini-pads during a menstrual period.
- Don't use superabsorbent tampons.
- Lubricate the tampon applicator with a water-soluble (nongreasy) lubricant like K-Y Jelly before insertion.
- Change tampons and sanitary pads every 4 to 6 hours or more often.

18. Women's Health Problems

84 Vaginal Yeast Infections

Yeast infections are the most common type of vaginal infections. Other names for this are Monilia, Candida, or fungus infection. Vaginal yeast infections result from the overgrowth of Candida albicans, which is normally present in harmless amounts in the vagina, the digestive tract, and the mouth.

Causes

- Hormonal changes that come with pregnancy or even before monthly periods
- Taking hormones or birth control pills
- Taking antibiotics
- Taking steroid medicines such as prednisone
- Having elevated blood sugar such as found in uncontrolled diabetes
- Vaginal intercourse, especially with inadequate lubrication
- Douching

Symptoms

- Itching, irritation, and redness around the outside of the genital area
- A thick, white discharge that looks like cottage cheese and may smell like yeast
- Burning and/or pain when you urinate or have sex

Prevention

- Practice good hygiene. Wash regularly to clean the inside folds of the vulva where germs are likely to grow. Dry the vaginal area thoroughly after you shower or bathe.
- Wipe from front to back after using the toilet.
- Wear all-cotton underpants and panty hose with cotton crotches.
- Don't wear slacks and shorts that are tight in the crotch and thighs, or other tight-fitting clothing such as panty girdles.
- Change underwear and workout clothes right away after exercising.
- Use unscented tampons or sanitary pads and change tampons and sanitary pads frequently.
- Don't use bath oils, bubble baths, feminine hygiene sprays or perfumed or deodorant soaps.
- Don't sit around in a wet bathing suit.
- Shower after you swim in a pool to remove the chlorine from your skin. Dry the vaginal area thoroughly.
- If you tend to get yeast infections whenever you take an antibiotic, ask your doctor to prescribe a vaginal antifungal agent or use an over-the-counter one.
- Eat well and include food products such as yogurt that contain live cultures of "lactobacillus acidophilus."
- Get plenty of rest to make it easier for your body to fight infections.

Treatment

Treatments for vaginal yeast infections are:

- Vaginal creams or suppositories that get rid of the Candida overgrowth. These can be over-the-counter ones (Examples: Monistat, Gyne-Lotrimin, etc.) or ones prescribed by your doctor, such as Terazol or Vagistat, etc.

Vaginal Yeast Infections, *Continued*

- Oral medicines, which include Diflucan (a pill taken once per episode of infection), Sporanox, Nystatin and Nizoral

- Gentian violet, a purple-colored solution applied to the vaginal area

Make sure that you have the right problem diagnosed. A burning sensation could be a symptom of a urinary tract infection caused by bacteria, which requires an antibiotic. Antibiotics will not help yeast infections. They make them worse. Know, too, that the STD trichomoniasis (see page 274) mimics yeast infections.

You should check with your doctor if:

- This is the first time you have symptoms of a yeast infection.

- You are not sure that your problem is a yeast infection.

- The infection does not respond to treatment or the infection you treat comes back within 2 months.

Chronic vaginal infections can be one of the first signs of diabetes, sexually transmitted diseases, or HIV/AIDS in women.

Questions to Ask

Do you have any other symptoms, such as vaginal swelling and/or unusual bleeding? Does the discharge have a foul-smelling odor? **YES** See Doctor

NO

Flowchart continued in next column

Do symptoms of a vaginal yeast infection worsen or continue 1 week or longer despite using Self-Care Tips or do they come back within 2 months after treatment? **YES** See Doctor

NO

Use Self-Care

Self-Care Tips

- Use an over-the-counter vaginal cream medicine or suppositories, such as Monistat, as directed. These used to be available only with a prescription. Women who have had yeast infections whenever they have taken antibiotics in the past should use this during the period of antibiotic treatment.

- Douche with a mild solution of 1–3 tablespoons of vinegar diluted in a quart of warm water. Repeat only once a day until the symptoms subside, but not longer than a week. Too much douching can lead to a flare-up of the infection.

- Limit your intake of sugar and foods that contain sugar, since sugar promotes the growth of yeast.

- Eat yogurt and other food items that contain live cultures of lactobacillus acidophilus several times daily, especially when taking an antibiotic. If you can't tolerate yogurt, ask your pharmacist for an over-the-counter product that contains this beneficial bacteria (lactobacillus acidophilus).

85 Bed-Wetting

The medical word for bed-wetting is enuresis. No one really knows why it happens. From the 1930s to the 1960s, people thought emotional problems caused bed-wetting. Many people think differently now. Bed-wetting may happen because the child is slow to get control over his or her bladder. Here are some facts on bed-wetting:

- Three out of four children stay dry all night by age 3½.

- Only 1 out of 5 five-year-olds wets the bed.

- Only 1 out of 10 six-year-olds wets the bed.

- Bed-wetting almost always stops by puberty.

- More boys than girls wet the bed.

- Your child may start wetting the bed again when he or she is upset.

- Bed-wetting runs in families.

Children don't wet their beds on purpose. A wet bed is uncomfortable, and it makes the child feel ashamed. Children more than 3 years old feel very bad when they wet their beds. Children who wet their beds may be afraid to go to pajama parties, friends' houses, or camp.

Sometimes bed-wetting means your child is sick. If your child has always stayed dry before, wetting the bed could be a sign of a urinary tract infection or diabetes. Sometimes the child's bladder is just too small. {*Note:* Bed-wetting after successful toilet training is sometimes associated with child sexual abuse.}

Questions to Ask

Does your child have these problems?
- Drinks a lot of liquids
- Goes to the bathroom more than normal in the day or night
- Acts very tired
- Eats a lot more than normal and gains weight
- Itches around the groin

YES → **See Doctor**

NO ↓

Does your child have these problems?
- A fever
- Stomach pain
- Burning when he or she goes to the bathroom

YES → **See Doctor**

NO ↓

Is your child older than 6 and has never been dry at night? Or has he or she started wetting the bed again after being dry for a long time?

YES → **Call Doctor**

NO ↓

 Use Self-Care

See Self-Care Tips on next page

Bed-Wetting, *Continued*

Self-Care Tips

It helps to be patient and give your child lots of love. Children who wet the bed can't help it. They don't do it on purpose. Getting mad only makes the problem worse.

Doctors say to just wait. Don't praise the child for a dry bed or punish the child for a wet bed.

Try these tips:

- Try to get your child to not drink more than 2 ounces of fluid during the 2 hours before going to bed.

- Make sure your child goes to the bathroom before bed.

- Help your child remember to do what the doctor tells them to do. (Sometimes the doctor can give your child exercises to do.)

- Have your child change the bed or pajamas during the night if they get wet. Or keep a flannel-covered rubber sheet near the bed. Your child can put this over a wet sheet.

- Set an alarm clock to wake your child 2 or 3 hours after they fall asleep. Then your child can get up and go to the bathroom.

- Consider getting a bed-wetting alarm if your child is 5 years old or older. The child wears the alarm on his or her underwear. The first drop makes the alarm buzz, so the child wakes up. After a while, the child learns to wake up when he or she has to urinate. Some of these alarms help prevent wet beds 85 to 90 percent of the time.

- You can get bed-wetting alarms and information from:

  - Nite Train'r Alarm: Koregon Enterprises, 9735 S.W. Sunshine Court, Suite 100 Beaverton, OR 97005 or call 1-800-544-4240.

  - Nytone Alarm: Nytone Medical Products, 2424 South 900 West Salt Lake City, UT 84119 or call 1-801-973-4090.

  - Wet-Stop Alarm: Palco Laboratories, 8030 Soquel Ave. Santa Cruz, CA 95062 or call 1-800-346-4488.

  - Check local home medical supply companies and drug stores, too.

19. Children's Health Problems

86 Chicken Pox

Chicken pox is a disease caused by a virus. It is very contagious. Someone can give you chicken pox by sneezing or coughing near you. You can also catch it from an infected person's clothes or from touching their blisters. You will know your child has chicken pox 7–21 days after they catch it.

Signs and Symptoms

A rash is usually the first sign that something is wrong. (See chart on skin rashes on page 113.) But some children feel tired, or get a fever or stomachache 1 to 2 days before the rash starts. The rash starts out flat and red. It usually starts on the head, face, and back. But the rash can go anywhere. Some children get small sores in their mouth, on their eyelids, or around the groin.

Soon the red spots turn into clear blisters that itch a lot. When your child scratches, the blisters break and make hard crusts. The crusts fall off in about 2 weeks. Your child will keep getting new sores for 2–6 days. Some children get chicken pox all over. Others don't. Children can give chicken pox to someone else before the rash develops and up until all of the blisters are crusted over.

Treatment

Most children get over chicken pox without any problems. Sometimes chicken pox can lead to encephalitis, a brain infection. Other problems are meningitis and pneumonia. But usually the biggest problem is infected blisters. (See the Self-Care Tips on pages 251 and 252 in this section.)

If your child gets chicken pox once, they will probably be immune to it. If they do get it again, it won't be as bad the second time.

Your child's doctor can give your child a prescription to control the chicken pox. But this is not a good idea most of the time. Also, your child has to take it during the first 24 hours of the illness. (Your child will still be immune to chicken pox later.) Ask your child's doctor for more information.

Prevention

A vaccine called Varivax can prevent chicken pox. (See "Immunization Schedule" on page 18.)

The only other way to prevent chicken pox is to keep your child away from people who have it. This is not a good idea, though. It is much better for people to get chicken pox when they are young. Chicken pox is much more serious in adults.

Take special care to keep your child with chicken pox away from adults, older people, and pregnant women who have never had chicken pox. And, keep your child away from people who are sick or taking medicines that make it harder for their bodies to fight off illnesses. If your child has cancer, or takes medicine that causes weakness, he or she may have more problems with chicken pox.

Chicken Pox, *Continued*

Questions to Ask

Does your child have these problems?
- Very bad headache
- Stiff neck and fever
- Convulsions
- Acts strange
- Throws up over and over

YES 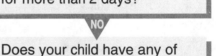 → Get Emergency Care

NO

Is it hard to wake up your child?
Is your child confused?
Is it hard for your child to breathe?

YES → Get Emergency Care

NO

Does your child have cancer or take medicine that makes it easier to get sick? And does your child have a fever higher than 102°F?

YES → Get Emergency Care

NO

Does your child have cancer or take medicine that makes it easier to get sick? And does your child have a fever of 102°F or less?

YES → See Doctor

NO

Flowchart continued in next column

Does your child have a fever higher than 103°F? Or has your child had a 102°F fever for more than 2 days?

YES → See Doctor

NO

Does your child have any of these problems?
- Red scabs
- Sores that bleed or have pus
- A red rash with tiny pink dots

YES → Call Doctor

NO

Is the person with the chicken pox an adult?

YES → Call Doctor

NO

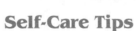
Use Self-Care

Self-Care Tips

The tips below will help you comfort your child. They will help with the itching so your child won't scratch so much. (Scratching the scabs can start another infection or leave scars.)

■ Keep your child busy. He or she can't scratch if his or her hands are busy. And he or she won't think about the itching so much.

■ Give your child a cool bath without soap every 3 or 4 hours. Do this the first 2 days. Keep your child in the bath for 15–20 minutes. Add ½ cup of baking soda or an oatmeal bath to the water. (Aveeno is one brand of oatmeal bath.) Pat your child dry. Don't rub.

19. Children's Health Problems

Chicken Pox, *Continued*

- Put a cool, wet washcloth on the itchy places.

- Put calamine lotion on the itchy places. Don't use Caladryl lotion.

- Keep your child's fingernails short so it is harder to scratch.

- If your child is a baby, cover the baby's hands with cotton socks to prevent scratching.

- Wash your child's hands 3 times a day. Use a soap that kills germs, like Safeguard or Dial. This helps keep germs away from the sores.

- Keep your child cool and calm. The itching gets worse when your child is hot and sweaty.

- Keep your child out of the sun. The sun makes the rash worse.

- You may choose to give your child Benadryl if the itching is very bad. Benadryl is an over-the-counter antihistamine. Use the liquid Benadryl that your child can take by mouth. Read the directions on the label.

- Give your child acetaminophen for the fever. Here are some brands: Tylenol, Tempra, Liquiprin, Datril, Anacin 3. Whatever brand you buy, be sure to buy the children's kind. {*Note:* Do not give aspirin to anyone under 19 years old. Aspirin and other medicines that have salicylates have been linked to Reye's Syndrome, a condition that can kill. This link has been noted when aspirin was taken during a viral infection such as chicken pox.}

- Give your child soft foods and cold drinks for mouth sores. Don't give your child salty foods, or fruits like oranges and grapefruit.

- Have your child gargle with salt water if his or her mouth itches. (Put $1/2$ teaspoon of salt in 1 cup of water.)

- Tell your child that the "bumps" will go away in a week or so. Tell your child not to worry.

87 Colic

When your baby cries and cries for no reason this may be due to colic. Your baby may pull his or her knees up to the stomach. Usually, colic attacks start in the evening. Colic is very hard on parents.

Nothing seems to help when your baby has colic – not feeding, changing the diaper, or cuddling. But don't worry. Colic is hardly ever dangerous. And it doesn't last long. Colic usually starts after the baby is 2 weeks old. It is worst at about 3 months. It usually goes away when the baby is 4 months old.

Causes

No one knows why babies get colic. It may be any or all of these problems:

- The baby can't digest its food.
- The baby has an allergy to some food.
- The baby has gas in its stomach.
- The baby doesn't get enough sleep.
- Noises in the house bother the baby.

When a colic attack is over, the baby may pass gas or have a full diaper.

Sometimes a colicky baby has a bigger problem. There may be something blocking the bowel, so the baby can't pass stool. A doctor can examine your baby and run tests for this and other medical problems.

Prevention

- Have your baby sit up at feeding time. This way, the baby will swallow less air.
- If you are breast-feeding, try these tips:
  - Cut down on cola, coffee, cocoa, and tea.

- Stop eating foods that have milk for a week. The baby's colic may go away. (Make sure you check with your doctor before you try this. He or she may want you to take extra calcium.)
- Don't make the baby's milk or formula too hot.
- Check the nipple on your baby's bottle. If the hole is too small, the baby will swallow air.
- Try a new formula.
- Try to make things quiet and calm when you feed your baby.
- Burp the baby more often.

Questions to Ask

Does your infant show any of these signs?
- Is hard to arouse or wake up
- Stares off into space
- Is unable to be normally active

YES → **Get Emergency Care**

NO ↓

Do you feel out of control and are you tempted to hit the baby?

YES → **See Doctor**

NO ↓

Is the baby doing any of these things?
- Throwing up
- Having diarrhea
- Passing black or bloody stool

YES → **See Doctor**

NO ↓

Flowchart continued on next page

19. Children's Health Problems

Colic, *Continued*

Flowchart continued

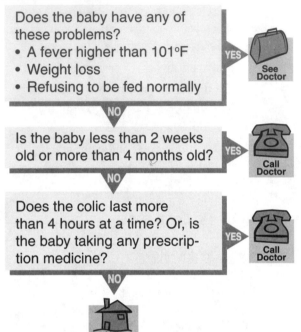

Does the baby have any of these problems?
- A fever higher than 101°F
- Weight loss
- Refusing to be fed normally

YES → See Doctor

NO ↓

Is the baby less than 2 weeks old or more than 4 months old?

YES → Call Doctor

NO ↓

Does the colic last more than 4 hours at a time? Or, is the baby taking any prescription medicine?

YES → Call Doctor

NO ↓

Use Self-Care

Self-Care Tips

Stay calm. Try to relax. It is hard to deal with a screaming baby. None of these tips will cure colic, but they may help.

- Be sure the baby has enough to eat. He or she may just be hungry.
- Try different bottle nipples. Make the hole bigger if it is too small. Cut across the hole that is already there. (You will make an X-shaped hole.) Here's how to find out if the hole is too small:
  - Put cold formula in the bottle.
  - Turn the bottle upside down and shake it or squeeze it.

  - Count the drops of formula that fall out. There should be 1 drop each second. If the drops come out slower than that, the hole is too small.
- Hold your baby up for feeding. Keep holding the baby up for a while after feeding.
- Burp your baby after each ounce of formula. Burp the baby every few minutes when breast-feeding.
- Use a pacifier. But never put a pacifier on a string around the baby's neck.
- Wrap the baby in a blanket and rock him or her. Or put the baby in a baby swing.
- Try the "colic carry." Lay the baby on its stomach across your arm. Put the baby's face in your hand and let the legs straddle your inner elbow. Hold the baby's back with your other hand so he or she won't fall. Walk around like this for a while.
- Carry the baby while you vacuum. Use a baby carrier that you wear on your back or chest.
- Play soft, gentle music. This may help you and the baby.
- Take your baby outside for a ride in the stroller or car.
- Run the dryer or dishwasher. Buckle your baby in a baby seat. Lean the seat against the side of the dryer or on the counter near the dishwasher. Stay with your baby. Make sure the heat or steam won't hurt the baby.
- Don't give the baby antacids like Maalox or simethicone drops unless a doctor tells you to.
- Let your baby cry him-or herself to sleep if nothing else helps. But call the doctor if the baby cries for more than 4 hours.
- Get someone else to take care of your baby if you get too stressed. Get some rest.

88 Croup

Croup is a viral infection that children can get between 3 months and 3 years old. The infection makes your child's throat give off mucus. The mucus gets dry and thick and makes it hard for your child to breathe. Your child gasps for air and makes a high, whistling sound like a seal's bark. Croup is scary, but not usually dangerous.

Steam can make the mucus soft and wet again. Sometimes you can make your child better with steam. (See the Self-Care Tips on page 256 of this section.) Children usually stop getting croup as they get older and their windpipe becomes wider.

Croup usually goes away in 3 to 7 days and is usually worse at night. Sometimes the doctor can give your child a prescription when the croup starts. This may help your child feel better.

Sometimes your child shows the signs of croup, but something else is wrong. Your child may have one of these problems:

- Epiglottitis. This looks like croup but is more serious. Children who are more than 3 years old can get it. Epiglottitis is when the piece of skin at the back of the throat swells up and blocks the throat. If the throat is blocked, it can also stop your child's breathing. Here are some signs of epiglottitis:

  - Drooling

  - Hanging the head down

  - Sticking out the jaw when breathing

  - Fever

- Something may be stuck in your child's windpipe. Get help right away if this happens.

Prevention

- Run a humidifier near your child's bed if he or she has croup. Do this many nights in a row. If your child has a fever, use a "cool-mist" vaporizer instead. Clean it every day.

- Buy a humidifier for your furnace. Change the filter often.

Questions to Ask

Does your child have any of these problems?
- Works very hard to breathe
- Can't swallow

YES → Get Emergency Care

↓ **NO**

Is your child doing these things?
- Drooling
- Breathing through the mouth
- Sticking the chin out
- Gasping for air

YES → Get Emergency Care

↓ **NO**

Are your child's lips and nails turning blue or dark?

YES → Get Emergency Care

↓ **NO**

Flowchart continued on next page

Croup, *Continued*

Flowchart continued

Does your child still make sounds like a barking seal and have trouble breathing after you have:
- Used steam for 15 minutes or more, or
- Taken your child out in the cold night air for 15 minutes

YES → **Get Emergency Care**

NO

Does your child make a high, whistling sound like a barking seal?

YES → **See Doctor**

NO

Use Self-Care

Self-Care Tips

■ Don't panic. You can help your child stay calm if you stay calm.

• Hold your child to comfort him or her. The windpipe may open up a little if your child relaxes.

■ Use a hot bath or shower:

• Go into the bathroom with your child and close the door.

• Turn on the hot water in the sink and shower. Let the steam fill the room.

• Don't put your child in the shower. Sit with your child on the toilet or in a chair. (Don't sit on the floor.) Read a book or play a game with your child. This will help pass the time.

• Open the window to let in cool air. This helps make more steam.

• Stay in the bathroom about 15 minutes. Or take your child outside if the air is cool. Let him or her breathe the cold night air. Get emergency care if this doesn't help.

■ Use a vaporizer in your child's room. "Cool-mist" vaporizers are safer than hot ones. Use distilled water, not tap water. Clean the vaporizer every day.

■ Give your child clear liquids, such as apple juice or tea. Warm the clear liquid first. Warm liquids may help loosen the mucus.

■ Crying is a good sign. It means your child is getting better.

19. Children's Health Problems

89 Lice

Head lice are bugs about the size of a sesame seed. They live on blood from people. Louse bites cause very bad itching and red spots that look like mosquito bites. You hardly ever see adult lice. Instead, you see "nits." Nits are lice eggs on the hair. Nits look like dandruff.

Nits on hair shaft (actual size)

Lice spread fast. No matter how clean your child is, he or she can get lice. Your child can get lice at school or from anyone who has lice. Lice lay about 6 eggs a day. The eggs hatch in 8–10 days. Then they start biting.

There are 3 kinds of lice:

- Head lice, which are the most common with children in day-care centers and schools
- Pubic lice, which live in the hair around the groin. They are called "crabs," because they look like crabs.
- Body lice, which live in dirty clothes and bedding

Prevention

Tell your child:

- Don't share hats, brushes, or combs.
- Don't lie on a pillow that another child uses.
- Wash your hair and bathe often.

You should:

- Change bed sheets often. Wash them in hot water and dry them in a dryer.
- Vacuum furniture, mattresses, rugs, stuffed animals, and car seats if anyone in your family has lice. Don't use bug spray on lice.

- As soon as you know your child has lice, call anyone who may have been close to your child. Be sure to call your child's school or child-care center, and neighbors and parents of your child's friends.
- Wash combs and brushes. Then soak them in hot (not boiling) water for 10 minutes.
- Check your children for head lice and nits once a week. Check more often if your child scratches his or her head. Look for nits behind the ears and on the back of the neck. Spread hairs apart with round toothpicks to look for the nits. Check your child's eyelashes if nits are found in the hair.

Questions to Ask

Does your child have any of these signs?
- Open sores on the head from scratching
- Lice or nits in the eyebrows or eyelashes, or on the skin
- Red bite marks
- Swollen lymph glands in the neck

YES →  Call Doctor

NO ↓

Does the child with lice have allergies or other health problems, or is your child under 2 years old?

YES → Call Doctor

NO ↓

Use Self-Care

See Self-Care Tips on next page

19. Children's Health Problems

Lice, *Continued*

Self-Care Tips

Only insecticidal shampoos, lotions, and creams kill lice. These products are made just for lice. You can buy them over-the-counter at your drug store. Your child's doctor can also give you a prescription for shampoo to treat lice and kill nits. Use them with caution and only as directed.

Check everyone in your home for lice and nits. But only treat those who have lice. The lice-killing products won't keep lice away.

To use an insecticidal shampoo:

■ Follow the directions, and:

- Take off your child's shirt.

- Give your child a towel to cover the eyes. Keep the shampoo away from the eyes.

- Lean your child over the sink. Don't put your child in the shower or bathtub. The shampoo is only for the head and neck.

■ Don't use too much shampoo. You will make your child's head too dry.

■ Wear gloves if you have open sores on your hands. Or have someone else shampoo your child's head and neck.

To take off the nits:

■ Shine a flashlight on the hair roots. Nits may be gray and hard to see. They are even harder to see in blond hair.

■ Start at one spot and go row by row, or even strand by strand.

■ Use tweezers, safety nail scissors, a nit comb, or your fingernails. (You can get a nit comb at the drug store.) Some products come with a nit-comb.

- Dip the comb in vinegar first. This will help loosen the nits.

- Comb the hair from the roots to the ends. Check the comb for nits after each pass.

- Or, divide the hair into 4 or 5 sections with hair clips. Lift about an inch of hair up and out. Put the comb against your child's head. Comb all the way to the tips of the hair. Keep going until you've done the whole head.

- Soak all combs, brushes, and barrettes for 1 to 2 hours in the insecticidal shampoo. Or, soak them 10 minutes in hot water.

■ Check for nits every day for 10 days.

■ Shampoo again a week later to kill any newly hatched nits. You don't have to remove nits after treatment is finished except for cosmetic reasons.

You should also:

■ Wash bedding and clothes right away in water hotter than 125°F. Heat kills the lice and nits. If you can't wash something, put it in a sealed plastic bag. Make sure no air gets in. Don't open it for at least 2 weeks. The lice will die without blood.

■ Dry-clean clothes and hats that you can't wash.

■ Vacuum all mattresses, pillows, rugs, and cloth-covered furniture. Do this especially where children play. Use the long, thin piece to suck the lice or nits out of car seats, toys, stuffed animals, etc. Put the vacuum cleaner bags outside in the trash.

19. Children's Health Problems

90 Measles

Measles is a very contagious disease caused by the rubeola virus. Also called red or seven-day measles, it mostly occurs in children, but can affect older persons, too. Persons who receive recommended immunizations will probably never get the measles. So make sure your child gets these shots. (See "Immunization Schedule" on page 18.)

Symptoms

When a child does get the measles, he or she has probably been exposed to someone else who had them 10–12 days earlier. The symptoms of measles usually take place in this order:

- Temperature of 102°F or higher
- Fatigue
- Loss of appetite
- Runny nose and sneezing
- Cough
- Red eyes and sensitivity to light
- Tiny white spots (called Koplik spots) in the mouth and throat
- Blotchy red rash that starts on the face and spreads to the rest of the body: to the chest and abdomen and then to the arms and legs. The rash usually lasts for up to 7 days.

The measles virus is spread by nose, mouth, or throat secretions, either on soiled articles or through coughing, sneezing, and so on. It can be picked up 3 to 6 days before the rash appears as well as up to several days after the rash starts.

If your child has been exposed to measles, but hasn't been immunized, contact his or her doctor or the public health department. If done early enough, a measles vaccine may prevent him or her from getting measles. An injection of gamma globulin can help protect your child against measles for 3 months. Let your child's school know if your child has measles. All cases of measles must be reported to the public health department.

When your child gets the measles, not much can be done to shorten the illness. Your child will probably start feeling better by the fourth day of the rash unless other problems occur. Possible problems include eye or ear infections, pneumonia, and meningitis.

Questions to Ask

Are any of these problems present:
- Blue or purple lips or nails
- Convulsion
- Extreme difficulty in breathing
- Inability to speak more than 3 or 4 words between breaths
- Confusion or excessive drowsiness
- Severe headache and stiff neck
- Bleeding from the nose or mouth or into the skin
- Dark purple splotches on the skin

YES → Get Emergency Care

NO

Flowchart continued on next page

Measles, *Continued*

Flowchart continued

Are any of these problems present?
- Sore throat
- Earache or tugging at the ears
- A yellow or green discharge from the eyes or nose
- Breathing that is labored, but not due to a stuffy nose
- Fever that comes back after temperature has been normal for a day or more or fever that is still present beyond the fourth day of the rash

YES → **See Doctor**

NO → **Use Self-Care**

Self-Care Tips

■ Keep a record of your child's temperature. Take it in the morning and the evening. Give the recommended dose of acetaminophen for fever and/or aches and pains. {*Note:* Do not give aspirin or any medication that has salicylates to anyone under 19 years of age, unless a doctor tells you to.}

■ Isolate your child from other people who have not had measles or a measles immunization. Any child who has come in contact with your child should be taken for a measles immunization unless he or she has already been immunized or had the measles.

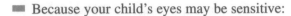

■ Because your child's eyes may be sensitive:
- Keep the lighting in the house dim. Draw the drapes, pull the shades down, and use low-wattage light bulbs.
- If your child must go outdoors, have him or her wear sunglasses.
- Keep the TV and video games turned off.
- Urge your child not to read or do close-up work.
- Wipe your child's closed eyes with a clean, wet cloth or wet cotton ball several times a day.

■ For a cough:
- Use a "cool-mist" vaporizer, especially at night. Use distilled, not tap, water in the vaporizer and change the water daily.
- If your child is 5 years of age or older, have him or her suck on cough drops, lozenges or hard candy.
- Give your child plenty of fluids. Water is helpful in loosening mucus and also soothes an irritated throat. Fruit juices and even tea and soda are also good.
- Give your child cough medicines as recommended by his or her doctor or pharmacist.
- You can make your own cough medicine at home by mixing 1 part lemon juice and 2 parts honey or corn syrup. (Do not give to children under 1 year of age.)

■ Have your child rest until the fever and rash go away.
- Keep your child home from school until 7–10 days after the fever and rash disappear and until his or her appetite, strength, and feeling of well-being are back to normal.

91 Tonsillitis

The tonsils are masses of tissue at the back of the throat. They act as a filter to help prevent infections in the throat, mouth, and sinuses from spreading to other parts of the body. They also produce antibodies that fight throat and nose infections. Tonsillitis occurs when the tonsils get inflamed. The cause for this is a bacterial or viral infection.

Symptoms

Symptoms of tonsillitis include:

- Mild to severe throat pain
- Swollen lymph glands on either side of the neck or jaw
- Ear pain
- Difficulty in swallowing
- Chills and fever
- Headache

A throat culture is necessary to diagnose the cause of tonsillitis. Antibiotics are prescribed for strep or other bacterial infections, but not for viral ones.

More often than not, having tonsillitis, even when it recurs up to 7 times a year, does not mean that the tonsils should be removed (in a surgical procedure called a tonsillectomy). Don't pressure your child's doctor to remove your child's tonsils just because this was commonly done years ago. Only under certain medical conditions should a tonsillectomy be done.

Questions to Ask

Is the tonsillitis severe and/or are these problems present?
- Extreme difficulty in swallowing
- Inability to swallow saliva
- Difficulty in breathing
- Inability to say more than 3 or 4 words between breaths
- Drooling

YES → Get Emergency Care

NO ↓

Is your child unable to fully open his or her mouth? **YES** → 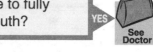 See Doctor

NO ↓

Does your child have large tonsils that:
- Touch each other when not infected, or
- Result in continued mouth breathing, or
- Muffle speech, which is due to no other cause

YES → See Doctor

NO ↓

Has the child with tonsillitis had rheumatic fever or a heart murmur? **YES** → See Doctor

NO ↓

Flowchart continued on next page

19. Children's Health Problems

261

Tonsillitis, *Continued*

Flowchart continued

Are any of the following present with the tonsillitis:
- Fever
- Swollen, enlarged, or tender neck glands
- Headache
- Ear pain or tugging at the ears
- Bad breath
- Loss of appetite
- Vomiting or abdominal pain

YES →  See Doctor

NO

Do the tonsils or back of the throat look bright red or have visible pus deposits?

YES → See Doctor

NO

Does someone else in the family have strep throat or does your child get strep throat often?

YES → Call Doctor

NO

Has your child's sore throat lasted more than 2 weeks even though it is mild?

YES → Call Doctor

NO

 Use Self-Care

Self-Care Tips

You can take some steps to relieve your child's discomfort from tonsillitis. Have him or her:

- Gargle every few hours with a solution of $1/4$ teaspoon of salt dissolved in 4 ounces of warm water, if your child is older than 8 years.

- Drink plenty of warm beverages such as tea (with or without honey) and soup, if tolerated. (Do not give honey to a child under 1 year of age.)

- Use a "cool-mist" vaporizer or humidifier in the room where he or she spends most of his or her time. (Use distilled water in it and clean after each use.)

- Eat foods that are soft and/or cold and easy to swallow (e.g., juices, popsicles, and ice cream). Avoid spicy foods.

- Suck on a piece of hard candy or medicated lozenge occasionally (if your child is 5 years of age or older). Corn syrup can be used periodically for younger children.

- Take the recommended dosage of acetaminophen for pain and/or fever. {*Note:* Do not give aspirin or any medication that has salicylates to anyone under 19 years of age, unless a doctor tells you to.}

- Avoid throat sprays. These may contain benzocaine, which could cause an adverse reaction.

- Avoid secondhand cigarette smoke.

92 Wheezing

Wheezing is a high purring or whistling sound. You hear it more on breathing out than in. Air flowing through swollen or tight breathing tubes usually causes wheezing.

Wheezing sounds like other problems. Croup sounds like wheezing. A high cough goes with croup. A stuffed nose makes a snorting sound. Mucus in the windpipe makes a rattling sound.

Wheezing means it is hard for your child to breathe. Check with the doctor if your child wheezes.

What Causes Wheezing?

- Asthma – This is the number 1 cause of wheezing. Most children grow out of asthma. But it sometimes comes back after they are grown up. Asthma attacks are scary. They can be serious, too. But they hardly ever kill. Here are some things that can cause an asthma attack:

  - Respiratory tract infection or bronchitis

  - Your child gets near something he or she is allergic to, like dust mites, pollen, mold, food, animals, perfume, etc.

  - Exercising too hard

  - Some medicines

  - Getting upset

  - A change in the weather

  - Smells from wet paint, cleaners, bug sprays, smoke, burning coals, car exhaust, wood smoke, etc.

- Ice-cold drinks or cold air. These can sometimes make breathing tubes close up.

- Respiratory tract infection

- Something caught in the windpipe

- A lung problem the child was born with

- Pneumonia

Questions to Ask

Is your child turning blue or not breathing?

YES → Get Emergency Care

NO

{*Note:* Do rescue breathing if your child has stopped breathing until emergency care comes or until your child starts breathing on his or her own. See "Airways and Breathing" on pages 285 and 286.}

Did your child's wheezing start during the last few hours? Is your child coughing up bubbly pink or white phlegm?

YES → Get Emergency Care

 NO

Does your child have any of these problems?
- Very bad wheezing
- Shortness of breath
- Can't talk

YES → Get Emergency Care

NO

Does your child have a fever over 101°F?

YES → 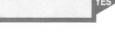 See Doctor

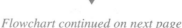 **NO**

Flowchart continued on next page

Wheezing, *Continued*

Flowchart continued

If your child has asthma, is the wheezing getting worse? Or is your child not getting better with treatment?

YES → Call Doctor

NO → Use Self-Care

Self-Care Tips

There is no cure for viral infections, allergies, or asthma. But you can help your child's wheezing:

■ Try to get your child to drink lots of liquids. These help thin the mucus. Get your child to sip juice, water, soup, or weak tea. Don't give your child ice-cold drinks.

■ Set up a "cool-mist" vaporizer. Clean it every day. Or take your child to the bathroom and turn on the hot water in the sink and shower. (See the Self-Care Tips for Croup on page 256.)

■ If your child has asthma, do what your child's doctor says, and:

• Stay calm. Use the bronchodilator the way the doctor told you.

• Keep your child away from things the child is allergic to.

• Mix 3/4 cup of bleach in a gallon of water. Wipe the bathroom tiles, kitchen stove, sink, woodwork, etc. Do this anyplace that fungus or mold grows. Then air out the room.

• Keep pets outside or away from your child if he or she is allergic to them. Be sure to keep pets out of your child's bedroom.

• Vacuum often to suck up dust mites, pollen, and pet dander. Put a filter mask on your child before you start to vacuum.

• Put a plastic cover on your child's mattress and pillow. Wash mattress pads in hot water every week.

• Quit smoking. Even old smoke in a room can make your child wheeze.

• Use throw rugs that you can wash instead of carpeting. Keep them clean.

• Put an air conditioner or electronic air filter on your furnace.

• Change or wash furnace and air conditioner filters often.

• Use a doctor-approved air purifier in your child's room.

• Use foam pillows, not feather pillows.

• Have your child shower, shampoo hair, and put on clean clothes after being near things the child is allergic to.

■ If exercise caused the wheezing, have your child:

• Avoid exercise in cold weather.

• Swim. Pool areas have moist air, which is easier to breathe.

• Start out any kind of exercise slowly and work up.

• Take prescribed medicine about 15 minutes before exercise.

■ Small children get things like small toy parts and foods like peanuts and popcorn stuck in their windpipe. Keep these things away from small children.

19. Children's Health Problems

93 Basic Facts about STDs

Infections that pass from one person to another during sexual contact are known as sexually transmitted diseases (STDs). Sexual contact includes vaginal, anal, and oral sex.

Sexually transmitted diseases include chlamydia, gonorrhea, genital herpes, syphilis, and trichomoniasis. These are presented separately on pages 266 through 275. HIV/AIDS is often classified as a sexually transmitted disease, but can be passed through means other than sexual contact. So, though mentioned at times, it is not defined here. (See "HIV/AIDS" on page 356.) Note, though, that the Self-Care/Prevention Tips on page 275 in this chapter can help prevent sexually acquired human immunodeficiency virus (HIV).

Signs and Symptoms

Each STD has its own set of symptoms, but a discharge from the penis or vagina, pain when urinating (in males), and open sores or blisters in the genital area are typical of most STDs. Unfortunately, early stages of STDs often have no detectable symptoms. In addition, you can also have more than one STD at the same time. Gonorrhea and chlamydia, for example, are often picked up at the same time.

How STDs Spread

STDs are transmitted through intimate sexual contact.

Fast Response Counts

If you suspect you have an STD, see a doctor as soon as possible. Your sexual partner(s) should also be contacted and treated.

Treatment

Some STDs can be treated and cured with antibiotics. For others, such as herpes and HIV/AIDS, there is no cure.

Possible Complications

Depending on the infection, STDs can cause serious, long-term problems like birth defects, infertility, diseases of the brain, or, in the case of HIV/AIDS, death.

No "Shots" for Prevention

At present, no vaccines exist to prevent STDs.

Repeat Episodes

Once you've had an STD, you can get it again. You can't develop an immunity once you've been exposed.

Parents Don't Have to Know

A minor does not need parental consent to receive treatment for an STD.

{*Note:* Medical treatment, not self-care treatment, is necessary for sexually transmitted diseases. One exception is genital herpes, for which many self-care measures can help alleviate the discomfort that occurs with recurrent attacks. Self-Care/Prevention Tips should be followed to lower the risk for contracting STDs, however. (See page 275.)}

94 Chlamydia

Chlamydia is now the most common nonviral sexually transmitted disease in the United States. It affects more men and women than syphilis and gonorrhea combined. In fact, chances are that persons who have had these other STDs are playing host to chlamydia as well. Chlamydia can also accelerate the appearance of AIDS symptoms for persons infected with HIV.

Signs and Symptoms

Symptoms of chlamydia in men include:

- Burning or discomfort when urinating
- Whitish discharge from the tip of the penis
- Pain in the scrotum

In women, symptoms include:

- Slight yellowish-green vaginal discharge
- Vaginal irritation
- Need to urinate often
- Pain when urinating
- Chronic abdominal pain and bleeding between menstrual periods

These symptoms can, however, be so mild that they often go unnoticed. It is estimated that 75% of women and 25% of men who have chlamydia have no symptoms until complications set in. If symptoms do appear, they usually do so 2–4 weeks after being infected. The only sure way to know whether or not you have chlamydia is to be tested.

Doctors recommend that sexually active people who are not involved in a long-term, monogamous relationship be tested periodically. You should be aware, though, that the most reliable test for chlamydia is a tissue culture that is expensive and not widely available. For that reason, many doctors use a simpler slide test instead. A small amount of fluid is collected from the infected site with a cotton swab. Sometimes the results are available the same day of the test.

Treatment

Anyone who has chlamydia should be treated with oral antibiotics such as tetracycline, erythromycin, or azithromycin. Doctors will treat the infected sexual partner even if he or she doesn't show any symptoms. Sex should be avoided until treatment is completed in both the person affected and in their sex partners. If left untreated, chlamydia can cause a variety of serious problems, including infection and inflammation of the prostate and surrounding structures in men and pelvic inflammatory disease (PID) and infertility in women. Infants born to mothers who have chlamydia are likely to develop pneumonia or serious eye infections in the first several months of life as well as permanent lung damage later on.

Chlamydia, *Continued*

Questions to Ask

For Men:

Do you have any of these problems?
- A whitish discharge from the penis, burning or discomfort when urinating, pain and swelling in the scrotum

YES  **See Doctor**

NO

For Women:

Do you have these problems?
- A yellowish-green vaginal discharge
- Frequent need to urinate
- Chronic abdominal pain
- Bleeding between menstrual periods

YES **See Doctor**

NO

Flowchart continued in next column

For Men and Women:

Does your sexual partner have, or do you suspect he or she might have a sexually transmitted disease? Does he or she have multiple sex partners?

YES **Call Doctor**

NO

Do you want to rule out the presence of chlamydia or other sexually transmitted diseases for any of these reasons:
- Because you or your sex partner have had multiple sex partners
- Because you are considering a new sexual relationship
- Because you are planning to get married or pregnant
- For peace of mind

YES **Call Doctor**

NO **Use Self-Care**

Use Self-Care/Prevention Tips on page 275.

20. Sexually Transmitted Diseases (STDs)

95 Genital Herpes

Genital herpes is caused by the herpes simplex virus. There are two types of this virus – type I and type II. Either type can cause genital herpes but type II is most often the culprit. Type I most often affects the oral area showing up as fever blisters or cold sores. Engaging in oral sex can spread oral herpes to the genitals and genital herpes to the mouth, lips, and throat. Both herpes simplex viruses are spread by direct skin-to-skin contact from the site of infection to the contact site. Once you are infected, the virus remains with you forever. It causes symptoms, though, only during flare-ups.

Signs and Symptoms

Symptoms include sores with blisters on the genital area and anus and sometimes on the thighs and buttocks. After a few days, the blisters break open and leave painful, shallow ulcers which can last from 5 days to 3 weeks. If infected for the first time, you may experience flu-like symptoms, such as swollen glands, fever, and body aches. Subsequent attacks are almost always much milder and much shorter in duration.

Genital herpes attacks may be triggered by emotional stress, fatigue, menstruation, other illnesses, or even by vigorous sexual intercourse. Itching, irritation, and tingling in the genital area may occur 1 to 2 days before the outbreak of the blisters or sores. (This period is called the prodrome.) Genital herpes is contagious during the prodrome, when blisters are present and up to a week or two after they have disappeared. If a pregnant woman has an outbreak of genital herpes when her baby is due, a Caesarean section may need to be done so the baby does not get infected during delivery.

Treatment

No cure exists for genital herpes. The prescription medication Zovirax and self-help measures only treat herpes symptoms. (See "Self-Care Tips for Genital Herpes" on the next page.) Medication can be helpful during the first attack of genital herpes. Self-help remedies may be all that is necessary during recurrent episodes.

{*Note:* Sores and blisters that look like herpes can be a side effect of taking certain prescription medicines in some people. One example is sulfa medications which are often used to treat urinary tract infections. Consult your doctor if you suspect this.}

Questions to Ask

Do you have sores and/or painful blisters on the genital area, anus, or tongue, and is this the first time you have had this? **YES** See Doctor

NO

Did these sores appear only after taking a recently prescribed medicine? **YES** See Doctor

NO

For persons who have already been diagnosed with genital herpes: Are you experiencing severe pain and blistering and/or are you having frequent attacks? **YES** See Doctor

NO

Flowchart continued on next page

Genital Herpes, *Continued*

Flowchart continued

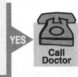

For pregnant women only: Are genital herpes sores present and are you close to your delivery date?

YES →  **Call Doctor**

NO ↓

Have you had sexual relations with someone who had sores or blisters on their genital area, anus, or tongue or had genital itching, irritation, and tingling?

YES → **Call Doctor**

NO ↓

 Use Self-Care

Self-Care Tips

■ Bathe the affected genital area twice a day with mild soap and water. Gently pat dry with a towel or use a hair dryer set on warm. Using Aveeno (colloidal oatmeal soap or bath treatments) may also be soothing.

■ Take a hot bath if you can tolerate it. This may help to inactivate the virus and promote healing.

■ Use sitz baths to soak the affected area. A sitz bath device fits over the toilet. You can get one at a medical supply store or at some pharmacies.

■ Apply ice packs on the genital area for 5–10 minutes. This may help relieve itching and inflammation.

■ Wear loose-fitting pants or skirts. Avoid wearing panty hose and tight-fitting clothing. These could irritate the inflamed area. Wear cotton, not nylon, underwear.

■ Squirt tepid water over the genital area while urinating. This may help decrease the pain.

■ Take an over-the-counter pain reliever. {*Note:* See "Pain relievers" in "Your Home Pharmacy" on pages 22 and 23.}

■ A local anesthetic ointment such as Lidocaine can help during the most painful part of an attack. (Check with your doctor before using.)

■ Ask your doctor about using the oral antiviral medicine acyclovir (brand name Zovirax).

■ To avoid spreading the virus to your eyes, don't touch your eyes during an outbreak.

■ Avoid sexual intercourse:

• At the first sign of a herpes outbreak (this may be evident by the feeling of tingling and itching in the genital area which takes place before blisters are noticeable). Note, though, that herpes can be contracted without visible blisters because viral lesions may be present on the female's cervix or inside the male's urethra.

• When active lesions are present

• Two to 3 days after lesions have disappeared

96 Gonorrhea

Gonorrhea is one of the most common infectious diseases in the world. Often called "the clap," "dose," or "drip," it is caused by a specific bacterium that is transmitted during vaginal, oral, or anal sex. A newborn baby can also get gonorrhea during childbirth if its mother is infected.

Signs and Symptoms

The signs of gonorrhea can, however, show up within 2–10 days after sexual contact with an infected person. In men, symptoms include pain at the tip of the penis, pain and burning during urination, and a thick, yellow, cloudy penile discharge that gradually increases. In women, symptoms include mild itching and burning around the vagina, a thick, yellowish-green vaginal discharge, burning on urination, and severe lower abdominal pain (usually within a week or so after their menstrual periods).

Gonorrhea can be symptom-free. In fact, about 60 to 80% of infected women have no symptoms.

Treatment

If ignored, gonorrhea can cause widespread infection and/or infertility. But gonorrhea can be cured with specific antibiotics. Since many strains of gonorrhea are resistant to penicillin, your doctor will almost always use another medicine.

To treat gonorrhea successfully, you should heed the following:

- Take prescribed medications.
- To avoid reinfection, be sure that your sexual partner is also treated.

- Have follow-up cultures to determine if the treatment was effective.

Questions to Ask

For Men:

Do you have any of these problems?
- A discharge of pus from the penis
- Discomfort or pain when urinating
- Irritation and itching of the penis
- Pain during intercourse

See Doctor

NO

For Women:

Do you have any of these problems?
- Itching and burning around the vagina
- A vaginal discharge (this could be slight, cloudy or greenish-yellow in color)
- Burning or pain when urinating
- The need to urinate often
- Discomfort in the lower abdomen
- Abnormal bleeding from the vagina

See Doctor

NO

Flowchart continued on next page

Gonorrhea, *Continued*

Flowchart continued

For Men and Women:

Are you symptom-free, but suspicious of having contracted gonorrhea or another sexually transmitted disease from someone you suspect may be infected?

YES → Call Doctor

NO ↓

Do you want to rule out the presence of gonorrhea or other sexually transmitted diseases for any of these reasons:

- Because you or your sex partner have had multiple sex partners
- Because you are considering a new sexual relationship
- Because you are planning to get married or pregnant
- For peace of mind

YES → Call Doctor

NO ↓

 Use Self-Care

Use Self-Care/Prevention Tips on page 275.

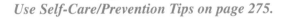

97 Syphilis

Syphilis is sometimes called "pox" or "bad blood". It is caused by a specific bacterium. Left untreated, syphilis is one of the most serious sexually transmitted diseases, leading to heart failure, blindness, insanity or death. Syphilis can progress slowly through 3 stages over a period of many years. When detected early, however, syphilis can be cured.

Signs and Symptoms

Primary Stage Symptoms

A large, painless, sore known as a chancre occurs 2 to 6 weeks after infection and generally appears around the area of sexual contact. The chancre disappears within a few weeks.

Secondary Stage Symptoms

Within a month after the end of the primary stage, a widespread skin rash may appear, cropping up on the palms of the hands, soles of the feet, and sometimes around the mouth and nose. The rash commonly has small, red, scaly bumps that do not itch. Other types of rashes, swollen lymph nodes, fever, and flu-like symptoms may also occur and small patches of hair may fall out of the scalp, beard, eyelashes, and eyebrows.

Latent Stage Symptoms

Once syphilis reaches this stage, it may go unnoticed for years, quietly damaging the heart, central nervous system, muscles, and various other organs and tissues. The resulting effects are often fatal.

Treatment

If you've been exposed to syphilis or have its symptoms, see a doctor or consult your county health department. For syphilis in its early stages, treatment consists of penicillin. If the disease has progressed further, you'll require 3 consecutive weekly injections. (If you're allergic to penicillin, you'll receive an alternative antibiotic taken orally for 2–4 weeks.) You should have a blood test 3, 6 and 12 months after treatment to be sure the disease is completely cured.

Once treatment is complete, you're no longer contagious. You can get syphilis again if you have sexual contact with an infected partner.

Questions to Ask

Do you have a large, painless ulcer-like sore (chancre) in the genital area, anus, or mouth?

YES →
See Doctor

NO ↓

Flowchart continued on next page

Syphilis, *Continued*

Flowchart continued

Did you have such a sore 6 or more weeks ago that healed, but now experience flu-like symptoms (fever, headache, general ill-feeling) and/or a skin rash of small, red, scaly bumps that do not itch?

YES See Doctor

NO

Are you suspicious of having contracted syphilis or another sexually transmitted disease from someone you suspect may be infected?

YES  Call Doctor

NO

Flowchart continued in next column

Do you want to rule out the presence of syphilis or other sexually transmitted diseases for any of these reasons:
- Because you or your sex partner have had multiple sex partners
- Because you are considering a new sexual relationship
- Because you are planning to get married or pregnant
- For peace of mind

YES Call Doctor

NO

 Use Self-Care

Use Self-Care/Prevention Tips on page 275.

98 Trichomoniasis

Unlike most sexually transmitted diseases, trichomoniasis is caused by a parasite rather than by bacteria or a virus. The trichomoniasis parasite can be present in the vagina for years without causing symptoms.

Signs and Symptoms

If they do occur, typical symptoms for women include vaginal itching and burning, a greenish-yellow vaginal discharge, and burning or pain when urinating. Sexual intercourse can be painful. In men, symptoms include mild itching and irritation of the penis, pain during intercourse, and discomfort when urinating. Men who have trichomoniasis usually don't experience any symptoms. They may infect their sexual partners and not know it.

Trichomoniasis is diagnosed by examining a drop of vaginal fluid under a microscope.

Treatment

The oral medication metronidazole (brand name Flagyl), is used to treat trichomoniasis. If you're a woman, don't take this drug during the first three months of pregnancy. Avoid drinking alcohol for 24 hours before, during, and 24 hours after taking the metronidazole. The combination causes vomiting, dizziness, and headaches.

Sexual partners of an infected person should also be treated to prevent getting infected again or spreading the infection further.

Questions to Ask

For Men:

Do you have any of these problems?
- Discomfort when urinating
- Pain during intercourse
- Irritation and itching of the penis

YES → See Doctor

NO ↓

For Women:

Do you have any of these problems?
- Itching and burning around the vagina
- A greenish-yellow vaginal discharge
- Burning or pain when urinating

YES → See Doctor

NO ↓

For Men and Women:

Are you suspicious of having contracted trichomoniasis or another sexually transmitted disease from someone you suspect may be infected?

YES → Call Doctor

NO ↓

Flowchart continued on next page

Trichomoniasis, *Continued*

Flowchart continued

Do you want to rule out the presence of Trichomoniasis or other sexually transmitted diseases for any of these reasons:
- Because you or your sex partner has had multiple sex partners
- Because you are considering a new sexual relationship
- Because you are planning to get married or pregnant
- For peace of mind

YES →
Call Doctor

NO ↓

Use Self-Care

Self-Care/Prevention Tips

- There's only one way to guarantee you'll never get a sexually transmitted disease: Never have sex.

- Limiting your sexual activity to one person your entire life is a close second, provided your partner is also monogamous and does not have a sexually transmitted disease.

- Avoid sexual contact with persons whose health status and practices are not known.

- Avoid sex if either partner has signs and symptoms of a genital tract infection.

- Don't have sex while under the influence of drugs or alcohol (except in a monogamous relationship in which neither partner is infected with an STD).

- Discuss a new partner's sexual history with him or her before beginning a sexual relationship. (Be aware, though, that persons are not always honest about their sexual history.)

- Latex condoms can reduce the spread of sexual diseases when used properly and carefully and for every sex act. They do not eliminate the risk entirely. Unless they are in a monogamous relationship in which neither partner has an STD, both women and men should carry latex condoms and insist that they be used every time they have sexual relations.

- Using spermicidal foams, jellies, creams (especially those that contain Nonoxynol-9), and a diaphragm can offer additional protection when used with a condom. Use water-based lubricants such as K-Y Brand Jelly. Don't use oil-based or "petroleum" ones such as Vaseline. They can damage latex condoms.

- Wash the genitals with soap and water before and after sexual intercourse.

- Seek treatment for a sexually transmitted disease if you know your sex partner is infected.

- Ask your doctor to check for STDs every 6 months if you have multiple sex partners, even if you don't have any symptoms.

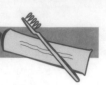

99 Abscess

A tooth abscess is formed when there is inflammation and/or infection in the bone and/or the tooth's canals. This generally occurs in a tooth that has a deep cavity, a very deep filling, or one that has been injured. The pain caused by an abscessed tooth can be persistent, throbbing, and severe. Other symptoms include fever, earache, and swelling of the glands on one side of the face or neck. It can also cause a general ill feeling, bad breath, and a foul taste in the mouth.

A tooth abscess is usually treated with either a root canal or by pulling the tooth. A root canal is done if the dentist thinks the tooth can be saved. This procedure relieves the pain and pressure caused by a tooth abscess. An antibiotic will also be prescribed.

Tooth abscesses, for the most part, can be prevented with regular dental care. This includes daily brushing (with a fluoride toothpaste) and flossing, and regular dental checkups and cleanings.

Questions to Ask

Do you have 1 or more of these problems with the toothache?
- Pain that lasts or throbs
- Fever
- Earache
- Neck or jaw tenderness or swollen glands in the side where the tooth aches
- General ill feeling
- Bad breath and/or foul taste in the mouth

YES
See Doctor
(Dentist)

NO

Flowchart continued in next column

Does the pain come and go or only occur when you are eating or drinking?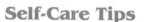

YES
Call Doctor
(Dentist)

NO

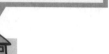
Use Self-Care

Self-Care Tips

- Take an over-the-counter medicine for pain. {*Note:* See "Pain relievers" in "Your Home Pharmacy" on pages 22 and 23.}

- Hold an ice pack on the jaw. This will relieve some of the pain.

- Never place a crushed aspirin on the tooth. Aspirin burns the gums and destroys tooth enamel.

- Do not drink extremely hot or cold liquids.

- Do not chew gum.

- Avoid sweets and hot or spicy foods. A liquid diet may be necessary for a day or two until the pain subsides.

- Gargle with warm salt water every hour.

- See a dentist even if the pain subsides.

100 Broken Or Knocked Out Tooth

Your teeth are meant to last a lifetime. They can, however, be vulnerable to nicks, chips and strains. To protect your teeth from damage and injury, take these precautions:

- Don't chew ice, pens, or pencils.
- Don't use your teeth to open paper clips or otherwise function as tools.
- If you smoke a pipe, don't bite down on the stem.
- If you grind your teeth at night, ask your dentist if you should be fitted for a bite plate to prevent tooth grinding.
- If you play contact sports like football or hockey, wear a protective mouth guard.
- Always wear a seat belt when riding in a car.
- Avoid sucking on lemons or chewing aspirin or vitamin C tablets. The acid wears away tooth enamel.

If a tooth does accidentally get knocked out, go to the dentist as soon as possible. Your dentist may be able to successfully put it back in. If this can be done within about a half an hour, there is a possibility that the interior pulp will survive. Even up to 6 hours, the outer tissue of the tooth may survive and allow successful reattachment. There is little chance that the tooth can be put back in 24 hours after it has been knocked out. It is important to keep the tooth moist until you get to the dentist.

Questions to Ask

Has 1 or more teeth been broken or knocked out?

YES → Get Emergency Care

{*Note:* See dentist as soon as possible. This is a dental emergency.}

NO ↓ Use Self-Care

Self-Care Tips

For a Broken Tooth:

- To reduce swelling, apply a cold compress to the area.
- Save any broken tooth fragments and take them to the dentist.

If Your Tooth has been Knocked Out:

- Rinse the tooth with clear water.
- If possible (and if you're alert), gently put it back in the socket or hold it under your tongue.
- Otherwise, put the tooth in a glass of milk or a wet cloth.
- If the gum is bleeding, hold a gauze pad, a clean handkerchief, or tissue tightly in place over the wound.
- Try to get to a dentist within 30 minutes of the accident.

101 Fractured Jaw

Jaw fractures can result from:

- Car accidents
- Sport and other recreational activity injuries
- Osteoporosis, the brittle bone disease (see page 363)

Signs and Symptoms

- Jaw pain, swelling, or numbness
- Not being able to close the jaw normally
- Difficulty in drinking, speaking, and swallowing
- Discoloration of the jaw area
- Jaw area is tender to touch

Treatment

A fractured jaw needs to be reset with surgery. After surgery the upper and lower teeth are wired together to let the jawbones heal. Recovery includes a liquid diet, pain relievers, and muscle relaxants, if needed. Your doctor will prescribe medicines that are best for you.

A physical exam and X-ray can be done to tell for certain if the jaw has been fractured. A CAT scan may be done.

Questions to Ask

Has an injury occurred that has caused pain, tenderness to touch, swelling, discoloration, and an inability to close the jaw? **YES** → Get Emergency Care

NO ↓

Have these symptoms occurred even in the absence of an injury? **YES** → Get Emergency Care

NO ↓

 Use Self-Care

Self-Care Tips

Do these things until you get emergency care.

- Try not to talk. Write notes instead.
- Close your mouth and secure the jaw with a necktie, towel, or scarf tied around your head and chin. Remove this if vomiting occurs. Rebandage when vomiting stops.
- Hold an ice pack against the fractured bone. This can reduce pain and swelling.

102 Gum (Periodontal) Disease

Plaque build-up, crooked teeth, illness, poorly fitting dentures, trapped food particles, and certain medications can irritate or destroy your gums. With good oral hygiene, however, you can prevent gum (periodontal) disease. If caught in the early stages, gum disease is easily treated. If ignored, the gums and supporting tissues wither, and your teeth may loosen and fall out.

Signs and Symptoms

Knowing the signs and symptoms of periodontal disease is important for early treatment. Pay attention to the following:

- Swollen, red gums that bleed easily (a condition called gingivitis)

- Teeth that are exposed at the gum line (a sign that gums have pulled away from the teeth)

- Permanent teeth that are close or separating from each other

- Bad breath and a foul taste in the mouth

- Pus around the gums and teeth

Treatment

Periodontal disease should be treated by a periodontist, a dentist who specializes in this area of dentistry. Material called tartar, or calculus (which is calcified plaque), can form even when normal brushing and flossing are done. The dentist or dental hygienist can remove tartar at regular intervals. When periodontitis (pockets of infection and areas of weakened bone) are established, the dentist can treat the problem with surgery or with a process known as "deep scaling."

Questions to Ask

Are 1 or more of the symptoms of gum disease present?
- Swollen gums
- Gums that bleed easily
- Teeth exposed at the gum line
- Loose teeth
- Teeth separating from each other
- Pus around the gums and teeth
- Bad breath and/or a foul taste in the mouth

YES
See Doctor
(Dentist)

NO

Use Self-Care

Self-Care Tips

- Brush and floss your teeth regularly. Have your dentist or hygienist show you how to brush and floss your teeth correctly. Ask what type of brush you should use.

- Eat sugary foods infrequently. When you eat sweets, do so with meals, not in between meals.

- Finish a meal with cheese, because this tends to neutralize acid formation.

- Include foods with good sources of vitamin A and vitamin C daily. Vitamin A is found in cantaloupe, broccoli, spinach, winter squash, liver, and dairy products fortified with vitamin A. Good vitamin C food sources include oranges, grapefruit, tomatoes, potatoes, green peppers, and broccoli.

103 Temporomandibular Joint Syndrome (TMJ)

Temporomandibular joint (TMJ) syndrome occurs when the muscles, joints, and ligaments of the jaw move out of alignment. Symptoms include earaches, headaches, pain in the jaw area that spreads to the face or the neck and shoulders, ringing in the ears, or pain when opening and closing the mouth. These TMJ symptoms frequently mimic other conditions, so the problem is often misdiagnosed. TMJ has a number of possible causes:

- Bruxism (grinding your teeth in your sleep)
- Sleeping in a way that misaligns the jaw or creates tension in the neck
- Stress-induced muscle tension in the neck and shoulder
- Incorrect or uneven bite

Treatment

TMJ may or may not require professional treatment. Many dentists specialize in the diagnosis and treatment of TMJ. They may prescribe anti-inflammatory medicine, tranquilizers, or muscle relaxants for a short period of time; braces to correct the bite; or a bite plate to wear when sleeping. Surgery may be needed.

Questions to Ask

Are you unable to open or close your mouth because of severe pain?

YES → Get Emergency Care

NO ↓

Flowchart continued in next column

Do you have 1 or more of these problems?
- Inability to open the jaw completely
- Pain when you open your mouth wide
- Headache, earache, or pain in the jaw area that is also felt in the face, neck or shoulders
- "Clicking" or "popping" sounds when you open your mouth and when you chew

YES → See Doctor

NO ↓

 Use Self-Care

Self-Care Tips

If you have TMJ, you may be able to minimize symptoms in the following ways:

- Don't chew gum.
- Try not to open your jaw wide. This includes yawning and taking big bites out of triple-decker and submarine sandwiches or other hard-to-eat foods.
- Massage the jaw area several times a day, first with your mouth open, then with your mouth closed.
- To help reduce muscle spasms that can cause pain, apply moist heat to the jaw area. Use a washcloth soaked in warm water.
- If stress is a factor, consider biofeedback and relaxation training.

104 Toothaches

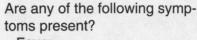

The pain of a toothache can be felt in the tooth itself or in the region around the tooth. Most toothaches are usually the result of either a cavity or an infection beneath or around the gum of a tooth. A lack of oxygen to the heart that comes with angina or a heart attack can also cause a toothache. A toothache is common after having corrective dental work on a tooth, but this should not last longer than a week. (If it does, inform the dentist.)

Toothaches can generally be prevented with regular visits to the dentist and daily self-care measures. Self-care includes proper daily brushing and flossing, good nutrition, and using fluoridated water, toothpaste, rinse, and fluoride supplement (if prescribed).

Tell your dentist if you notice any of the following. (They may lead to a toothache if left unchecked.)

- Sensitivity to hot, cold, or sweet foods
- Brown spots or little holes on a tooth
- A change in your bite – the way your teeth fit together
- Loose teeth in an adult

Questions to Ask

Do you have any of these problems with the tooth pain?
- Gnawing pain in the lower teeth or neck
- Chest discomfort beneath the breast bone
- Pain that travels to or is felt in the arm or neck
- Sweating

YES Get Emergency Care

NO

Flowchart continued in next column

Are any of the following symptoms present?
- Fever
- Red, swollen, or bleeding gums
- Swollen face
- Foul breath even after thorough brushing and flossing
- Constant toothache even when sleeping at night
- Toothache only when eating or just after eating

YES  See Doctor (Dentist)

NO

 Use Self-Care

Self-Care Tips

- Take an over-the-counter pain reliever. {*Note:* See "Pain relievers" in "Your Home Pharmacy" on pages 22 and 23.}
- Hold an ice pack on the jaw.
- Never place a crushed aspirin on the tooth. Aspirin burns the gums and destroys tooth enamel.
- Do not drink extremely hot or cold liquids.
- Do not chew gum.
- Avoid sweets, soft drinks, and hot or spicy foods. (These can irritate cavities and increase pain.) It may be best not to eat at all until you see your dentist.
- Gargle with warm salt water every hour.
- For a cavity, pack it with a piece of sterile cotton soaked in oil of cloves (available at pharmacies.)
- See a dentist even if the pain subsides.

21. Dental Problems & Injuries

SECTION III
Emergencies

Introduction

Would you know what to do in a medical crisis? Can you tell:

- If a problem needs emergency care?
- When you should see or call your doctor?
- If you can do first aid measures to take care of the problem?

This section can help you answer these questions.

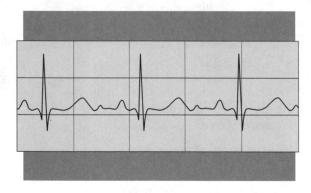

Emergency Procedures

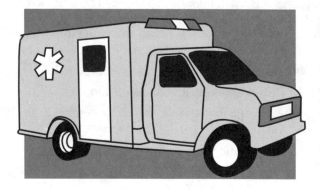

Emergency Conditions

Recognizing Emergencies

How do you tell the difference between a true emergency and a minor problem? Certain symptoms are so alarming that the need for emergency care – or even an ambulance – is obvious. But what should you do about more common illnesses and injuries?

Only a doctor can diagnose medical problems. But you can protect your family's health by learning to recognize certain symptoms.

Know which symptoms to watch for. According to the American College of Emergency Physicians, the following are warning signs of a medical emergency:

- Difficulty breathing, shortness of breath
- Chest or upper abdominal pain or pressure
- Fainting
- Sudden dizziness, weakness, or change in vision
- Change in mental status (such as unusual behavior, confusion, difficulty arousing)
- Sudden, severe pain anywhere in the body
- Bleeding that won't stop
- Severe or persistent vomiting
- Coughing up or vomiting blood
- Suicidal or homicidal feelings

You should also be familiar with the symptoms of common illnesses and injuries.

Talk to your regular doctor before you have an emergency. Ask what you should do if you think someone in your family needs emergency care. Should you call the doctor's office first? Should you go straight to the emergency department? What should you do when the doctor's office is closed?

Trust your instincts. Parents are usually very good at recognizing signs of unusual behavior or other symptoms that indicate an emergency. Many other factors, including the time of day, other medical problems, or state of mind, can make an otherwise minor medical problem an "emergency."

"Recognizing Emergencies" is reprinted from the *Home Organizer for Medical Emergencies*. Copyright © 1992 by the American College of Emergency Physicians. Used with permission.

Being Ready for Medical Emergencies

Things to Do Before an Emergency Happens:

- Learn basic first-aid skills. Take a course in cardiopulmonary resuscitation (CPR) and first aid. These courses give hands-on practice in doing first aid the right way. What you learn can save a life. Find out about first-aid courses from your local
  - Red Cross
  - American Heart Association
  - National Safety Council
  - Hospital
  - Police and/or fire department
  - Community education department
- Find out what services your health insurance company covers.
- Find out what procedures you have to follow to get emergency care.
- Carry this information with you at all times: {*Note:* Give this information to people who care for your children, too.}
  - Your name, address, and phone number and the name and phone number of the person to call if you need emergency care
  - Your health insurance information
  - Important medical information. This could be on a medical alert bracelet or necklace. It could be on a wallet card or on the back of your driver's license.
  - Emergency telephone numbers

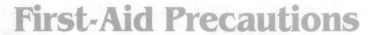

First-Aid Precautions

You can get organisms carried in blood that cause diseases such as hepatitis B virus (HBV) and human immunodeficiency virus (HIV) from an infected victim's blood or other body fluids if they enter your body. These organisms can enter through cuts or breaks in your skin or through the lining of your mouth, nose, and eyes. When you give first aid, take these precautions:

- Wear latex gloves that you can throw away whenever you touch a victim's body fluids, blood, or other objects that may be soiled with his or her blood. If latex gloves are not available, put some type of waterproof material, such as a plastic bag, on top of the wound when you apply direct pressure. Or have the victim apply pressure to the wound with his or her own hand, if possible.

- Cover the victim's open wounds with dressings, extra gauze, or waterproof material.

- Use a mouth-to-mouth barrier device when you do rescue breathing. The victim could have blood in the mouth.

- Wash your hands with soap and water right away.

- Report every incident in which you are exposed to a victim's blood or other body fluids. Do this whether or not you use the precautions listed above.

- Before you give any medicine to a victim:

  - Find out if the victim has medicine prescribed for him or her to take for the medical condition at hand. An example of this is nitroglycerin for a heart condition. Ask where the victim keeps the medicine.

  - Ask the victim for permission to give him or her the medicine.

  - Find out if the victim is allergic to any medicine.

106 CPR (Rescue Breathing/ Chest Compressions)

These emergency procedures for cardiopulmonary resuscitation (CPR), which are based on procedures recommended by the American Heart Association, are reprinted from *Home Organizer for Medical Emergencies*. Copyright © 1992 by the American College of Emergency Physicians. Used with permission.

The information below is designed as a reminder of and not a substitute for formal training in CPR (cardiopulmonary resuscitation). The American Heart Association and the American Red Cross offer courses in CPR. All family members should take one of these courses. You should have both your skill in and your knowledge of CPR tested at least once a year.

A. Airway

1. If you find a collapsed person, determine if the victim is unconscious. If there is no response, shout for help. Call 9-1-1 or your local emergency number.

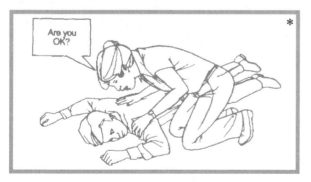

2. If the victim is not lying flat on his or her back, roll the victim over, moving the entire body at one time as a unit.

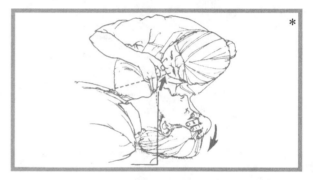

3. Open the victim's airway. Lift up the chin gently with one hand while pushing down on the forehead with the other to tilt the head back.

NECK INJURY: If the victim may have suffered a neck injury – in a diving or automobile accident for example – open the airway using the chin-lift without tilting the head back. If the airway remains blocked, tilt the head slowly and gently until the airway is open.

4. Once the airway is open, check to see if the person is breathing.

5. If opening the airway does not cause the victim to begin to breathe, you must provide rescue breathing.

CPR (Rescue Breathing/Chest Compressions), *Continued*

B. Breathing (Rescue Breathing)

1. Pinch the victim's nose shut using your thumb and forefinger. Keep the heel of your hand on the victim's forehead to maintain the head-tilt. Your other hand should remain under the victim's chin, lifting up.

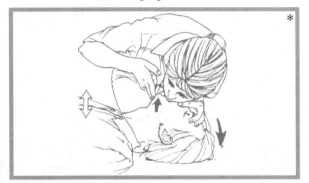

2. Immediately give two full breaths while maintaining an air-tight seal with your mouth on the victim's mouth.

C. Circulation (Chest Compressions)

1. After giving the two full breaths, locate the victim's pulse to see if the heart is beating. To find the pulse, use the hand that is supporting the chin to locate the Adam's apple (voice box). Slide the tips of your fingers down into the groove beside the Adam's apple. Feel for the pulse.

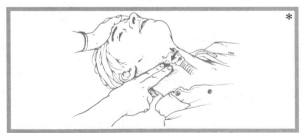

If you cannot find the pulse, you must provide artificial circulation in addition to rescue breathing.

2. Kneel at the victim's side near the chest.

3. With the middle and forefingers of the hand nearest the legs, locate the notch where the bottom rims of the rib cage meet in the middle of the chest.

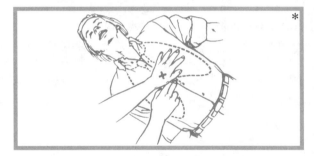

4. Place the heel of the hand on the breastbone (sternum) next to the notch. Place your other hand on top of the one that is in position. Be sure to keep your fingers up off the chest wall. You may find it easier to do this if you inter-lock your fingers.

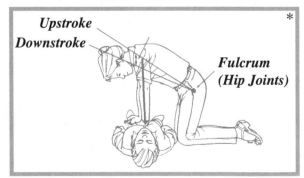

Upstroke
Downstroke
Fulcrum (Hip Joints)

* Illustrations are reproduced with permission from <u>Basic Life Support Heartsaver Guide</u>, 1993. Copyright © American Heart Association.

CPR (Rescue Breathing/Chest Compressions), *Continued*

5. Bring your shoulders directly over the victim's sternum. Press downward, keeping your arms straight. For an adult victim, depress the sternum about $1\frac{1}{2}$ to 2 inches. Then relax pressure on the sternum completely.

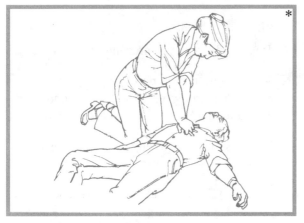

Do not remove your hands from the victim's sternum, but do allow the chest to return to its normal position between compressions. Relaxation and compression should be of equal duration.

6. If you must provide both rescue breathing and external chest compressions, the proper ratio is 15 chest compressions to 2 breaths. You must compress at the rate of 80 to 100 times per minute.

7. Continue CPR until advanced life support is available.

For Infants (Birth to 1 year) and Children (1 to 8 years)

A. Airway

With infants, be careful that you do not tilt the head backward too far. An infant's neck is so pliable that forceful backward tilting might block breathing passages instead of opening them.

B. Breathing

Do not try to pinch the nose of an infant who is not breathing. Cover both the mouth and the nose with your mouth and breathe slowly (1 to $1\frac{1}{2}$ seconds/breath), using enough volume and pressure to make the chest rise. With a small child, pinch the nose closed, cover the mouth with your mouth and breathe at the same rate as for an infant.

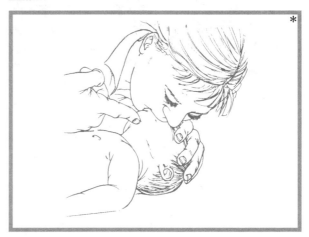

22. Emergency Procedures

---

* Illustrations are reproduced with permission from <u>Basic Life Support Heartsaver Guide</u>, 1993.
Copyright © American Heart Association.

CPR (Rescue Breathing/Chest Compressions), *Continued*

C. Circulation

PULSE

In an infant, check for a pulse by feeling on the inside of the upper arm midway between the elbow and the shoulder. The pulse check in the small child is the same as in the adult.

Chest Compressions
Infants:

1. Use only the tips of the middle and ring fingers of one hand to compress the chest at the sternum (breastbone) as described in the table below. The other hand may be slipped under the back to provide a firm support.

2. Depress the sternum between $\frac{1}{2}$ to 1 inch at a rate of at least 100 times a minute.

3. Breaths should be given during a pause after every fifth chest compression.

4. Continue CPR until advanced life support is available.

Small Children (ages 1-8):

1. Use only the heel of one hand.

2. Depress the sternum between 1 and $1\frac{1}{2}$ inches, depending on the size of the child. The rate should be 80 to 100 times per minute.

3. Breaths should be given during a pause after every fifth chest compression.

4. Continue CPR until advanced life support is available.

Chest Compression Chart					
	Part of Hand	Hand Position	Depress Sternum	Rate of Compression	Ratio of Breaths to Compression
Infants	tips of middle and ring fingers	1 finger's width below line between nipples*	$\frac{1}{2}$ to 1 inch	at least 100 per minute	five compressions to one breath
Children	heel of hand	sternum (same as in adults)	1 to $1\frac{1}{2}$ inches	80–100 per minute	five compressions to one breath
Adults	both hands (see illustration)	sternum	$1\frac{1}{2}$ to 2 inches	80–100 per minute	fifteen compressions to two breaths

* Make sure not to depress the tip of the sternum

107 Choking (Heimlich Maneuver)

These emergency procedures for choking, which are based on procedures recommended by the American Heart Association, are reprinted from the *Home Organizer for Medical Emergencies*. Copyright © 1992 by the American College of Emergency Physicians. Used with permission.

Adults: Conscious Victim

1. Choking is indicated by the Universal Distress Signal (hands clutching the throat).

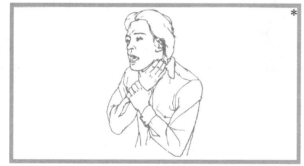

2. If the victim can speak, cough or breathe, do not interfere.

   If the victim cannot speak, cough or breathe, give abdominal thrusts (the Heimlich maneuver).

Reach around the victim's waist. Position one clenched fist above navel and below rib cage. Grasp fist with other hand. Pull the clenched fist sharply and directly backward and upward under the rib cage 6 to 10 times quickly.

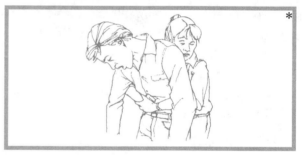

In case of extreme obesity or late pregnancy, give chest thrusts. Stand behind victim. Place thumb of left fist against middle of breastbone, not below it. Grab fist with right hand. Squeeze chest 4 times quickly.

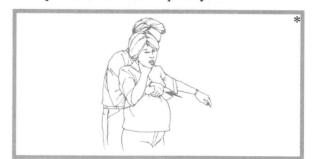

3. Continue uninterrupted until the obstruction is relieved or advanced life support is available. In either case, the victim should be examined by a physician as soon as possible.

* Illustrations are reproduced with permission from <u>Basic Life Support Heartsaver Guide</u>, 1993. Copyright © American Heart Association.

Choking (Heimlich Maneuver), *Continued*

If Victim Becomes Unconscious

1. Position victim on back, arms by side.

2. Shout for "Help". Call 9-1-1 or the local emergency number.

3. Perform finger sweep to try to remove the foreign body.

4. Perform rescue breathing. If unsuccessful, give 6–10 abdominal thrusts (the Heimlich maneuver).

5. Repeat sequence: perform finger sweep, attempt rescue breathing, perform abdominal thrusts, until successful.

6. Continue uninterrupted until obstruction is removed or advanced life support is available. When successful, have the victim examined by a physician as soon as possible.

7. After obstruction is removed, begin the ABC's of CPR, if necessary.

Conscious Infant (Under 1 year old)

1. Support the head and neck with one hand. Straddle the infant face down over your forearm, head lower than trunk, supported on your thigh.

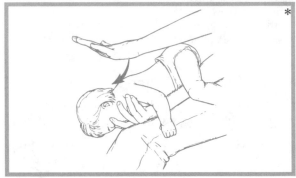

2. Deliver four back blows, forcefully, with the heel of the hand between the infant's shoulder blades.

3. While supporting the head, immediately sandwich the infant between your hands and turn onto its back, head lower than trunk.

4. Using 2 or 3 fingers (see illustration for finger position), deliver four thrusts in the sternal (breastbone) region. Depress the sternum $1/2$ to 1 inch for each thrust. Avoid the tip of the sternum.

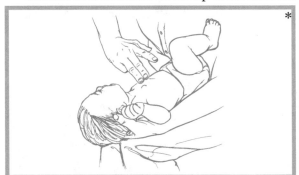

Choking (Heimlich Maneuver), *Continued*

5. Repeat both back blows and chest thrusts until foreign body is expelled or the infant becomes unconscious.

ALTERNATE METHOD: Lay the infant face down on your lap, head lower than trunk and firmly supported. Perform 4 back blows. Turn infant on its back as a unit and perform 4 chest thrusts.

Unconscious Infant

1. Shout for help. Call 9-1-1 or the local emergency number.

2. Perform tongue-jaw lift. If you see the foreign body, remove it.

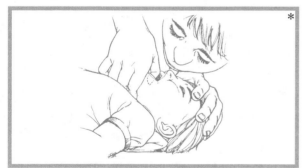

3. Attempt rescue breathing.

4. Perform the sequence of back blows and chest thrusts as described for conscious infant.

5. After each sequence of back blows and chest thrusts, look for the foreign body and, if visible, remove it.

6. Attempt rescue breathing. Repeat steps 4 and 5.

7. If foreign body is removed and victim is not breathing, begin the ABC's of CPR.

Conscious Child (Over 1 year old)

To dislodge an object from the airway of a child:

▬ Perform abdominal thrusts (the Heimlich maneuver) as described for adults. Avoid being overly forceful.

Unconscious Child (Over 1 year old)

If the child becomes unconscious, continue as for an adult except:

▬ Do not perform blind finger sweep in children up to 8 years old. Instead, perform a tongue-jaw lift and remove foreign body only if you can see it.

{*Note:* Abdominal thrusts are not recommended in infants. Blind finger sweeps should not be performed on infants or small children.}

22. Emergency Procedures

108 Recovery Position

The recovery position may need to be used in many conditions that need first aid such as unconsciousness. It should <u>not</u> be used when a person:

- Is not breathing
- Has a head, neck, or spinal injury
- Has a serious injury

The recovery position:

- Allows the victim to breathe freely
- Protects the victim's airway. It allows fluids such as vomit and blood to drain so the victim doesn't choke on them.
- Promotes good circulation
- Supports the body
- Puts the victim in a comfortable position.

To put a person in the recovery position:

1. Kneel at his or her side.
2. Turn the victim's face toward you. Tilt the head back to open the airway. Check the mouth if the victim is unconscious and remove false teeth or any foreign matter.

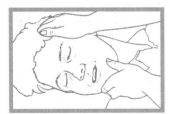

3. Place the victim's arm nearest you by his or her side and tuck it under the victim's buttock.

4. Lay the victim's other arm across his or her chest.

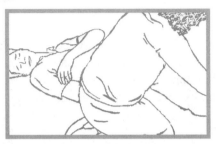

5. Cross the victim's leg that is farthest from you over the one nearest you at the victim's ankles.

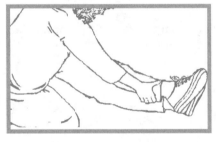

6. Support the victim's head with one hand and grasp his or her clothing at the hip farthest from you. Have him or her rest against your knees.

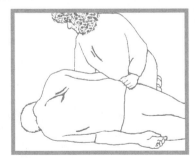

22. Emergency Procedures

Recovery Position, *Continued*

7. Bend the victim's upper arm and leg until each forms a right angle to the body. This position helps to support the victim. Don't let the victim roll onto his or her face.

8. Pull the other arm out from under the victim's body. Ease it out toward the back from the shoulder down. Position it parallel to the victim's back to keep him or her from rolling over on their back.

9. Make sure the head is tilted back to keep the airway open.

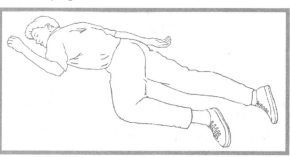

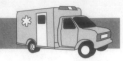

109 Animal/Insect Bites

The most common animal bites in the United States are from dogs, cats, and other humans in that order. Less common but often more dangerous are bites from skunks, raccoons, bats and other animals that live in the wild. The health problems from a bite depend on the animal/insect and how severe the bite is. Problems include:

- Rabies–a serious and often fatal viral infection of the central nervous system. The virus is transmitted to humans through the saliva of the infected animal. Only warm-blooded animals can carry rabies.

- Poison–from these snakes: rattlesnake, copperhead, coral, and water moccasin; from spiders–the worst ones are black widows and the brown recluse. The "poison" from tarantulas is due to an allergic reaction to the tarantula's hairs.

- Bleeding

- Infection

- Tissue loss if the wound is disfiguring

- Lyme Disease–a bacterial infection spread by deer tick bites

- Lockjaw–painful, persistent stiffness of the jaw due to a toxin which can be prevented with up-to-date tetanus immunizations. (See "Immunization Schedule" on page 18.)

- Allergic reaction, such as with insect bites

In the United States, particularly in the northeastern states, skunks, raccoons, bats, and foxes are the main carriers of rabies.

Most house pets are vaccinated for rabies and are unlikely to carry the virus. Abandoned kittens and puppies may be at risk if not vaccinated. Rabid animals can show these signs:

- Strange behavior such as activity by day for animals that are normally active by night

- Agitation and/or lack of fear of humans

- Foaming at the mouth

Rabies shots can prevent transmission to humans if the series of shots is begun soon after a bite from an infected animal.

Antivenom is available for poisonous snake bites at emergency medical facilities. It should be given within four hours of the bite.

Prevention

Here are some ways to prevent animal bites:

- Never leave a small child alone with a dog or cat, even if it's a puppy or kitten. Teething and/or excited pets have been known to bite.

- Teach children not to tease animals. Tell them not to wave sticks, throw stones, or pull an animal's tail.

- Do not move suddenly or scream around an animal. Don't rush up to a dog until you know for sure that it is friendly. Sudden movements and loud noises can scare animals and cause them to attack.

- Be very cautious when separating fighting animals.

Animal/Insect Bites, *Continued*

- Leave pet dogs and cats alone while they are eating or sleeping.
- Do not feed wild animals with your hands.
- Be careful when you handle your sick or injured pet.
- Do not pick up a sick or injured animal that you don't know.
- Do not run from a strange dog.
- Do not keep wild animals as pets.
- Wear heavy boots when walking in areas where snakes live.

To Prevent Lyme Disease:

- Wear long pants, tucked into socks, and long-sleeve shirts when walking through fields or forests, and when camping. Wear light-colored, tightly-woven clothing.
- Inspect for ticks after these activities.
- Use an insect repellent that is approved for deer ticks.

Questions to Ask

Is the skin severely mangled by the animal bite, or has the face been bitten? **YES**

NO

{*Note:* See "First Aid for Major Bleeding" Under Self-Care Tips on page 97.}

Flowchart continued in next column

Does the person show signs of shock? These include:
- Pale or bluish lips, skin, or fingernails
- Cool, moist skin
- Rapid or slow heartbeat and/or breathing
- Weakness, trembling
- Restlessness, anxiety, confusion
- Enlarged pupils
- Vomiting
- Unconsciousness

YES

{*Note:* See "First Aid for Shock Until Emergency Care Arrives" under Self-Care Tips on page 328.}

NO

Has the victim been bitten by a snake known to be poisonous or are you unsure whether or not the snake is poisonous? **YES**

NO

{*Note:* See "First Aid for Shock Until Emergency Care Arrives" under Self Care Tips on page 328.}

Has the victim been bitten by a spider known to be poisonous or do any of these symptoms result from the bite?
- Painful cramps and muscle stiffness in the abdomen or shoulders, chest and back
- Nausea, vomiting
- Restlessness, dizziness, problems with breathing, convulsions
- Fever, chills, heavy sweating

YES

{*Note:* See "First Aid for Poisonous Spider Bites Until Emergency Care Arrives" under Self-Care Tips on page 296.}

NO

Flowchart continued on next page

23. Emergency Conditions

295

Animal/Insect Bites, *Continued*

Flowchart continued

Has the skin been punctured or has the bite caused a lot of bleeding? **YES** → **See Doctor**

↓ **NO**

{*Note:* See "Cuts, Scrapes & Punctures" on page 96.}

Was the bite over a joint and does it cause painful movement? **YES** → **See Doctor**

↓ **NO**

Is the animal wild or a pet that has not been immunized against rabies? **YES** → **See Doctor**

↓ **NO**

Are there any signs of infection 24 hours or more after the animal bite? These include:
• Fever   • Severe swelling
• Redness   • Pus
YES → **See Doctor**

↓ **NO**

Use Self-Care

Self-Care Tips

First Aid for Poisonous Snake Bite Until Emergency Care Arrives

- Carefully move the victim (or yourself) away from the snake. Carry the victim if necessary.

- Calm the victim and have the victim rest as much as possible. Moving about can help the venom spread.

- Gently wash the bite area with soap and water.

- Keep the limb of the bite site level with or just below the level of the heart.

- Apply a splint to the limb of the bite site to keep it from moving.

- Observe the snake carefully, if you can. Be able to describe the shape of its eyes and pupils, head shape, color scheme, and the presence of rattles.

- Don't try to kill the snake. You could get bitten.

- Don't apply cold or ice to the bite

- Don't cut the fang mark

- Don't try to suck out the venom

- Don't apply a tourniquet or a bandage

First Aid for Poisonous Spider Bites Until Emergency Care Arrives

- Perform rescue breathing, if needed. (See "Airway and Breathing" on pages 285 and 286.)

- If you can, keep the bitten area lower than the level of the heart.

- Calm the victim and keep him or her warm.

- Gently clean the site of the bite with soap and water or rubbing alcohol.

- Put an ice pack over the bite site for pain relief.

- If you can, catch the spider in a closed container for identification.

Animal/Insect Bites, *Continued*

For Dog and Cat Bites:

- Wash the bite area right away with soap and warm water for 5 minutes. This helps to remove any saliva and other debris. If the bite is deep, flush the wound with water for ten minutes. This helps to protect against infection. Dry the wound with a clean towel.

- If the wound is swollen, apply ice wrapped in a towel for 10 minutes.

- Have the victim get a tetanus shot if his or her tetanus immunizations are not up-to-date. (See "Immunization Schedule" on page 18.)

- If the bite hurts, take an over-the-counter medicine for pain. {*Note:* See "Pain relievers" in "Your Home Pharmacy" on pages 22 and 23.}

- Observe the wound for a few days, checking it for infection.

- Report the incident to the animal control department.

- If you know the pet's owner, find out the date of the pet's last rabies vaccination. If its immunizations are not current, arrange with the animal control department for the pet to be observed for the next 10 days to be sure it does not develop rabies.

For Non-Poisonous Snake Bites:

- Gently wash the site with soap and water.

- Treat the bite as a minor wound. (See "Cuts, Scrapes & Punctures" on page 96.)

- Consult a health care provider if you notice signs of infection.

For Deer Tick Bites:

- Remove any ticks found on the skin. Use tweezers to grasp the tick as close to the skin as possible. Pull gently and carefully in a steady upward motion at the point where the tick's mouthpart enters the skin. Try not to crush the tick because the secretions released may spread disease.

- Wash the wound area and your hands with soap and water after removing ticks.

- Save the tick. Put it in a closed jar with rubbing alcohol. Being able to show the tick could help in diagnosing Lyme Disease.

For Human Bites Without Heavy Bleeding

- Wash the wound area with soap and water for at least 5 minutes but don't scrub hard.

- Rinse with running water or with an antiseptic solution such as Betadine.

- Cover the wound area with sterile gauze. Tape only the ends of the gauze in place.

{*Note:* Contact your doctor if you notice signs of infection such as redness, swelling, pus, and/or fever. Find out, too, if a tetanus shot is needed.}

23. Emergency Conditions

110 Choking

Choking happens when the airway is blocked partly or completely. Things that block the airway include:

- Food that goes down the windpipe

- Small objects that get stuck in the throat and airway

- Fluids that block the airway, such as mucus, blood, vomit, or liquids swallowed the wrong way

- Snoring, when the tongue blocks the airway

When the airway is completely blocked, the brain doesn't get oxygen. Without oxygen, the brain can begin to die in 4–6 minutes. A few thousand Americans, many of them young children, die from choking each year. Knowing what to do when you or someone else is choking can be life-saving. It's also good to know how to prevent choking.

Prevention

- Teach your child to chew all foods thoroughly before swallowing. Do the same yourself. Eat at a slow pace.

- Go easy on alcoholic beverages before you eat, to lessen the chance of swallowing large pieces of food.

- Try not to laugh and eat at the same time. Laughing can draw food into the windpipe.

- If you wear dentures, make sure they fit well.

- Never run or play sports with objects in the mouth.

- Don't give these things to children under 5 years of age:
  - Small beads
  - Nuts of any kind
  - Popcorn
  - Foods with pits, such as watermelon, grapes, cherries
  - Chewing gum (especially bubble gum)
  - Hard candy, throat lozenges, cough drops

- Hot dogs, sausages, grapes (seedless ones), and caramels are common causes of choking in children. Chop them up before you give them to children under 5.

- Don't let your child chew or suck on rubber balloons or pieces of rubber balloons.

- Keep small, solid objects such as paper clips and buttons away from children 3 years old and younger. Make sure, too, that they don't get their hands on toys that have small parts, such as eyes on stuffed animals, game pieces, dice, etc.

- Put childproof latches on cupboards that contain harmful items.

- Make sure that all medicines and vitamins are stored in containers with childproof lids. Keep them out of your child's reach. Put them in locked cabinets, if necessary.

- Remove plastic labels and decals from baby walkers and other kiddy furniture before youngsters can peel them off.

Choking *Continued*

Questions to Ask

Is the choking victim unconscious or is the victim unable to breathe?

YES **Get Emergency Care**

NO

{*Note:* Perform Heimlich Maneuver before emergency care. See "Choking (Heimlich Maneuver)" on page 289.}

Does the choking victim have fast and/or labored breathing?

YES **Get Emergency Care**

NO

Are any of these things present after a choking incident?
- Wheezing
- Cough that doesn't go away
- Symptoms of pneumonia such as chest pain when breathing in, and/or fever

YES **See Doctor**

NO

 Use Self-Care

Self-Care Tips

If you or someone else is choking, but able to breathe and speak:

■ Cough to clear the airway.

■ Take a slow, deep breath to get a lot of air into the lungs.

■ Give a deep, forceful cough. (Try to breathe in deeply enough to be able to cough out 2 or 3 times in a row before taking a second breath.)

{*Note:* Choking can be a sign of other problems such as allergic reactions, breathing problems, and some heart attacks. See "Insect Stings" on page 105, "Breathing Problems" on page 78, and "Chest Pain" on page 150.}

23. Emergency Conditions

111 Drowning

Drowning occurs when a person is submerged in water or other liquid and breathing stops. If the airway is not cleared, the victim will die. Near-drowning is when a person is in danger of drowning

Drowning is the fourth leading cause of accidental death. Each year, over 4,000 people drown and about one-third of them are children under 14 years of age.

It takes very little water for a child to drown. In fact, as little as 2 inches of water in a bathtub, sink, or shower can kill a toddler. Toilet bowls are unsafe, too, if a small child falls into one head-first.

Adults drown under different conditions. When the weather is hot, for example, adults are tempted to cool off with alcoholic beverages while swimming and boating. This is not a good idea. Alcohol interferes with good judgment and is a major factor in adult drownings.

Causes

- Leg or stomach cramps
- Loss of consciousness
- Playing in water too deep and too rough for one's ability to swim
- Falling in deep water such as drainage ditches or any area that collects rain water
- Not knowing how to swim
- Stroke
- Heart attack
- Breaking through thin ice
- Falling through the ice while fishing, skating, or snowmobiling during the winter
- Not wearing a life preserver

Prevention

A child could drown or get seriously injured in the seconds it takes to answer a phone or go to the door.

To Prevent a Child from Drowning:

- Never turn away from an infant in a baby bathtub or one sitting in a bathtub "supporting ring."
- Keep young children out of the bathroom unless supervised by an adult. Put childproof handles on door knobs, if necessary.
- Put up a secure fence around your swimming pool and install self-closing and self-latching gates. Make sure the gates are always locked.
- Make sure neighbors also have high fences with locked gates around their pools.
- Consider using a cordless phone out-of-doors so you can call for emergency help right away.
- Never leave a child alone near water, swimming pools, or any large container of water.
- Teach your child to swim. Classes for children as young as 6 months teach them how to kick so if they fall in the water, they can break through the water surface.
- Tell your children never to swim alone and never to swim too far from shore without the company of an experienced adult swimmer.

Drowning, *Continued*

- Warn your children to always check the depth of water before diving in. It should be at least 9 feet deep.

- Do not go on untested ice.

- Take cardiopulmonary resuscitation (CPR) and water safety courses.

To Prevent an Adult from Drowning:

- Learn to swim. Take classes at your local YMCA or in adult education programs offered at city schools.

- Swim in sight of a lifeguard, when possible.

- Never swim alone at the beach or in a swimming pool. Someone should be nearby in case you suffer a leg cramp or other potential emergency.

- If you can't swim, always wear a personal flotation device when you enter a lake or pool or ride in a boat.

- Always check the depth of the water before diving. It should be at least 9 feet deep. Never dive into an above-ground pool.

- Do not use a hot tub or jaccuzi if you've had any alcoholic drinks. You could fall asleep in the warm, relaxing water, slip under the surface, and drown.

- Take a cardiopulmonary resuscitation (CPR) and water safety course.

Questions to Ask

Is the person unconscious, not breathing, and has no pulse? **YES** **Get Emergency Care**

NO

{*Note:* See "First Aid for Drowning" under Self-Care Tips on page 302.}

Is the person not breathing, but has a pulse? **YES** **Get Emergency Care**

NO

{*Note:* See "First Aid for Drowning" under Self-Care Tips on page 302.}

Does the person have blue lips and ears, and is the skin cold and pale? **YES** **Get Emergency Care**

NO

{*Note:* See "First Aid for Drowning" under Self-Care Tips on page 302.}

Does the person in the water show these signs of near-drowning?
- Waving, shouting for help
- Uneven swimming motions
- Inability to stay above water

YES **Get Emergency Care**

NO

{*Note:* See "First Aid for Near Drowning" under Self-Care Tips on page 302.}

After a near-drowning incident, does the person have a fever, cough, or muscle pain? **YES** **See Doctor**

NO

Use Self-Care

See Self-Care Tips on next page

23. Emergency Conditions

Drowning, *Continued*

Self-Care Tips

First Aid for Drowning

(Before emergency care arrives)

- Get the victim out of the water if you can do so safely. (See "Neck/Spine Injuries" on page 319 if you suspect the victim has injured his or her neck in a diving or other water accident.)

- Monitor for breathing and pulse. If there is no breathing and no pulse, do CPR. (See "CPR" on page 285.) If there is no breathing, but there is a pulse, do rescue breathing. (See "Airway and Breathing" on pages 285 and 286.) If victim is breathing and has a pulse, put him or her in the recovery position (see page 292). This position keeps the airway clear and allows swallowed water or vomit to drain.

- Take cold, wet clothes off the victim and cover him or her with something warm to prevent hypothermia.

First Aid for Near-Drowning

(Before emergency care arrives)

{*Note:* Saving a person who is in danger of drowning carries risk. Before swimming out to someone in trouble, be sure you can handle the situation. Many people drown in the brave effort of trying to save someone else because they are not well trained and have not properly thought through the risks of the situation.}

- First try to reach the person with a pole or extended hand. If you can't reach him or her, use a life preserver or rope.

- If the person is further than you can reach and you decide to enter the water, approach the person carefully and from behind. Talk to the person, trying to calm him or her as you slowly move closer. Get the person to talk. Ask if everything is all right and tell him or her to do as you instruct.

- Grab a piece of clothing or cup one hand under the person's chin and pull the person on his or her back to shore.

{*Note:* During the rescue, monitor for breathing and pulse. If there is no pulse and/or breathing do "First Aid for Drowning." See "First Aid for Drowning" on this page.}

- Tell the person to extend his or her arms away from you. Continue talking to the person to reassure him or her.

- Put the victim in the recovery position (see page 292). This position keeps the airway clear and allows swallowed water or vomit to drain.

- Take cold, wet clothes off the victim and cover him or her with something warm to prevent hypothermia.

{*Note:* All near-drowning victims should see their health care provider because lung problems are common following a near-drowning episode.}

112 Electric Shock

Electric shocks can result in:

- Slight shocking sensations
- Muscle spasms, or muscle and tissue damage under the skins surface
- Seizures
- Interrupted breathing
- Irregular heartbeats or cardiac arrest
- Third-degree burns (at the spots where the electricity enters and exits the body)
- Unconsciousness
- Death

People can be electrocuted when they touch high-tension wires that fall during a storm or are struck by lightning. A bolt of lightning carries as many as 30 million volts, more than 250,000 times the voltage of ordinary household current. July is the most dangerous month for lightning in the Northern Hemisphere.

Take care when rescuing someone who has been electrocuted so you do not become a victim as well.

Prevention

- Take a first-aid course that covers electrical burns, electric shocks, and cardiopulmonary resuscitation (CPR).
- Install ground-fault circuit-interrupters (GFCIs) in wall outlets located in bathrooms, kitchens, basements, garages, and outdoor boxes. These act as circuit breakers. When an electrical appliance falls into water, the current is instantly cut off.
- Replace worn cords and wiring.

- Cover all electric sockets with plastic safety caps so children can't stick their fingers or a metal object in the sockets.
- Never use an electrical appliance like a radio or curling iron near water. Only buy hair dryers and curling irons that have built-in shock protectors.
- Never turn electrical switches on or off or touch an electric appliance while your hands are wet, while standing in water, or when sitting in a bathtub.
- Know the location of fuse boxes and circuit breakers in your home and place of work. Remove the appropriate fuse or switch off the circuit breaker before doing household electrical repairs. Turning off the appliance or light switch is not enough.
- Pay attention to weather warnings. A weather warning means severe weather is coming your way.
- To avoid being harmed by lightning:
  - Take shelter in a building, if you can.
  - Stay in your car (if it is not a convertible) rather than out in the open.
  - If you are caught outside, avoid tall trees, open water, and high ground. Look for a ravine or other low-lying place and crawl in. If you are out in the open, curl up on the ground, head to knees, with your head touching the ground. Don't touch items that contain metal, such as golf clubs.
  - If you are indoors, stay away from windows, appliances, waterpipes, and telephones with cords.

Electric Shock, *Continued*

Questions to Ask

Has the person received a shock from a high-voltage wire? **YES** Get Emergency Care

NO

{*Note:* Do not try to remove the person from the wire, and stay at least 20 feet away. Act fast. Call 911 or the operator and state the problem and the location of the high-voltage wire.}

Has the person been struck by lightning? **YES** Get Emergency Care

 NO

{*Note:* You will not get an electric shock from someone who has been struck by lightning.)
• If the person has no heartbeat and is not breathing, do CPR. (See "CPR" on page 285.)
• If the person has a heartbeat but is not breathing, start rescue breathing. (See "Airway and Breathing" on page 285 and 286.)}

Has the person received a shock from low-voltage current? **YES**   Get Emergency Care

NO

{*Note:* See "First Aid Tips" for Shock from Low-Voltage Current" under Self-Care Tips in next column.)

Has the person received a mild shock and does his or her heart keep skipping beats? **YES** Get Emergency Care

NO

After getting an electric shock, does the person have a fever or cough up sputum? **YES** See Doctor

 NO

Use Self-Care

Self-Care Tips

First Aid for Shock from Low Voltage Current

Do these things until emergency care arrives:
■ Switch off the current, if possible, by removing the fuse or switching off the circuit breaker.
■ Do not touch the person who is in contact with electricity.
■ If you can't turn off the source of current, use a board, wooden stick, rope, or other non-conducting device to pull the victim away from the source of the electric current. Make sure your hands and feet are dry and you are standing on a dry surface.

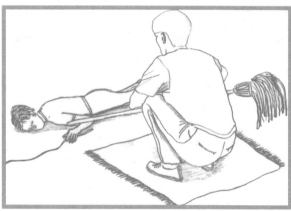

■ If it is safe for you to touch the victim:
• Check for heartbeat and breathing. Feel for a pulse along the neck, under the earlobe, on the chest, or on the wrist. Watch the rise and fall of the chest to see if the person is breathing. If you find no heartbeat and no breathing, do CPR. (See "CPR" on page 285.)
• If there is a heartbeat but no breathing, immediately start rescue breathing. (See "Airway and Breathing" on pages 285 and 286.)
• Check for burns and treat as third-degree burns. (See "Burns" on page 91.)

113 Eye Injuries

There are many causes of eye injuries. These include:

- A physical blow to the eye, or a blast exposure, such as from a firecracker.

- Harsh chemicals like lye, bleach, and acids, which can burn eye tissue and permanently damage the eyes

- A grain of sand, fleck of paint, sliver of metal, or splinter of wood, which can scratch the cornea and induce infection

- Excessive exposure to the sun, very low humidity, or a strong wind, which may dry the eyes so much they feel like sandpaper rubbing against your lids

- Insect bites

- Exposure to bright sunlight, tanning-booth light, or welder's arc

- Scratches from contact lenses

Prevention

- Wear safety glasses during any job or activity that exposes your eyes to sawdust, metal flecks, etc.

- Be careful when using harsh chemicals. Wear rubber gloves and protective glasses. Don't rub your eyes if you've touched harsh chemicals. Wash your hands. Turn your head away from chemical vapors so as not to let any get into your eyes.

- Don't allow a child to stick his or her head out of the window of a moving vehicle. Sand, insects, and other flying objects can strike the eye and irritate or damage the cornea.

- Avoid alcohol, use a humidifier, and limit exposure to smoke, dust, and wind to help prevent dry eyes.

- Use artificial tear drops with your doctor's okay.

- Never stare directly at the sun, especially during a solar eclipse.

- Wear sunglasses that block UV rays anytime you're in the sun or in a tanning booth.

All eye injuries should be taken seriously. All should be checked by a physician.

Questions to Ask

Is there a foreign body sticking into the eye?

YES Get Emergency Care

NO

{*Note:* See "First Aid for Foreign Body Sticking into the Eye" under Self-Care Tips on page 306.}

Is there a severe blow to the eye, with or without a broken bone of the face?

YES Get Emergency Care

NO

Is there a cut to the eye or eyelid?

YES Get Emergency Care

NO

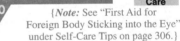

Have harmful chemicals gotten into the eye(s)?

YES Get Emergency Care

NO

{*Note:* Before emergency care flush the eyes with water immediately! See "First Aid for Harmful Chemicals in the Eye(s)" under Self-Care Tips on page 306.}

Flowchart continued on next page

23. Emergency Conditions

Eye Injuries, *Continued*

Flowchart continued

Has a bee sting or insect bite to the eye caused a severe allergic reaction with any of these symptoms?
- Wheezing, shortness of breath, and breathing difficulties
- Severe swelling in the eye and in other parts of the body such as the tongue, lips, throat
- Bluish lips and skin
- Collapse

YES **Get Emergency Care**

{*Note:* Give shot from and follow other instructions in emergency insect sting kit, if available.}

NO

Do any of these problems occur after an eye injury?
- Blurred or double vision
- Blood in the pupil

YES **Get Emergency Care**

NO

Is eye pain present?

YES **See Doctor**

NO

 Use Self-Care

Self-Care Tips

First Aid for Foreign Body Sticking into the Eye

- Do not try to remove the object.
- Do not press on, touch, or rub the eye(s).

- Cover the affected eye with a paper cup or other clean object that will not touch the eye or the foreign object. Hold the paper cup in place with tape without putting pressure on the eye or the foreign object.

- Gently cover unaffected eye as well with a clean bandage and tape. This will help to keep the affected eye from moving

First Aid for Harmful Chemicals in the Eye(s)

Flush the eye(s) with water immediately!

- Hold the affected eye open with your thumb and forefinger.

- Using a pitcher or other clean container, pour large amounts of water over the entire eye. Start at the inside corner and pour downward to the outside corner. This lets the water drain away from the body and keeps it from getting in the other eye. Keep pouring the water for 10 to 30 or more minutes. It is best to flush the eye with water until you get medical help.

- Loosely bandage the eye with a sterile cloth and tape. Do not touch the eye.

- If both eyes are affected, pour water over both eyes at the same time or quickly alternate the above procedure from one eye to another.

- Or, place the victim's face in a sink or container filled with water. Tell the victim to keep his or her eyes open and to come out of the water at intervals so he or she can breathe. Do this procedure on yourself if you are the victim and are alone.

Eye Injuries, *Continued*

To Remove a Foreign Object in the Eye:

- Wash your hands.

- Twist a piece of tissue, moisten the tip with tap water (not saliva) and gently try to touch the speck with the tip. Carefully pass the tissue over the speck, which should cling to the tip.

- If the foreign object is under the upper lid, have the person look down and pull the upper lid away from the eyeball by gently grabbing the eyelashes. Press a cotton-tipped swab down on the skin surface of the upper eyelid and pull the upper eyelid up and toward the brow. The upper lid will invert. Touch and remove the debris with the tip of the tissue.

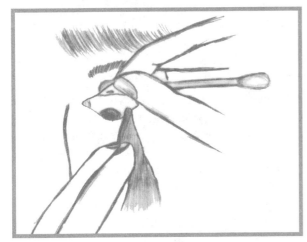

- Do not rub the eye. And never use tweezers or anything sharp to remove a foreign object. Doing so can scratch the cornea.

- Gently wash the eye with cool water.

To Treat a Black Eye from a Minor Injury:

- Put a cold compress over the injured area right away.

- Take an over-the-counter medicine for the pain and inflammation. Acetaminophen will help the pain, but not the inflammation. {*Note:* See "Pain relievers" in "Your Home Pharmacy" on pages 22 and 23.}

- Later, put a warm compress over the injured area.

- Seek medical attention if these measures do not help.

To Ease the Discomfort of Dry Eyes:

- Try an over-the-counter artificial tear product such as Ocu-Lube, Refresh or Liquifilm. Check the label. If there are no preservatives, keep the solution refrigerated. Always wash your hands before putting drops in the eyes.

To Treat an Insect Bite Without a Severe Allergic Reaction:

- Gently wash the eye(s) with warm water.

- Call the victim's doctor and ask if an antihistamine should be taken. Have the doctor recommend one. Tell the doctor what has happened and ask if anything else should be done.

23. Emergency Conditions

114 Fainting

Fainting is a brief loss of consciousness. Someone who faints may pass out for several seconds or up to one half an hour.

There are many reasons people faint. Medical reasons include:

- Low blood sugar (hypoglycemia), which is common in early pregnancy, or if a person is on a severe diet

- Anemia

- Any condition in which there is a rapid loss of blood. This can be from internal bleeding such as with a peptic ulcer, or a tubal pregnancy or ruptured ovarian cyst in females.

- Heart and circulatory problems such as abnormal heart rhythm, heart attack, or stroke

- Heat stroke or heat exhaustion

- Eating disorders such as anorexia, bulimia

- Toxic shock syndrome

- Head injury

Other things that can lead to feeling faint or fainting include:

- A sudden change in body position like standing up too quickly (postural hypotension)

- Extreme pain

- Any procedure in women that stretches the cervix, such as having an IUD inserted, especially in women who have never been pregnant

- Sudden emotional stress or fright

- Anxiety

- Standing a long time in one place

- Taking some prescription medicines. Examples are some that lower high blood pressure, tranquilizers, antidepressants, or even some over-the-counter medicines when taken in excessive amounts.

Know, also, that the risk for fainting increases if you are in hot, humid weather, or in a stuffy room or have consumed excessive amounts of alcohol.

Just before fainting, a person may:

- Feel a sense of dread

- Feel dizzy

- See spots before his or her eyes

- Feel nauseous

Here are some dos and don'ts to remember if someone is about to faint or faints:

Dos:

- Catch the person before he or she falls.

- Have the person lie down with the head below the level of the heart. {*Note:* Check for breathing and a pulse. (See Questions to Ask on the next page.)} Raise the legs 8 to 12 inches. This promotes blood flow to the brain. If a victim who is about to faint can lie down right away, he or she may not lose consciousness. If the person can't lie down, have him or her sit down, bend forward, and put his or her head between his or her knees.

- Turn the victim's head to the side so the tongue doesn't fall back into the throat.

- Loosen any tight clothing.

- Apply moist towels to the person's face and neck.

Fainting, *Continued*

■ Keep the victim warm, especially if the surroundings are chilly.

Don'ts:

■ Don't force the person to stay standing.

■ Don't slap or shake anyone who's just fainted.

■ Don't try to give the person anything to eat or drink, not even water, until they are fully conscious.

■ Don't allow the person who fainted to get up until the sense of physical weakness passes. Then be watchful for a few minutes to be sure he or she doesn't faint again.

Questions to Ask

Is the person who fainted not breathing and does he/she not have a pulse? **YES** Get Emergency Care

{*Note:* See "CPR" on page 285.}

Are signs of a heart attack also present with the fainting?
• Chest pressure or pain (may spread to the arm, neck, or jaw)
• Chest discomfort with any of these problems: Shortness of breath or trouble breathing; nausea or vomiting; sweating; uneven heartbeat or pulse; or sense of doom **YES** Get Emergency Care

NO

Flowchart continued in next column

Did the person who fainted have sudden, severe back pain? **YES** Get Emergency Care

NO

Are signs of a stroke also present with the fainting?
• Numbness or weakness in the face, arm or leg
• Temporary loss of vision or speech, double vision
• Sudden, severe headache **YES** Get Emergency Care

NO

Did the fainting come after an injury to the head? **YES** Get Emergency Care

NO

{*Note:* See "Head Injuries" on page 313.}

Are any of these conditions present with the fainting?
• Being more than 40 years old and this is the first fainting episode
• A known heart problem
• Being a young person and the fainting took place during a sports activity
• Fainting for no apparent reason **YES** Get Emergency Care

NO

Are one or both of these problems present?
• Pelvic pain
• Black stools **YES** See Doctor

NO

Flowchart continued on next page

23. Emergency Conditions

Fainting, *Continued*

Flowchart continued

Do any of these apply to the person who fainted?
- He/she is taking high blood pressure medicine and:
  - started taking a new medicine, or
  - increased the dose of a medicine

YES →  Call Doctor

NO ↓

 Use Self-Care

Self-Care Tips

{*Note:* A doctor should be consulted for any episode of fainting. Self-Care Tips can help for the following situations, though.}

Do these things when you feel faint:

- Sit down, bend forward, and put your head between your knees, or
- Lie down and elevate both legs 8–12 inches.

If You Faint Easily:

- Get up slowly from bed or from a sitting position.
- Follow your doctor's advice to treat any medical condition which may lead to fainting. Take medicines as prescribed, but let your doctor know about any side effects.
- Avoid any strenuous activities until heart-related causes of fainting are ruled out.

- Don't wear tight-fitting clothing around your neck.
- Avoid turning your head suddenly.
- Avoid excessive exercise in hot, humid conditions. Drink a lot of liquids when you do exercise.
- Stay out of stuffy rooms and hot, humid places. If you can't, use a fan.
- Avoid activities that can put your life in danger if you have frequent fainting spells. Examples include: driving and climbing to high places.
- Drink alcoholic beverages in moderation.

For Women Who are Pregnant:

- Talk to your doctor about your specific symptoms.
- Get out of bed slowly.
- Keep crackers at your bedside and eat a few before getting out of bed. Try other foods such as dry toast, graham crackers, bananas, etc.
- Eat small, frequent meals instead of a few large ones. Avoid sweets. Don't skip meals or go for a long time without eating.
- Don't sit for long periods of time.
- Keep your legs elevated when you sit.
- When you stand for a long time (e.g. in a line) don't stand still. Move your legs or contract your leg muscles to pump blood up to your heart.
- Take vitamin and mineral supplements as your doctor prescribes.
- Never lie on your back during the third trimester of pregnancy. It is best to lie on your left side. If you can't, lie on your right side.

115 Frostbite

Frostbite looks like a serious heat burn, but it's actually body tissue that's frozen and, in severe cases, dead. Most often, frostbite affects the toes, fingers, earlobes, chin, and tip of the nose. These body parts are often left uncovered and can freeze quickly. Danger signs are pain (at first), swelling, white skin, then numbness. Loss of function and absence of pain follow. The skin feels hard and solid. Blisters may also develop.

Frostnip is a less serious problem. The skin turns white or pale and feels cold but the skin does not feel hard and solid.

Frostbite and frostnip can happen when temperatures drop below freezing, but wind chill speeds up heat loss and can add to the risk. Both can set in very slowly, or very quickly. This will depend on how long the skin is exposed to the cold and how cold and windy it is.

Prevention

Frostbite can be prevented. Here are some ways to keep warm if you expect to spend any length of time in the cold:

■ Layer your clothing. Many layers of thin clothing are warmer than one bulky layer. Air spaces trap body warmth close to the skin, insulating the body against the cold. Wear 2 or 3 pairs of socks instead of 1 heavy pair, for example, and wear roomy shoes.

■ Don't drink alcohol or smoke cigarettes. Alcohol causes blood to lose heat quickly. Smoking slows down blood circulation to the extremities.

■ Stay indoors as much as possible when it is very cold and windy.

■ When you are outside, shield your face, etc. from the wind.

Questions to Ask

After being in cold temperature, do you have any of these problems?
- Skin that swells and feels hard and solid
- Loss of function and absence of pain
- Skin color changing from white to red to purple
- Blisters
- Slurred speech
- Memory loss

YES → **Get Emergency Care**

{*Note:* See "First Aid Before Emergency Care" under Self-Care Tips below.}

NO → **Use Self-Care**

Self-Care Tips

First Aid Before Emergency Care

■ If victim is not breathing and has no pulse, do CPR. (See "CPR" on page 285.) If victim is not breathing but has pulse, do rescue breathing. (See "Airway and Breathing" on pages 285 and 286.)

■ Get victim out of the cold and into a warm place.

Frostbite, *Continued*

- Loosen or remove wet and/or tight clothing. Remove jewelry.

- Don't rub the area with snow or soak it in cold water.

- Warm the affected area by soaking it in a tub of warm water (101°F–104°F) and an antiseptic solution, such as betadine.

- Stop when the affected area becomes red, not when sensation returns. (This should take about 45 minutes. If done too fast, thawing can be painful and blisters may develop.)

- If warm water is not available, cover victim with blankets, coats, sweaters, etc., or place the frostbitten body part in a warm body area such as an armpit or on the abdomen.

- Keep exposed area elevated but protected.

- Never rub or massage a frostbitten area.

- Protect exposed area from the cold. It is more sensitive to reinjury.

- Don't break blisters.

First Aid for Frostnip

- Warm the affected area. This can be done a number of ways:

  - Place cold fingers in armpits.

  - Place cold feet onto another person's warm stomach

  - Put the affected area in warm water (101°F–104°F).

{*Note:* After warming the area, the skin may be red and tingling. If not treated, frostnip can lead to frostbite.}

- Protect the exposed area from the cold. It is more sensitive to reinjury.

116 Head Injuries

Any blow to the head can result in a head injury. Head injuries can cause damage to the:

- Scalp–such as a minor bump on the head or scalp wound that bleeds

- Skull–such as a skull fracture (a break or crack in the bone that surrounds the brain)

- Brain itself–such as a concussion, a contusion (the brain tissue is bruised), or a hematoma (blood collects in an area of the brain from a broken blood vessel)

Blood from broken vessels may seep into the brain even though you may not be able to see any bumps, cuts, or bruises. The blood has nowhere to go because skull bones don't expand. This puts pressure on the vital areas of the brain. This can cause serious problems.

Bleeding within the skull often starts within the first 24 hours after a head injury and can last for 3 days or longer. It is very important that you watch for signs and symptoms of a serious head injury during the first 24 hours. Also, be aware that symptoms may not occur for as long as several weeks later. {*Note:* Also, suspect a neck injury when there is a blow to the head. See "Neck/Spine Injuries" on page 319.}

Signs and symptoms of head injuries that indicate the need for medical care include:

- Loss of consciousness, confusion, drowsiness, or personality change

- Inability to move any part of the body, or weakness in an arm or leg

- Dent, bruise, cut, or blood on the scalp

- Severe headache

- Stiff neck

- Vomiting

- Blood or fluid that comes from the mouth, nose, or ear

- Loss of vision, blurred or double vision, pupils of unequal size

- Convulsions

- Loss of consciousness

{*Note:* Some of these signs can happen at the time of the injury. Or they come later.}

Prevention
Ways to Prevent Head Injuries:

- Wear a helmet when biking, motorcycling, roller-blading, horseback riding, riding in an all-terrain vehicle, or boxing. Insist that your child does, too.

- Use child safety seats and/or seatbelts in any car, van, or truck.

- Teach your child:

  - To stop and look both ways before crossing a street

  - About the dangers of running into the street without looking first

  - Not to run under the garage door as it closes

  - Not to bang his or her head against something hard during a temper tantrum

23. Emergency Conditions

313

Head Injuries, *Continued*

- To protect your child:
  - Don't leave him or her alone in a shopping cart. When available, use carts with seat belts or child safety seats.
  - Don't leave a baby or toddler alone on a high place like a sofa, changing table, or bed.
  - Don't use baby walkers because they tip over easily.
  - Install window locks or guards on windows on upper floors. Don't rely on screens. A child can fall through a screen.
  - Place a sturdy gate at the top of the stairs.
  - Lock the basement door or put a childproof cover on the doorknob.
- Keep stairs free of clutter.
- Don't walk on wet floors or other slippery surfaces.
- Avoid the use of throw rugs unless they have rubber backing.

{*Note:* If you suspect a head, neck, or back injury in yourself or someone else, you must keep the head, neck, and back perfectly still until an emergency crew arrives. Do not move someone with a suspected head, neck, or spine injury unless the person must be moved because his or her safety is in danger. Any movement of the head, neck, or back could result in paralysis or death. Hold the head, neck, and shoulders perfectly still. Use both hands, one on each side of the head.}

Questions to Ask

With head injury, does the victim have any of these signs?
- No pulse
- No breathing
- Neck injury

YES Get Emergency Care

NO {*Note:* See "CPR" on page 285, but do not tilt the head back or move the head or neck when you do the "Airway and Breathing" part of CPR. Instead, pull the lower jaw (chin) forward to open the airway. Place your thumb(s) or fingers on the jawbones, just in front of and below the earlobes to do this.}

Is the victim of a head injury bleeding?

YES  Get Emergency Care

NO {*Note:* See "First Aid for Bleeding from the Scalp" under Self-Care Tips on page 97.}

Is the head injury victim unconscious longer than 5 minutes or confused as to time and place?

YES Get Emergency Care

NO {*Note:* See "Unconsciousness" on page 329.}

Was the head injury victim unconscious for any period of time but is okay now?

YES Get Emergency Care

NO

Flowchart continued on next page

Head Injuries, *Continued*

Flowchart continued

Do any of these problems occur after a head injury?
- Convulsions
- Drowsiness or it is hard to awaken the victim

YES Get Emergency Care

{*Note:* See "First Aid for Seizures with Convulsions" on page 325.}

NO

Do any of these problems occur after a head injury?
- Headache that lasts longer than 1 or 2 days or gets worse with time
- Inability to move arms or legs, weakness in limbs
- Blurred or double vision, pupils of unequal size
- Slurred speech
- Nausea, vomiting, dry heaves
- Memory loss, confusion, disorientation, personality change

YES Get Emergency Care

NO

Did the head injury victim see stars or feel unusual in any way?

YES See Doctor

NO

 Use Self-Care

Self-Care Tips

{*Note:* See also "First Aid for Bleeding from the Scalp" under Self-Care Tips on page 98.}

First Aid for Minor Head Injuries:

- Apply an ice pack to the injured area to reduce swelling or bruising. Change it every 15 to 20 minutes for an hour or two. Do not put ice directly on the skin. To make an ice pack:
  - Put ice cubes into a plastic bag with a little cold water and seal it. Wrap it in a clean towel and apply to the bump or bruise. Or cover a bag of frozen vegetables with a towel and place on the injured area.

- Cover an open small cut with gauze and first-aid tape or a band-aid.

- Resume normal activities once you know there is no serious head injury.

- Take an over-the-counter medicine for pain. {*Note:* See "Pain relievers" in "Your Home Pharmacy" on pages 22 and 23.}

117 Heat Exhaustion & Heat Stroke

Sweat acts like our natural air conditioner. As sweat evaporates from our skin, it cools us off. Our personal cooling system can fail, though, if we overexert ourselves on hot and humid days. This can result in heat exhaustion or a heat stroke, which is lifethreatening.

Heat exhaustion takes time to develop. Fluids and salt are vital for health. They are lost as children and adults sweat a lot during exercise or other strenuous activities. It is very important to drink lots of non-alcoholic liquids before, during, and after exercise in hot weather. As strange as it seems, people suffering from heat exhaustion have low, normal, or only slightly elevated body temperatures.

Signs and Symptoms

Signs and symptoms of heat exhaustion include:

- Cool, clammy, pale skin
- Sweating
- Dry mouth
- Fatigue, weakness
- Dizziness
- Headache
- Nausea, sometimes vomiting
- Muscle cramps
- Weak and rapid pulse

Signs of heat stroke include:

- Very high temperature (104°F or higher)
- Hot, dry, red skin
- No sweating
- Deep breathing and fast pulse, then shallow breathing and weak pulse
- Dilated pupils
- Confusion, delirium, hallucinations
- Convulsions
- Loss of consciousness

Heat stroke, unlike heat exhaustion, strikes suddenly, with little warning. When the body's cooling system fails, the body's temperature rises fast. This creates an emergency condition.

A chronic medical condition such as diabetes, use of alcohol, and vomiting or diarrhea can put children and adults at risk for heat stroke during very hot weather. Heat stroke in children is not only due to high temperatures and humidity, but also to not drinking enough fluids.

Prevention

Heat exhaustion and heat stroke can be prevented if you:

- Do not stay in or leave anyone in closed, parked cars during hot weather.
- Use caution when you must be in the sun. At the first signs of heat exhaustion, get out of the sun or your body temperature will continue to rise.
- Do not exercise vigorously during the hottest times of the day. Instead, run, jog, or exercise closer to sunrise or sunset. If the outside temperature is 82°F or above and the humidity is high, do your activity for a shorter time.

Heat Exhaustion & Heat Stroke, *Continued*

- Wear light, loose-fitting clothing, such as cotton, so sweat can evaporate. And put on a wide-brimmed hat with vents.

- Drink lots of liquids, especially if your urine is a dark yellow, to replace the fluids you lose from sweating. Thirst is not a reliable sign that your body needs fluids. When you exercise, it is better to sip rather than gulp the liquids.

- Drink water or water with salt added if you sweat a lot. (Use $\frac{1}{2}$ teaspoon salt in 1 quart of water.) Sport drinks such as Gatorade, All Sport and PowerAde are good, too.

- If you feel very hot, try to cool off. Open a window, use a fan, or turn on an air conditioner.

- Limit your stay in hot tubs or heated whirlpools to 15 minutes. Don't use them when you are alone.

- Do not drink alcohol or beverages with caffeine, because they speed up fluid loss.

- Stay out of the sun if you are taking water pills (diuretics), mood altering, or antispasmodic medications. Check with your doctor which ones are safe.

- Do not bundle a baby in blankets or heavy clothing. Infants don't tolerate heat well because their sweat glands are not well developed.

- Some people perspire more than others. Those who do should drink as much fluid as they can during hot, humid days.

- Know the signs of heat stroke and heat exhaustion and don't ignore them.

Questions to Ask

Are any signs of heat stroke present?
- Body temperature 104°F or higher
- Skin that is red, dry, and/or hot
- Pulse that is rapid and then gets weak
- No sweating
- Confusion, hallucinations, loss of consciousness, or convulsions

YES Get Emergency Care

NO

{*Note:* Do CPR if the person is not breathing and has no pulse. (See "CPR" on page 285.) Do rescue breathing if the person is not breathing but does have a pulse. (See "Airway and Breathing" under CPR on pages 285 and 286.) See also "First Aid Before Emergency Care" under Self-Care Tips in this section.}

Does the person have any of these signs?
- Too dizzy or weak to stand
- Non-stop vomiting
- Pale, cool, and clammy skin

YES Get Emergency Care

NO

{*Note:* See "First Aid Before Emergency Care" under Self-Care Tips on the next page.}

Flowchart continued on next page

23. Emergency Conditions

Heat Exhaustion & Heat Stroke, *Continued*

Flowchart continued

Are 2 or more of these signs of heat exhaustion present?
- Dry mouth
- Fatigue and weakness
- Headache
- Nausea
- Weak and rapid pulse
- Muscle cramps
- Feeling lightheaded or faint

YES

See Doctor

NO

Use Self-Care

Self-Care Tips

First Aid Before Emergency Care

- It is important to lower the body temperature. To do this:

  - Move the person to a cool place indoors or under a shady tree. Place the feet higher than the head.

  - Remove the clothing and either wrap the person in a cold, wet sheet, sponge the person with towels or sheets that are soaked in cold water; or spray the person with cool water. Fan the person. If using an electric fan, use caution. Make sure your hands are dry when you plug the fan in and turn it on. Keep the person with wet items far enough away from the fan so as not to cause electric shock.

  - Put ice packs or cold compresses on the neck, under the armpits, and on the groin area.

- Place the person in the recovery position once his or her temperature reaches 101°F. (Do not lower the temperature further.) (See "Recovery Position" on page 292.)

First Aid for Heat Exhaustion

{*Note:* These apply to you or anyone else who has heat exhaustion}

- Move to a cool place indoors or in the shade.

- Loosen clothing.

- Take fluids such as cool or cold water. If available, add $1/2$ teaspoon of salt to 1 quart of water and sip it, or drink sport drinks such as Gatorade, All Sport, or PowerAde.

- Have salty foods such as saltine crackers, if tolerated.

- Lie down in a cool, breezy place.

118 Neck/Spine Injuries

Anything that puts too much pressure or force on the neck or back can result in a neck and/or spinal injury.

Causes

Accidents with cars, motorcycles, snowmobiles, toboggans, roller blades, etc.

- Falls–especially from high places
- Diving mishaps–from diving into water that is too shallow
- A hard blow to the neck or back while playing a contact sport such as football
- Violent acts such as a gunshot wound that penetrates the head, neck, or trunk

Suspect a neck injury, too, if a head injury has occurred.

Some neck and spinal injuries can be serious because they could result in paralysis. These need emergency medical care. Others, such as whiplash, can be temporary, minor injuries.

A mild whiplash typically causes neck pain and stiffness the following day. Some people, though, have trouble raising their heads off the pillow the next morning. Physical therapy and a collar to support the neck are the most common types of treatment. It often takes 3 to 4 months for all symptoms to disappear.

Prevention

- Use padded headrests in your car to prevent whiplash.
- Drive carefully and defensively.
- Wear seat belts, both lap belts and shoulder harnesses.

- Buckle children into approved car seats appropriate for their age.
- Wear a helmet whenever you ride a bicycle or motorcycle, or when you roller-skate or roller-blade.
- Wear the recommended safety equipment for contact sports.
- Take care when jumping up and down on a trampoline, climbing a ladder, or checking a roof.
- Check the water's depth before diving into it. Do not dive into water that is less than 9 feet deep. Never dive into an above-ground pool.

{*Note:* If you suspect a neck or back injury in yourself or someone else, you must keep the neck and/or back perfectly still until an emergency crew arrives. Do not move someone with a suspected neck or spine injury unless the person must be moved because his or her life is in danger. Any movement of the head, neck or back could result in paralysis or death. Hold the head, neck and shoulders perfectly still. Use both of your hands, one on each side of the head.}

Questions to Ask

Is the injured person not breathing and has no pulse? **YES** Get Emergency Care

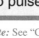 **NO**

{*Note:* See "CPR" on page 285, but do not tilt the head back or move the head or neck when you do the "Airway and Breathing" part of CPR. Instead, pull the lower jaw (chin) forward to open the airway. Place your thumb(s) or fingers on the jawbones, just in front of and below the earlobes to do this. Also See "To Immobilize the Neck and/or Spine" under Self-Care Tips on the next page.}

Flowchart continued on next page

23. Emergency Conditions

Neck/Spine Injuries, *Continued*

Flowchart continued

Is the injured person not breathing, but has a pulse? **YES** Get Emergency Care

NO

{*Note:* See "Airway and Breathing" on pages 285 and 286. But do not tilt the head back or move the head or neck. Instead, pull the lower jaw (chin) forward to open the airway. Place your thumb(s) or fingers on the jawbones, just in front of and below the earlobes, to do this. Also see "To Immobilize the Neck and/or Spine" under Self-Care Tips on this page.}

Does the injured person have any of these signs or symptoms?
• Paralysis
• Inability to open and close his or her fingers or move his or her toes
• Feelings of numbness in the legs, arms, shoulders, or any other part of the body
• Appearance that the head, neck, or back is in an odd position
• Immediate neck pain

YES Get Emergency Care

{*Note:* See "To Immobilize the Neck and/or Spine" under Self-Care Tips on this page.}

NO

Are any of these present following a recent injury to the neck and/or spine that did not get treated with emergency care at the time of the injury?
• Severe pain
• Numbness, tingling, or weakness in the face, arms, or legs
• Loss of bladder control

YES Get Emergency Care

NO

Flowchart continued in next column

Do you suspect a whiplash injury, or has pain from any injury to the neck or back lasted longer than 1 week? **YES** See Doctor

NO

 Use Self-Care

Self-Care Tips

To Immobilize the Neck and/or Spine:

■ Tell the victim to lie still and not move his or her head, neck, back, etc.

■ Place rolled towels, articles of clothing, etc. on both sides of the neck and/or body. Tie and wrap in place, but don't interfere with the victim's breathing. If necessary, use both of your hands, one on each side of the victim's head, to keep the head from moving.

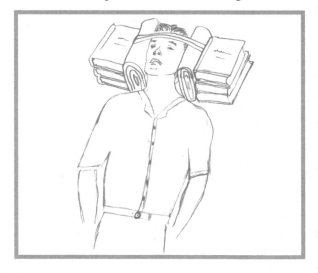

23. Emergency Conditions

Neck/Spine Injuries, *Continued*

To Move Someone with a Suspected Neck or Spinal Injury

Follow the above procedures and:

- Select a stretcher, door, or other rigid board.

- Several people should carefully lift and move the person onto the board, being very careful to align the head and neck in a straight line with the spine. The head should not rotate or bend forward or backward.

- Make sure one person uses both of his or her hands, one on each side of the victim's head, to keep the head from moving. If you can, immobilize the neck and/or spine by placing rolled towels, articles of clothing, etc., on both sides of the neck and/or body. Tie and wrap in place, but don't interfere with the victim's breathing.

To Move Someone You Suspect has Injured His or Her Neck in a Diving or Other Water Accident:

Before emergency care arrives:

- Protect the neck and/or spine from bending or twisting. Place your hands on both sides of the neck and keep in place until help arrives.

- If the person is still in the water, help the person float until a rigid board can be slipped under the head and body, at least as far down as the buttocks.

- If no board is available, several people should take the person out of the water, supporting the head and body as one unit, making sure the head does not rotate or bend in any direction.

If You Suspect a Whiplash Injury:

- See your doctor as soon as you can so he or she can assess the extent of injury.

- For the first 24 hours, apply ice packs to the injured area for up to 20 minutes every hour.

  - To make an ice pack, wrap ice in a face towel or cloth.

- After 24 hours, use ice packs or heat, whichever works best, to relieve the pain. Ways to apply heat:

  - Take a hot shower for 20 minutes a few times a day.

  - Use a hot-water bottle, heating pad (set on low), or heat lamp directed to the neck for 10 minutes several times a day. (Use caution not to burn the skin.)

- Use a cervical pillow or a small rolled towel placed behind your neck instead of a regular pillow.

- Wrap a folded towel around the neck to help hold the head in one position during the night.

- If your arm or hand is numb, ask your doctor about a cervical-traction device.

- Take an over-the-counter medicine for pain. {*Note:* See "Pain relievers" in "Your Home Pharmacy" on pages 22 and 23.}

- Get plenty of rest.

119 Poisoning

Each year, millions of cases of accidental poisoning occur. Most of them are in children aged 1 to 6.

Poisoning most often occurs from swallowing harmful substances, such as strong lyes, like drain cleaners.

The kitchen between 4 p.m. and 6 p.m. is the time and place when most accidental poisonings occur. The bathroom is the next most likely site.

The most common potential poisons include:
- Medicines such as aspirin, tranquilizers, sleeping pills
- Household cleaners such as bleach, dishwasher detergent, floor and furniture polishes and waxes, drain cleaners
- Ammonia, lye
- Insecticides and rat poison
- Vitamins
- Alcoholic beverages
- Rubbing alcohol, iodine, hair dye, mouthwash, mothballs
- Some indoor plants
- Some outdoor plants and berries
- Gasoline, antifreeze, oil, and other chemicals for the car
- Lighter fluid
- Paint thinner

Some substances are toxic when they are inhaled or absorbed through the skin. Examples are:
- Airplane glue
- Gasoline
- Auto exhaust
- Formaldehyde and other chemicals

Prevention

To prevent poisoning:
- Keep all harmful substances out of the reach of children. Better yet, keep them locked up.
- Buy and put childproof latches on cabinet doors.
- Do not store hazardous materials or medications in food containers. It's best to keep these items in their original containers, out of reach and out of sight.
- Place plants where children cannot pull off a leaf or berry for tasting.
- Store all medications and vitamins in containers with child-resistant tops. Even vitamins with iron can be deadly to a small child.
- Read warning labels on pesticides, household cleaners, and other potentially poisonous products so you know what to do in the event of an accidental poisoning. Some label instructions may be outdated, so always call the Poison Control Center when poisoning occurs.
- Flush unused medications down the toilet and rinse the containers before throwing them away.
- Buy a 1-ounce bottle of syrup of ipecac and replace it with a new one each year. Syrup of ipecac is used to induce vomiting after certain poisons have been swallowed.
- Also, keep activated charcoal on hand. This may be necessary to give when certain chemicals are swallowed.
- Teach your child never to touch anything with a skull-and-crossbones on it. This is the standard symbol for poison.
- Never call medications or vitamins "candy" in front of a child.

Poisoning, *Continued*

- Wear protective clothing, masks, etc., when using chemicals that could cause harm if inhaled or absorbed by the skin.

- Only use volatile substances such as gasoline and wood stain in areas that are well ventilated. Product labels tell you if ventilation is needed.

- Post the phone number of your local Poison Control Center next to the phone. And keep the numbers of the closest hospital emergency room, your doctor and ambulance service near the phone as well. Find out what these numbers are now. Write them on page 1 of this booklet. Write the telephone number for the Poison Control Center below:

_____

If and when you need to call the Poison Control Center, your doctor, or nearby hospital, be ready to give this information:

- The name of the substance taken
- The amount
- When it was taken
- A list of ingredients on the product label
- Information about the person who took the poison:
  - His or her age, gender, and weight
  - How he or she is feeling and reacting
  - Any medical problems he or she has

Questions to Ask

Is the person not breathing and has no pulse? **YES** → 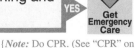 Get Emergency Care

NO

{*Note:* Do CPR. (See "CPR" on page 285.}

Flowchart continued in next column

Is the person not breathing, but has a pulse? **YES** → Get Emergency Care

NO

{*Note:* Do rescue breathing. (See "Airway and Breathing" on pages 285 and 286.}

Is the person unconscious or having convulsions? **YES** → Get Emergency Care

NO

{*Note:* See "Unconsciousness" on page 329; "First Aid for Seizures with Convulsions" on page 325.}

Has any substance been swallowed, inhaled, or absorbed by the skin that:
- Has a "Harmful or fatal if swallowed" warning on the label?
- Has a skull-and-crossbones sign on the container?
- You suspect is poisonous

YES → Get Emergency Care

{*Note:* Call the Poison Control Center first.}

NO

 Use Self-Care

Self-Care Tips

See items under "Prevention" on page 322 of this section to prevent poisoning.

23. Emergency Conditions

120 Seizures

A seizure is an out-of-control misfire between nerve cells in the brain. Normal brain functions are impaired with a seizure.

Things known to cause seizures are:

- High fevers in children. This kind of seizure is called a fever fit. A temperature higher than 102°F can set off a fever fit. High fevers are the most common cause of seizures in children ages 6 months to 4 years. These seizures are generally harmless.
- Epilepsy, a brain disorder. Seizure is the most common symptom of epilepsy.
- Brain injury, tumor, or stroke
- Electric shock
- Heat stroke
- Poisons
- Infections
- Reactions or overdoses to medicines or drugs
- Reye's Syndrome
- Snakebites
- Vaccinations
- Breath-holding

Sometimes the cause of a seizure is not known.

Seizures fall in 2 general groups: general and partial. A partial seizure affects small areas of the brain. A general seizure affects the whole brain and can cause loss of consciousness and/or convulsions. This is the type most people associate with a seizure. This type of seizure is also called a tonic-clonic or a grand mal seizure. First aid can be helpful for this type of seizure.

Symptoms of seizures with convulsions are:

- Crying out
- Falling down
- Losing consciousness
- Entire body stiffening
- Uncontrollable jerks and twitches

The sufferer's muscles relax after the seizure. He or she may lose bowel and bladder control and may be confused, sleepy and have a headache.

Most seizures last 1–5 minutes. A fever fit can last from 1–10 minutes.

Fever Fit Prevention

The best way to prevent a fever fit is to reduce the fever fast. This is especially important for a child who has had a fever fit in the past. He or she is more likely to have another one with future fevers. When your child has a fever:

- Dress him or her in lightweight clothes or remove most of his or her clothes. Don't use more than a top sheet or one blanket on your child when he or she sleeps.
- Apply washcloths rinsed in lukewarm (not cold) water to your child's forehead and neck. Sponge the rest of his or her skin with lukewarm water. Don't use rubbing alcohol.
- Give the dose of acetaminophen the label states for your child's weight or age. {*Note:* Do not give aspirin or any medication that has salicylates to anyone under 19 years of age unless your doctor tells you to.}
- Continue trying to reduce the fever until it is 101°F or less.

Seizures, *Continued*

■ Ask your child's doctor about suppositories that lower fevers if your child has had a fever fit in the past. Using one at the first sign of a fever may prevent a seizure.

Questions to Ask

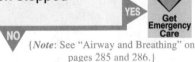

Has the person stopped breathing?

YES — Get Emergency Care

NO

{*Note*: See "Airway and Breathing" on pages 285 and 286.}

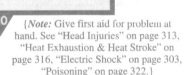

Does the seizure occur with another serious problem such as?
• Head injury
• Heat stroke
• Electric shock
• Poisoning

YES — Get Emergency Care

NO

{*Note:* Give first aid for problem at hand. See "Head Injuries" on page 313, "Heat Exhaustion & Heat Stroke" on page 316, "Electric Shock" on page 303, "Poisoning" on page 322.}

Are any of the following also present?
• The seizure lasts longer than 5 minutes.
• The person has a second seizure soon after the first one
• The person has a hard time breathing
• The person is pregnant

YES — Get Emergency Care

{*Note:* See "First Aid for Seizures with Convulsions" under Self-Care Tips on this page.}

NO

Flowchart continued in next column

In a Child:

Are one or both of these things true?
• This is the child's first seizure
• The seizure occurred in a child less than 6 months old or older than 4 years of age

YES — Get Emergency Care

NO

Use Self-Care

{*Note*: See "First Aid for Seizure in a Child" under Self-Care Tips in this section. Do this until emergency care arrives.}

Self-Care Tips

{*Note:* Some seizures in people who have epilepsy and in children with high fevers do not need immediate medical care. If you see someone having a convulsive seizure without other problems, do "First Aid for Seizures with Convulsions" on this page. (A person with epilepsy may wear a medic-alert bracelet or neck chain with "epilepsy" written on it or he or she may have "epilepsy" written on a card or driver's license in his or her wallet or purse. Look for this.) Also, inform your child's doctor whenever he or she has a seizure.}

First Aid for Seizures with Convulsions:

■ Stay calm.

■ Protect the victim from injury. Cushion the head with a soft object such as a pillow, coat, or blanket.

■ Move sharp objects out of the way.

■ Loosen tight clothes around the neck.

■ Place the person on his or her side.

23. Emergency Conditions

Seizures, *Continued*

- Clear the mouth of vomit if there is any.

- Do not try to hold the victim down.

- Do not put a spoon or anything into the mouth to prevent tongue biting.

- Do not give anything to eat or drink.

- Do not give medication.

- Do not throw water on the victim's face.

- Note how many minutes the seizure(s) lasts and observe the symptoms that take place so you can report these to the doctor.

- Offer to help the victim when the seizure is over. Do not embarrass the victim.

First Aid for a Seizure in a Child

- Prevent injury to the child during the seizure:

  - Keep the child from falling and hitting his or her head on a table edge or any sharp object.

  - Cushion the child's head.

  - Move furniture and toys and such out of the way.

- Make sure his or her air passage is open. Gently pull the jaw forward as you extend the neck backwards.

- Roll the child on his or her side to allow saliva to drain from the mouth.

- Following the seizure, the child will likely be sleepy and not remember what has happened. This is normal. Consult your child's doctor and follow instructions.

- Dress the child in light, loose-fitting clothing and put him or her to sleep in a cool room.

- If the seizure in a child is due to a fever, lower the child's temperature as soon as the seizure stops:

  - Sponge the body with lukewarm water.

  - Do not use rubbing alcohol.

  - Do not use ice because it drops the temperature too fast.

  - Do not put the child in a bathtub.

121 Shock

Shock is an emergency condition. It occurs when the circulation system fails to send blood to all parts of the body. With shock, areas of the body are deprived of oxygen because blood flow or blood volume is too low to meet the body's needs. The result is damage to parts of the body such as the limbs, lungs, heart, and brain.

Some causes for shock are:

- Heart attack
- Severe or sudden blood loss from an injury or serious illness
- Large drop in body fluids, such as following a severe burn or severe vomiting and/or diarrhea
- Blood poisoning from major infections
- Exposure to extreme heat or cold for too long

Other things that lead to shock are:

- Fractures of a large bone
- A severe allergic reaction
- Very low blood sugar such as occurs with diabetes (insulin shock)
- Excessive drinking of alcohol
- Drug overdose

Signs and Symptoms

- Weakness, trembling
- Restlessness, confusion
- Pale or blue-colored lips, skin, and/or fingernails
- Cool and moist skin
- Weak but fast pulse
- Rapid, shallow breathing
- Nausea, vomiting
- Enlarged pupils
- Extreme thirst
- Loss of consciousness

Questions to Ask

Is the person not breathing and has no pulse? **YES** Get Emergency Care

NO

{*Note:* See "CPR" on page 285.}

Is the person not breathing, but does have a pulse? **YES** Get Emergency Care

NO

{*Note:* See "Airway and Breathing" on page 285 and 286.}

Is the person?
- Bleeding
- Suffering from an injury
- Having a hard time breathing
YES Get Emergency Care

NO

{*Note:* See "First Aid for Major Bleeding" under Self-Care Tips on page 98. Also, see other injury topics such as "Head Injuries" on page 313, "Broken Bones" on page 136, "Cuts, Scrapes, & Punctures" on page 96, etc.}

Is the person unconscious? **YES** Get Emergency Care

NO

{*Note:* See "Unconsciousness" on page 329.}

Flowchart continued on next page

Shock, *Continued*

Flowchart continued

Does the person show any of these signs of shock?
- Weakness, confusion
- Pale or blue-colored lips, skin and/or fingernails
- Cool and moist skin
- Weak but fast pulse
- Rapid, shallow breathing
- Nausea, vomiting
- Enlarged pupils
- Extreme thirst

YES ➤ **Get Emergency Care**

{*Note:* See "First Aid for Shock Until Emergency Care Arrives" under Self-Care Tips on this page.}

NO ⬇ **Use Self-Care**

Self-Care Tips

First Aid for Shock Until Emergency Care Arrives:

- Lay the person down, face up.

- Elevate the feet about 1 foot with a box or rolled blankets. This causes blood to flow from the legs to the head and vital organs in the body. {*Note:* Do not raise the feet or lower the head if you suspect the person has a head, neck, back, or leg injury.}

- Do not raise feet or move legs if hip or leg bones are broken. Keep the victim lying flat.

- Loosen tight clothing. Then cover the person with a coat or blanket to prevent heat loss. If necessary, lie down next to and hug the person to share your body heat until help arrives. Place insulation between the person and the ground. {*Note:* Do not use hot-water bottles or electric blankets to try to warm the person.}

- Monitor for breathing and pulse every so often.

- Do not give any food or liquids. If the person asks for water, moisten the lips, but do not allow him or her to drink any fluids.

- Reassure the person. Make him or her as comfortable as you can.

- If the person vomits, roll him or her on the side so the vomit does not back up into the windpipe and lungs.

122 Unconsciousness

Someone who is unconscious is not sleeping. Rather, an unconscious person is hard to rouse or can't be made aware of his or her surroundings. Unconsciousness is caused by illness, injury, or emotional shock.

Signs and Symptoms

There are many levels of unconsciousness. Some are more serious than others. Levels include unconscious episodes that are:

- Brief. Examples are fainting or blacking out.

- Longer. The victim is incoherent when roused.

- Prolonged. A person in a coma, for example, can be motionless and not at all aware of his or her surroundings for a very long time.

Causes

- Carbon monoxide poisoning

- Hypothermia (low body temperature, usually caused by overexposure to cold temperatures or cold water)

- Stroke

- Shock

- Epilepsy

- Heat exhaustion

- Diabetic coma

- Excessive bleeding

- Alcohol abuse

- Drug overdose

- Poisoning

- Head injury/concussion

- Low blood sugar

- Too fast, too slow, and/or irregular heartbeats

- Heart attack

- Medications

- Underactive thyroid

- Heart valve disease

Look for medic alert information if you find a person unconscious. It could be on a bracelet or a neck chain. It could be in his or her wallet on a card or on a sticker on the back of his or her driver's license. Each of these can identify a known medical condition.

Questions to Ask

Is the person not breathing and has no pulse?

YES → Get Emergency Care

{*Note:* See "CPR" on page 285.}

NO

Has the person stopped breathing?

YES → Get Emergency Care

{*Note:* See "Airway and Breathing" on page 285 and 286.}

NO

Does the person have a head or neck injury?

YES → Get Emergency Care

{*Note:* See "Head Injuries" on page 313 and "Neck/Spine Injuries" on page 319.}

NO

Flowchart continued on next page

Unconsciousness, *Continued*

Flowchart continued

Is the person bleeding a lot? YES → **Get Emergency Care**

NO

{Note: See "First Aid for Major Bleeding" under Self-Care Tips on page 96.}

With or without a medic alert tag for diabetes: Did the person have these signs of a diabetic coma before the unconsciousness?
- Fast and weak pulse
- Rapid, deep breathing
- Red, dry, warm skin
- Fruity breath odor (can smell like grape juice or nail polish remover)
- Vomiting

YES → **Get Emergency Care**

NO

Did the person show these signs of an insulin reaction or low blood sugar before unconsciousness?
- Lack of coordination
- Bad temper, angry outburst
- Confusion
- Pale skin
- Sweating
- Trembling
- Seizure

YES → **Get Emergency Care**

{Note: See "First Aid for Low Blood Sugar Reaction" under Self-Care Tips on this page.}

NO

Flowchart continued in next column

Has the person been stung by an insect? YES → **Get Emergency Care**

NO

{Note: Give shot from "emergency insect sting" kit, if available. Follow other instructions in kit.}

When you shake the person, does he or she not respond after 2 minutes, but is still breathing and has not been seriously injured? YES → **Get Emergency Care**

NO *{Note:* Put the victim in the "Recovery Position." See "Recovery Position" on page 292.}

Has the person fainted or blacked out for no apparent reason? YES → **Get Emergency Care**

NO

{Note: See "Fainting" on page 308.}

 Use Self-Care

Self-Care Tips

First Aid for Low Blood Sugar Reaction:

■ Check the victim's pocket or purse for something sweet. He or she may have a tube of glucose paste (a sweet source) for emergencies. If so, squeeze some under his or her tongue. Or place a small amount of sugar under the victim's tongue.

■ Keep the victim's airway open.

■ Place victim on his or her side.

■ Do not give liquids.

SECTION IV
Major Medical Conditions

Introduction

Section IV presents common chronic illnesses. Each of the conditions is divided into 3 parts:

- Information about the condition
- Signs and symptoms of the condition
- Care and treatment for the condition

Unlike the common health problems in Section II, which you may be able to treat with Self-Care Tips alone, these chronic medical conditions need diagnosis and medical treatment from health care professionals. If you have one or more of these conditions, you will still need to do things to take care of yourself.

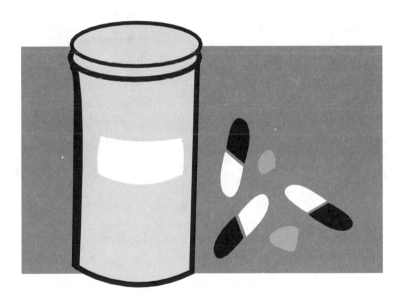

Chronic Illnesses

123 Alzheimer's Disease

Alzheimer's disease afflicts nearly 4 million Americans. It strikes over 45 percent of the population over age 85 and about 10 percent of those over age 65. In rare instances, Alzheimer's comes earlier than age 65.

No one knows what causes Alzheimer's disease. Some research hints that a virus or infectious agent is the culprit. Other studies point to a genetic link, environmental toxins, such as aluminum, and/or brain chemical deficits. Two brain chemicals are known to be produced less in Alzheimer's disease. These chemicals (acetylcholine and somatostatin) are needed for normal communication between nerve cells. Whatever the cause, the end result is the death of brain cells that control intellect (the way your brain receives and processes information).

Signs and Symptoms

Alzheimer's disease has a gradual onset. The signs and symptoms may progress in stages. How quickly they occur varies from person to person. The course of the disease averages 8 years from the time symptoms start.

Stage One

- Forgetfulness
- Disorientation of time and place
- Increasing inability to do routine tasks
- Impairment in judgement
- Lessening of initiative
- Lack of spontaneity
- Depression and fear

Stage Two

- Increasing forgetfulness
- Increasing disorientation
- Wandering
- Restlessness and agitation, especially at night
- Repetitive actions
- Muscle twitching and/or convulsions may develop

Stage Three

- Disorientation
- Inability to recognize either themselves or other people
- Speech impairment (may not be able to speak at all)
- Develop need to put everything into their mouths
- Develop need to touch everything in sight
- Become emaciated
- Complete loss of control of all body functions

{*Note:* The stages very often overlap.}

Treatment and Care

If someone you care about shows signs of Alzheimer's disease, see that they get medical attention to confirm (or rule out) the diagnosis. Not everything that looks like Alzheimer's is Alzheimer's.

Alzheimer's Disease, *Continued*

There are many diseases or other problems that can cause dementia (severe problems with memory and thinking). These include:

- Brain tumors
- Blood clots in the brain
- Severe vitamin B12 deficiency
- Hypothyroidism
- Depression
- Side effects of some medicines

Unlike Alzheimer's, these problems can be treated.

There is no known cure for Alzheimer's disease. Good planning and medical and social management are necessary to help both the victim and caregivers cope with the symptoms and maintain the quality of life for as long as possible. An advance directive should be drafted in the early stages to allow for the victim's wishes. (See Advance Directives" on page 28.) It's especially helpful to put structure in the life of someone who's in the early stages of Alzheimer's. Some suggestions include:

- Maintain daily routines.
- Post reminders on a large calendar that can be easily seen.
- Make "to do" lists of daily tasks for the person with Alzheimer's to do, and ask him or her to check them off as they are completed.
- Put things in their proper places after use, to help the person with Alzheimer's find things when he or she needs them.

- Post safety reminders (like "Turn off the stove") at appropriate places throughout the house.
- See that the person with Alzheimer's eats well-balanced meals, goes for walks with family members, and continues to be as active as possible.

Two prescription medications, tacrine (Cognex), and donepezil (Aricept) may help some persons with mild to moderate Alzheimer's disease. Sometimes medications to treat depression, paranoia, and agitation, etc., can minimize symptoms, but they will not necessarily improve memory.

At late stages, providing a safe environment is very important. Alzheimer's victims should wear identification bracelets or necklaces so they can be identified should they be separated from their home environment. Seeking adult foster care or nursing home care for those who require supervision or medical management may be necessary.

Most persons with Alzheimer's disease eventually need 24-hour care. Caregivers of Alzheimer's victims should also be given "care." They must deal with a number of financial, social, physical, and emotional issues. Care for caregivers can be provided by professionals of home care, day care, respite care, service programs, and self-help groups.

(See "Places to Get Information & Help" under "Alzheimer's Disease" on page 375.)

124 Angina

Angina is a common term shortened for the medical term "angina pectoris." The word angina itself means pain; pectoris means chest. Angina is the chest pain or discomfort brought on by decreased circulation in the heart and heart muscle itself. It results from a shortage of oxygen and other nutrients to any part of the heart muscle.

Signs and Symptoms

- Squeezing pressure, heaviness, or mild ache in the chest (usually behind the breastbone)

- Aching in a tooth with or without squeezing pressure or heaviness in the chest

- Aching into the neck muscles or jaw

- Aching into one or both arms

- Aching into the back

- A feeling of gas in the upper abdomen and lower chest

- A feeling that you're choking or shortness of breath

- Paleness and sweating

These symptoms may not be extreme, so are often neglected. It is better for you to report an episode of angina to your doctor than not to, even if you might feel foolish later if something minor is the cause. Episodes of angina are usually associated with:

- Anger or excitement

- Emotional shock

- Exertion or physical work, especially if it strains the muscles of the chest or arms

- Walking rapidly uphill

- Waking up at night with discomfort due to decreased blood flow to the heart

In all of these situations, there is relief from the distress when the activity is stopped. Moderate daytime activity helps relieve nighttime angina, though.

Many people who experience angina for the first time fear they're having a heart attack. Here's why angina and heart attack are mistaken for each other:

- Both can be caused by a buildup of fatty plaque (atherosclerosis) in the heart arteries (coronary arteries). These plaques cause a decrease in blood flow to the heart muscle beyond the partial obstruction. In both, the pain can be felt in the chest, arms, shoulders, and/or neck.

- Both may be brought on by physical exertion.

- Both are most prevalent in men who are 50 and older and women who are past menopause.

The difference between angina and a heart attack is that a heart attack results in a damaged or injured heart muscle. Angina does not. Rather, anginal pain is a warning sign of a potential heart attack. The pain indicates that the heart muscle isn't getting enough blood.

Angina, *Continued*

It is hard, sometimes, to tell the difference between angina and a heart attack. A person may have to be given tests and be observed for a day in the hospital or emergency room to tell the difference.

A doctor can diagnose angina as stable or unstable based on your description of the painful episode, but he or she may need to confirm it with a stress test (a measurement of heart function taken while you exercise on a treadmill). Unstable angina, a symptom of coronary artery disease, needs immediate attention. This serious medical condition affects many Americans, some of whom may not know they have heart disease. Although unstable angina can precede a heart attack, prompt treatment can lower the risk of death or serious cardiac events.

Factors like high blood pressure, obesity, diabetes, high cholesterol, smoking, or a family history of atherosclerotic heart disease increase the odds of angina.

Treatment and Care

Seek emergency care for any chest pain which is suspicious for angina. Contact your physician or a cardiologist, who should insist on close follow-up, appropriate studies to diagnose your condition, and therapy to treat it. The keystones to treatment are:

- Medications such as:
  - Nitroglycerin (or other medication to temporarily dilate or widen the coronary arteries), which eases blood flow to the heart. Nitroglycerin takes effect within a minute or two.
  - Medicine(s) to control high blood pressure
  - Low-dose daily aspirin

- Daily physical exercise for endurance. This should be prescribed just for you by an exercise physiologist to whom a cardiologist has referred you. Exercise must be maintained below the onset of any discomfort. Exercise may not be a part of treatment for some individuals.

- Don't smoke. Nicotine in cigarettes constricts the arteries and prevents proper blood flow.

- Avoid large, heavy meals. Instead, eat lighter meals throughout the day.

- Rest after eating, or engage in some quiet activity.

- Minimize exposure to cold, windy weather.

- Lower your cholesterol level, if high, by eating a low-saturated-fat diet and/or taking lipid (fat)-lowering medication, if necessary and prescribed.

- Avoid sudden physical exertion, such as running to catch a bus.

- Avoid anger and frustration whenever possible.

(See "Places to Get Information & Help" under "Heart Disease/High Blood Pressure" on page 376.)

125 Arthritis

Arthritis robs some 40 million Americans of their freedom of movement by breaking down the protective cartilage in the joints. By destroying cartilage, arthritis results in pain and decreased movement.

Many forms of arthritis exist. Four of the most common are osteoarthritis, rheumatoid arthritis, ankylosing spondylitis, and gout (see page 353).

Osteoarthritis is a painful degeneration of the cartilage in the weight-bearing and frequently used joints. This kind of arthritis is typically brought on by genetics, activity, and wear and tear on the joints. It can also follow an injury to the joint. Osteoarthritis usually affects older people and is the most common type of arthritis.

Rheumatoid arthritis (RA) is caused by a chronic inflammation of the fingers, wrists, ankles, elbows, and/or knees, causing pain, swelling, and tenderness. Morning stiffness lasting longer than an hour is very common. RA affects women more often than men, striking in their thirties and forties.

Ankylosing spondylitis generally affects young men between the ages of 15 and 45. Symptoms are stiff backbone and low back pain.

Signs and Symptoms

Symptoms of arthritis depend upon the type of arthritis that is present. Symptoms generally include:

- Stiffness
- Swelling in one or more joints
- Deep, aching pain in a joint
- Pain that comes with joint movement
- Tenderness, warmth, or redness in affected joints

Treatment and Care

The goal of treatment is to reduce pain and improve joint mobility. Your doctor may prescribe medication (usually aspirin or a nonsteroidal anti-inflammatory medicine), rest, heat or cold treatment, weight-reduction (if you are overweight) and some physical therapy or exercise.

Exercise is perhaps the most important of these, whether it is some form of stretching, isometrics, or simple endurance exercise. Exercise prevents the muscles from shrinking. Inactivity encourages both loss of muscle tone and bone deterioration. Too much exercise, however, will cause more pain in those with rheumatoid arthritis or osteoarthritis. So if you have arthritis, consult your physician, a physical therapist, or a physiatrist (a doctor who specializes in rehabilitative treatment) to help you set up an exercise program.

One form of exercise that's effective and soothing is hydrotherapy, or movement done in water. Doctors highly recommend swimming, too. But remember, hydrotherapy, or any form of exercise, should never produce pain. If you begin to hurt, stop and rest or apply ice packs.

The following exercise suggestions may provide relief:

- Choose exercise routines that use all affected joints.
- Keep movements gradual, slow, and gentle.
- If a joint is inflamed, don't exercise it.
- Don't overdo it. Allow yourself sufficient rest.
- Concentrate on freedom of movement, especially in the water, and be patient.

(See "Places to Get Information & Help" under "Arthritis" on page 375.)

126 Cancer

Cancer refers to a broad group of diseases in which body cells become abnormal, grow out of control, and are or become malignant (harmful).

Cancer is the second leading cause of death in the United States (heart disease is first). Current estimates say that about 1 in 3 of all Americans will develop some kind of cancer in their lifetime. The most common forms are cancer of the skin, lungs, colon and rectum, breast, prostate, urinary tract, and uterus.

Exactly what causes all cancers has not yet been found. Evidence suggests, however, that cancer could result from complex interactions of viruses, a person's genetic makeup, their immune status, and their exposure to other risk factors that may promote cancer.

These risk factors include:

- Exposure to the sun's ultraviolet rays, nuclear radiation, X-rays, and radon
- Use of tobacco and/or alcohol (for some cancers)
- Use of certain medicines such as DES (a synthetic estrogen)
- Polluted air and water
- Dietary factors such as a high-fat diet; specific food preservatives, namely nitrates and nitrites; char-broiling and char-grilling meats
- Exposure to a variety of chemicals such as asbestos, benzenes, VC (vinyl chloride), wood dust, some ingredients of cigarette smoke, etc.

Signs and Symptoms

Symptoms of cancer depend on the type of cancer, the stage that it is in, and whether or not it has spread to other parts of the body (metastasis). The following signs and symptoms should always be brought to your doctor's attention because they could be warning signals of cancer:

- Any change in bladder or bowel habits
- A lump or thickening in the breast, testicles, or anywhere else
- Unusual vaginal bleeding or rectal discharge or unusual bleeding from any part of the body
- Persistent hoarseness or nagging cough
- A sore that doesn't heal
- Noticeable change in a wart or mole
- Indigestion or difficulty swallowing

Treatment and Care

Cancer is not necessarily fatal and is, in many cases, curable. Early detection and proper treatment increase your chances for surviving cancer. Early detection is more likely if you:

- Know the above warning signs for cancer and report any of these warning signs to your doctor if they occur
- Do regular self-examinations such as monthly breast self-examination if you are a woman, (see page 224) and a testicular self-exam monthly or as directed by your doctor if you are a man (see page 221). {*Note:* Men can also get breast cancer and should check with their doctor for signs to look for.}
- Look at yourself in the mirror for any noticeable changes in warts or moles or for any wounds that have not healed

Cancer, *Continued*

■ Ask your doctor to perform routine tests that can help detect early signs of cancer. Examples are pap tests, breast exams, and mammograms, for women. See the common health tests on page 17 for other tests, including digital rectal exam, sigmoidoscopy, and stool blood test.

If and when cancer is diagnosed, treatment will depend on the type of cancer present, the stage it is in, and your body's response to treatment.

Cancer treatment generally includes one or more of the following:

■ Surgery to remove the cancerous tumor(s) and clear any obstruction to vital passageways caused by the cancer

■ Radiation therapy

■ Chemotherapy

■ Possibly immunotherapy, hormonal therapy, or bone-marrow transplant

Prevention

Measures can be taken to lower the risk for certain forms of cancer.

Dietary:

■ Reduce the intake of total dietary fat to no more than 30% of total calories and reduce the intake of saturated fat to less than 10% of total calories.

■ Eat more fruits, vegetables, and whole grains, especially:

• Broccoli and other cabbage-family vegetables, including cabbage and brussels sprouts. These contain cancer-fighting chemicals, such as sulforaphane antioxidants.

• Deep yellow-orange fruits and vegetables such as cantaloupe, peaches, tomatoes, carrots, sweet potatoes and squash, and very dark-green vegetables like spinach, greens, and broccoli for their beta-carotene and cancer-fighting chemical content

• Strawberries, citrus fruits, broccoli, and green peppers for vitamin C

• Whole-grain breads, cereals, fresh fruits and vegetables, and legumes for their dietary fiber content

■ Consume salt-cured, salt-pickled, and smoked foods only in moderation.

■ Drink alcoholic beverages only in moderation, if at all.

Lifestyle:

■ Do not smoke, use tobacco products, or inhale secondhand smoke.

■ Limit your exposure to known carcinogens such as asbestos, radon, and other workplace chemicals, as well as pesticides and herbicides.

■ Have X-rays only when necessary.

■ Limit your exposure to the sun's ultraviolet (UV) rays, sun lamps, and tanning booths. Protect your skin from the sun's UV rays with sunscreen (applied frequently and containing a sun protection factor [SPF] of 15 or higher) and protective clothing (sun hats, long sleeves, etc.).

■ Reduce stress. Emotional stress may weaken the immune system, which fights off stray cancer cells.

(See "Places to Get Information & Help" under "Cancer" on page 375.)

127 Cataracts

A cataract is a cloudy area in the lens or lens capsule of the eye. A cataract blocks or distorts light entering the eye. This causes problems with glare from lamps or the sun. Vision gradually becomes dull and fuzzy, even in daylight. Most of the time, cataracts occur in both eyes, but only one eye may be affected. If they form in both eyes, one eye can be worse than the other, because each cataract develops at a different rate. When cataracts are forming, vision can be helped with frequent changes in eyeglass prescriptions.

There are several causes of cataracts:

- Senile cataracts are the most common form. These cataracts result from aging. This is probably due to changes in the chemical state of lens proteins. About half of Americans aged 65 to 74 have cataracts. About 70 percent of those over 75 have this condition.

- Traumatic cataracts. These develop after a foreign body enters the lens capsule with enough force to cause specific damage.

- Complicated cataracts. These occur secondary to other diseases (e.g., diabetes mellitus) or other eye disorders (e.g., detached retinas, glaucoma, and retinitis pigmentosa). Ionizing radiation or infrared rays can also lead to this type of cataract. Also, a baby can be born with cataracts in one or both eyes if its mother had German measles (rubella) when she was pregnant.

- Toxic cataracts can result from medicine or chemical toxicity. Smokers have an increased risk for developing cataracts.

Signs and Symptoms

- Cloudy, fuzzy, foggy, or filmy vision

- Sensitivity to light and glazed nighttime vision. This can cause problems when driving at night because headlights seem too bright.

- Double vision

- Pupils which are normally black appear milky white

- Halos which may appear around lights

- Changes in the way you see colors

- Problems with glare from lamps or the sun

- Better vision for awhile, only in farsighted people. This is called "second sight."

Prevention

- Limit exposing your eyes to X-rays, microwaves, and infrared radiation.

- Use sunglasses that block ultraviolet (UV) light–both UVA and UVB rays.

- Wear a wide-brimmed hat or baseball cap to keep direct sunlight from your eyes while outdoors.

- Avoid overexposure to sunlight.

- Wear glasses or goggles that protect your eyes whenever you use strong chemicals, power tools, or other instruments that could result in eye injury.

- Don't smoke.

- Avoid heavy drinking.

Cataracts, *Continued*

- Eat a lot of foods high in beta-carotene and/or vitamin C, which are thought to help prevent or delay cataracts. Carrots, cantaloupes, oranges, and broccoli are examples of such foods.

- Follow your doctor's advice to keep other illnesses such as diabetes under control.

- For females: Get a vaccination for German measles if you haven't had them and if you plan on getting pregnant.

Treatment and Care

If the vision loss caused by a cataract is only slight, surgery may not be needed. A change in your glasses, stronger bifocals, or the use of magnifying lenses and taking measures to reduce glare may help improve your vision and be enough for treatment. To reduce glare, wear sunglasses that filter both UVA and UVB rays when you are outdoors. When indoors, make sure your lighting is not too bright or pointed directly at you. Use soft, white light bulbs instead of clear ones, for example, and arrange to have light reflect off walls and ceilings. When cataracts interfere with your life, however, surgery should be considered.

Modern cataract surgery is safe and effective in restoring vision. Ninety-five percent of operations are successful. For the most part, surgery can be done on an outpatient basis or involve no more than an overnight hospital stay.

A person who has cataract surgery usually gets an artificial lens at the same time. A plastic disc called an intraocular lens is placed in the lens capsule inside the eye. Other choices are contact lenses and cataract glasses. Your doctor will help you to decide which choice is best for you.

It takes a couple of months for an eye to heal after cataract surgery. Experts say it is best to wait until your first eye heals before you have surgery on the second eye if it, too, has a cataract.

Following surgery, continue to protect your eyes by wearing sunglasses that filter both UVA and UVB rays.

(See "Places to Get Information & Help" under "Visual Problems" on page 377.)

128 Chronic Fatigue Syndrome

Until about 1983, doctors knew next to nothing about chronic fatigue syndrome. Its exact cause is still unknown. Some researchers used to think it was caused by the Epstein-Barr virus. Others suggest its cause could be a virus that has not yet been found. Most experts now lean toward a theory of multiple causes.

Signs and Symptoms

Symptoms of chronic fatigue syndrome are:

- Fatigue for at least 6 months
- Sore throat
- Swollen glands
- Low-grade fever
- Headaches
- Depression
- Muscle aches
- Mild weight loss
- Short-term memory problems
- Sleep disturbances (insomnia or hypersomnia)
- Confusion, difficulty thinking, inability to concentrate

These symptoms can signal a number of health conditions. Chronic fatigue syndrome can be diagnosed, therefore, only after other illnesses, such as HIV/AIDS, tuberculosis, chronic inflammatory diseases, autoimmune diseases (such as lupus), Lyme disease or psychiatric illnesses have been ruled out. As yet, no specific laboratory tests can diagnose the syndrome.

For some, the symptoms are so debilitating that a normal working life is impossible. Yet others experience only a vague sense of feeling ill. In some cases, symptoms never let up, while in others they come and go.

Treatment and Care

Until more is known, people with chronic fatigue syndrome are encouraged to do the following:

- Get plenty of rest.
- Learn to manage stress.
- Take good care of their general health.
- Try to lead as normal a life as possible.
- Join a support group of others who have this problem.

Medicines may be prescribed to relieve pain and muscle aches and to control fever. These include over-the-counter medicines such as acetaminophen, aspirin, ibuprofen, naproxen sodium, or prescription, nonsteroidal, anti-inflammatory drugs (NSAIDs). Antidepressant medicine may also be prescribed. A gradual exercise program, if tolerated, may also be beneficial.

129 Cirrhosis

Cirrhosis is a chronic disease of the liver. It can be caused by any injury, infection, or inflammation of the liver. With cirrhosis, normal, healthy liver cells are replaced with scar tissue. This prevents the liver from doing its many functions.

The liver is probably the body's most versatile organ. Among its many tasks are the following:
- Makes bile (a substance that aids in the digestion of fats)
- Produces blood proteins
- Helps the blood to clot
- Metabolizes cholesterol
- Helps maintain normal blood sugar levels
- Forms and stores glycogen (the body's short-term energy source)
- Makes more than 1,000 enzymes needed for various bodily functions
- Detoxifies substances (e.g., alcohol and certain drugs)

The liver can handle a certain amount of alcohol without much difficulty. But too much alcohol, too often, and for too long, causes the vital tissues in the liver to break down. Fatty deposits accumulate and scarring occurs. Cirrhosis is most commonly found in men over 45. Yet, the number of women getting cirrhosis is on the rise.

To make matters worse, people who regularly overindulge in alcohol generally have poor nutritional habits. When alcohol replaces food, essential vitamins and minerals can be missing from the diet. Malnutrition makes cirrhosis worse.

Alcohol abuse is the most common cause of cirrhosis. Hepatitis, taking certain drugs, or exposure to certain chemicals can also produce this condition.

Signs and Symptoms

Early signs and symptoms are vague, but generally include:
- Poor appetite
- Nausea
- Indigestion
- Vomiting
- Weight loss
- Constipation
- Dull abdominal ache
- Fatigue

Doctors recognize the following as signs of advanced cirrhosis:
- Enlarged liver
- Yellowish eyes and skin and tea-colored urine (indicating jaundice)
- Bleeding from the gastrointestinal tract
- Itching
- Hair loss
- Swelling in the legs and stomach
- Tendency to bruise easily
- Mental confusion
- Coma

Treatment and Care

Cirrhosis can be life-threatening. Get medical attention if you have any of the above symptoms. And needless to say, you (or anyone you suspect of having cirrhosis) should abstain from alcohol and get treatment for alcoholism. If you suspect some toxic substance (e.g., medicines or industrial poisons) has caused the cirrhosis, discuss the possibility with your doctor so that you can identify and get rid of the culprit.

(See "Places to Get Information & Help" under "Liver Diseases" on page 376.)

130 Coronary Heart Disease

The coronary arteries supply blood to the heart muscle. When they became narrowed or blocked (usually by fatty deposits and/or blood clots), the heart muscle can be damaged.

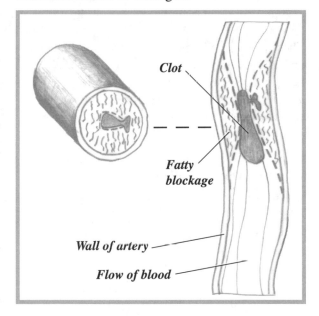

Clot

Fatty blockage

Wall of artery

Flow of blood

This is coronary heart disease. Two conditions of coronary heart disease are angina pectoris (see angina on page 334) and acute heart attacks. Every day, about 4,000 Americans have heart attacks, one every 20 seconds. And each year, nearly 600,000 people die of coronary artery disease, making it the nation's number 1 killer. Fortunately, heart disease claims fewer and fewer lives each year, thanks to advances in medical treatment of heart disease and growing public awareness of the benefits of exercise and good nutrition. Prevention is of utmost importance.

Prevention

To help avoid coronary heart disease, follow these steps:

■ Have your blood pressure checked regularly. To control high blood pressure, follow your doctor's advice.

■ Don't smoke. If you smoke, quit. Nicotine constricts blood flow and decreases oxygen supply to the heart.

■ Be aware of the signs and symptoms for diabetes, which is associated with hardening of the arteries. (See "Diabetes" on page 345.) Follow your doctor's advice if you have diabetes.

■ Maintain a normal body weight. People who are 30% or more above their ideal body weight are more prone to high blood pressure and diabetes, and therefore coronary heart disease.

■ Follow a diet low in saturated fats and cholesterol. (Saturated fats are found in meats, dairy products with fat, hydrogenated vegetable oils, and some tropical oils, like coconut and palm kernel oils.) High-saturated fat, high-cholesterol diets contribute to the fatty sludge that collects inside artery walls.

■ Reduce your intake of salt and foods high in salt if you are "salt-sensitive." Salt-sensitive persons' blood pressure goes up if they eat too much salt.

Coronary Heart Disease, *Continued*

■ Get some form of aerobic exercise at least 3 times a week for 20 minutes at a time. Sitting around hour after hour, day after day, week in and week out with no regular physical activity may cause circulation problems later in life. Start new exercise programs gradually. Report symptoms of chest pain and/or shortness of breath to your doctor.

■ Practice relaxation techniques. These can reduce the harmful effects of stress and improve your outlook on daily events. Stress has been linked to elevated blood pressure, among other health problems.

■ Get regular medical checkups.

■ Take medication to lower your cholesterol and/or triglycerides (another blood fat) if prescribed by your doctor.

■ Know the signs of a heart attack. Get immediate medical attention if you have any of the following:

• Chest pressure or pain. The pain may spread to the arm, neck, or jaw.

• Feelings of tightness, burning, squeezing, fullness, or heaviness in the chest that last more than a few minutes, or go away and come back

• Chest discomfort with:

 – Rapid or irregular heartbeat

 – Sweating; pale, gray colored or clammy skin; dizziness, nausea, and/or vomiting

 – Shortness of breath or trouble breathing

 – Lightheadedness, fainting, or sense of doom

Treatment and Care

If you think you're having a heart attack, get to a hospital as soon as possible. If given within 4 hours, an injection that dissolves clots can reduce the risk of death and severity of damage to the heart muscle. Other emergency procedures can also prevent damage to the heart muscle.

The type of care after a heart attack will depend on the amount of damage done to the heart muscle. Specific medical tests and procedures can assess the damage. Your doctor will decide the course of treatment. This could include 1 or more of the following:

■ Medication (cardiac, blood pressure, cholesterol-lowering medicines, etc.)

■ Hospitalization for treatment and recovery from the heart attack

■ Cardiac rehabilitation for lifestyle changes. These include:

• Smoking cessation

• Weight loss

• Low-fat, cholesterol-controlling diet

• Behavior modification, stress management, and relaxation techniques

■ Surgery if indicated: angioplasty, coronary artery bypass grafts, etc.

■ Long-term maintenance and medical follow-up

(See "Places to Get Information & Help" under "Heart Disease/High Blood Pressure" on page 376.)

131 Diabetes

Diabetes is a condition which results when a person's body doesn't make any insulin, enough insulin, or doesn't use insulin the right way. Insulin is a hormone made in the pancreas gland that helps your cells use blood sugar for energy. When insulin is in short supply, the glucose (sugar) in the blood can become dangerously high. Someone who is diabetic may have to take insulin by injection, or pills by mouth to help the body secrete more of its own insulin or make better use of the insulin it does secrete. Some diabetics, however, require no medication. All persons with diabetes must follow a controlled diet and exercise regularly to prevent their blood sugar from getting too high.

There are 2 forms of diabetes:

Type 1 – this type (sometimes called insulin-dependent diabetes mellitus [IDDM] or juvenile diabetes) is more severe and usually shows up before the age of 30 (but may occur at any age). Daily insulin injections are needed as well as dietary control and exercise.

Type 2 – this type (sometimes called noninsulin- dependent diabetes mellitus [NIDDM] or adult-onset diabetes) is less severe, usually affecting persons who are 40 years of age or older and overweight. This type is most often treated with diet and exercise and sometimes oral medicine. Occasional insulin injections may be required as well.

When untreated, diabetes can lead to hardening of the arteries, strokes, kidney problems, blindness, and limb amputations.

Signs and Symptoms

The American Diabetes Association uses the acronyms DIABETES and CAUTION to help identify the warning signs of diabetes.

- Drowsiness
- Itching
- A family history of diabetes
- Blurred vision
- Excessive weight
- Tingling, numbness, or pain in extremities
- Easy fatigue
- Skin infection, slow healing of cuts and scratches, especially on the feet

Other signs are:

- Constant urination
- Abnormal thirst
- Unusual hunger
- The rapid loss of weight
- Irritability
- Obvious weakness and fatigue
- Nausea and vomiting

Diabetes, *Continued*

You don't need to have all of these warning signs to be diabetic. Only 1 or 2 may be present. Some people show no warning signs and find out they're diabetic after a routine blood test. If you have a family history of diabetes, you should be especially watchful of the signs and symptoms above. If you notice any of these signs, report them to your doctor. Being overweight increases your risk a lot. A diet high in sugar and low in fiber may increase your risk if you are prone to developing diabetes. Pregnancy can trigger diabetes in some women.

Treatment and Care

Treatment for diabetes will depend on the type and severity of the disorder. Both forms, however, require a treatment plan that maintains normal, steady blood-sugar levels. This can be done through:

- Proper dietary measures that:
  - Promote weight reduction, if necessary
  - Give prescribed amounts of protein, fat, and carbohydrates
  - Are set up in regular meals
  - Give 20–35 grams of dietary fiber per day
  - Limit dietary cholesterol to 300 milligrams per day
  - Limit saturated fat to no more than 9% of total calories

- Regular exercise
- Medicine:
  - Oral pills that inhibit enzymes from breaking down complex carbohydrates into simple sugars in the gut. These lower blood sugar because they delay absorption of glucose into the blood. (Example: Precose) The pills must be taken at the start of each meal. They can be used alone or with other kinds of oral pills that lower blood sugar.
  - Oral pills that lower blood sugar and don't stimulate the pancreas to secrete more insulin. (Example: Glucophage)
  - Oral pills that stimulate the pancreas to secrete more insulin. (Examples: DiaBeta, Micronase, and Tolinase)
  - Insulin by injection
- Home monitoring of blood sugar levels

With either type of diabetes, routine care and follow-up treatment are important. Careful control of blood sugar levels can allow a person with diabetes to lead a normal, productive life. Persons with a family history of diabetes should watch their weight, control their eating habits, and exercise regularly to reduce their risk of getting the disease. They should also see their doctor every 1–3 years to get checked for diabetes.

(See "Places to Get Information & Help" under "Diabetes" on page 375.)

132 Diverticulosis

Sometimes small saclike pockets protrude from the wall of the colon. This is called diverticulosis. The pockets (called diverticuli) can fill with intestinal waste. Increased pressure within the intestines seems to be responsible. This may be caused by many years of a diet low in fiber.

When the intestinal pouches become inflamed, the condition is called diverticulitis.

Many older persons have diverticulosis. The digestive system becomes sluggish as a person ages. Things that increase the risk for diverticulosis include:

- Not eating enough dietary fiber. (See "Say Yes to Dietary Fiber" on page 45.) Diverticulosis is common in nations where fiber intake is low.

- Continual use of medicines that slow bowel action. (Examples: painkillers and anti-depressants.)

- Overuse of laxatives

- Having family members who have diverticulosis

- Having gallbladder disease

- Being obese

Signs and Symptoms

In most cases, diverticulosis causes no discomfort. When there are symptoms, they are usually:

- Tenderness, mild cramping, or a bloated feeling usually on the lower left side of the abdomen

- Sometimes constipation or diarrhea

- Occasionally, bright red blood in the stools

With diverticulitis, you can experience severe abdominal pain, nausea, and fever. The pain is made worse with a bowel movement. If these things occur, you should see your doctor.

Treatment and Care

Diverticulosis disease can't be cured, but you can reduce the discomfort and prevent complications. Follow these tips:

- Eat a diet high in fiber throughout life. You can add more fiber to your diet with fresh fruits and vegetables and whole-grain foods. Check with your doctor about adding wheat bran to your diet.

- Avoid corn, nuts, seeds, and foods with seeds, like figs. These seeds are easily trapped in the troublesome pouches.

- Drink 1½–2 quarts of water every day.

- If you are not able to eat a high-fiber diet, ask your doctor about taking bulk-producing laxatives like Metamucil. These are not habit-forming.

- Avoid the regular use of laxatives that make your bowel muscles contract, such as Ex-Lax. You should consult your doctor before taking any laxatives, though.

- Try not to strain when you have bowel movements.

- Get regular exercise.

{*Note:* Diverticulitis needs medical treatment. This includes antibiotics, pain relievers, bed rest, and a stay in the hospital, if needed. Fluids and medicine may need to be given by vein.}

133 Emphysema

Over 1 million Americans are forced to lead restricted lives because they have emphysema, a chronic lung condition. With emphysema, the air sacs (alveoli) in the lungs are destroyed. The lung loses its elasticity, along with its ability to take in oxygen. The vast majority of people with emphysema are cigarette smokers aged 50 or older. In fact, emphysema is sometimes called "the smoker's disease" because of its strong link with cigarettes. Exposure to irritants in the workplace and environment can also cause the disease. Only 3 to 5 percent of all cases of emphysema are caused by genetic factors.

Signs and Symptoms

Emphysema takes a number of years to develop. Early symptoms can be easily missed. Symptoms to look out for include:

- Breathing through pursed lips
- Shortness of breath on exertion
- Wheezing
- Fatigue
- Slight body build with marked weight loss and barrel chest

Emphysema is often accompanied by chronic bronchitis. Together they are called chronic obstructive pulmonary disease (COPD). Persons with chronic bronchitis have symptoms of coughing and excess sputum.

Treatment and Care

A doctor can diagnose emphysema based on your medical history, a physical exam, a chest X-ray, and a lung-function test (spirometry). By the time emphysema is detected, however, anywhere from 50–70 percent of your lung tissue may already be destroyed. At that point, your doctor may recommend the following:

- A program to help you stop smoking
- Avoidance of secondhand smoke
- Avoidance of dust, fumes, pollutants, and other irritating inhalants
- Physical therapy to help loosen mucus in your lungs (if chronic bronchitis accompanies the emphysema)
- Daily exercise
- A diet that includes adequate amounts of all essential nutrients
- Prescription medication which may include a bronchodilator, steroids, and antibiotics
- Annual flu vaccinations
- A pneumonia vaccination given once as recommended by your doctor
- Supplemental oxygen as needed

Emphysema can't be reversed, so prevention is the only real way to avoid permanent damage.

{*Note:* Persons with emphysema having severe symptoms may need emergency care.}

(See "Places to Get Information & Help" under "Lung Diseases" on page 376.)

134 Epilepsy

Epilepsy is a disorder of the brain. For some reason, with epilepsy there is excessive electrical activity in nerve cells in the brain. Some of the known causes of epilepsy include:

- Brain damage, either at birth or from a severe head injury
- Alcohol or drug abuse
- Abrupt withdrawal of alcohol or drugs in heavy users
- Brain infection
- Brain tumor

More often than not, however, the cause is not known. Epilepsy affects people of all ages, male and female. It often begins in childhood or adolescence. The disorder tends to run in families but is not contagious.

Signs and Symptoms

The most common symptom is a seizure, of which there are many types. The type depends on the part of the brain the seizure starts in, how fast it takes place, and how wide an area of the brain it involves.

Types of seizures fall in 2 general groups: general and partial. Involvement is confined to small areas of the brain with a partial seizure. A general seizure affects the whole brain and can cause loss of consciousness and/or convulsions.

Types of General Seizures are:

- **Nonconvulsive.** These are also called absence or petit mal seizures. Symptoms include staring into space and repeated blinking. The person is not aware of the seizure. Someone else may think he or she is daydreaming or not paying attention. These types of seizures can occur once a day or more than 100 times a day. They occur most often in children and can result in learning problems.

- **Convulsive.** These are also called tonic-clonic or grand mal seizures. There can be many symptoms, including crying out, falling down, losing consciousness, entire body stiffening, then uncontrollable jerks and twitches. The person's muscles relax after the seizure. He or she may lose bowel and bladder control and may be confused, sleepy, and have a headache.

Types of partial seizures are:

- Simple ones, in which symptoms include tingling feelings, twitching, seeing flashing lights, hallucination of smell and/or taste

- Complex ones, involving episodes (e.g., sitting motionless or moving or behaving in strange or repetitive ways) called automatisms. Examples include lip smacking, chewing, and fidgeting with the hands. There is usually no loss of consciousness, but the person who has this type of seizure may be confused and not remember details of it.

If a partial seizure spreads, it could lead to a general seizure.

Epilepsy, *Continued*

Treatment and Care

A medical diagnosis is necessary and will include:

- Information about the attacks. This may need to be given by someone else, because the sufferer is often not aware of what has happened.

- A complete neurological exam that includes a test to measure the electrical activity of the brain (EEG). Specialized imaging tests (e.g., computerized tomography [CAT] scans and magnetic resonance imaging [MRI] scans). Blood tests may also be done.

Persons who have seizures that recur are usually given anticonvulsant drugs. These prevent or lessen the chance for future seizures. Epileptics can lead normal lives once the seizures are controlled by medicine or do not occur for several years. This depends on the type of seizure, however. Persons with general convulsive seizures may have restrictions on driving and high-risk activities (e.g., certain jobs, sports, or anything that involves heights, using dangerous machinery or being in a potentially hazardous situation). Surgery may be performed if medication is not effective and the seizures are confined to a specific single area of the brain. (See also "Seizures" on page 324.)

(See "Places to Get Information & Help" under "Epilepsy" on page 376.)

135 Gallstones

Gallstones are stone deposits of a mixture of cholesterol (the same fatlike substance that clogs arteries), bilirubin, and protein that are found in the gallbladder or bile ducts. These stones can range in size from less than a pinhead to 3 inches across. Over 16 million Americans (most of them women) have gallstones. Depending on their size and location, gallstones may cause no symptoms or may require medical treatment.

Doctors aren't sure why gallstones form, but some people are clearly more prone to them than others. Factors that invite gallstones to form include:

- A family history of gallbladder disease
- Obesity
- Middle age
- Being female
- Pregnancy
- Taking estrogen
- Diabetes
- Eating a diet high in cholesterol-rich foods
- Diseases of the small intestine

Signs and Symptoms

Symptoms of gallstones include:

- Feeling bloated and gassy, especially after eating fried or fatty foods
- Steady pain in the upper-right abdomen that lasts from 20 minutes to 5 hours
- Pain between the shoulder blades or in the right shoulder
- Indigestion, nausea, vomiting
- Severe abdominal pain with fever and sometimes yellow skin and/or eyes (jaundice)

Treatment and Care

Treatments for gallstones include:

- Dietary measures (e.g., a low-fat diet) to reduce contractions of the gallbladder and limit pain
- Medications to dissolve the stones
- Lithotripsy (the use of shock waves to shatter the stones)
- Surgery to remove the gallbladder

136 Glaucoma

Glaucoma happens when the pressure of the liquid in the eye gets too high and causes damage. Glaucoma tends to run in families and is one of the most common major eye disorders in people over the age of 60. In fact, the risk of getting glaucoma increases with age. It can also be triggered or aggravated by some medicines like antihistamines and antispasmodics.

Signs and Symptoms

There are two types of glaucoma:

- **Chronic or open-angle glaucoma**. This type takes place gradually. It usually causes no pain and no symptoms early on. When signs and symptoms begin, they include:
  - Loss of side (peripheral) vision
  - Blurred vision

  In the late stages, symptoms include:
  - Vision loss in larger areas (side and central vision), usually in both eyes
  - Blind spots
  - Seeing halos around lights
  - Poor night vision
  - Blindness, if not treated early enough

- **Acute or angle-closure glaucoma**. This type can occur suddenly and is a medical emergency! Signs and symptoms include:
  - Severe pain in and above the eye
  - Severe, throbbing headache
  - Fogginess of vision, halos around lights
  - Redness in the eye, swollen upper eyelid
  - Dilated pupil
  - Nausea, vomiting, weakness

Treatment and Care

Glaucoma may not be preventable, but the blindness that may result from it is. Things you can do:

- Ask to be tested for glaucoma whenever you get a regular vision checkup. It's a simple, painless procedure. If pressure inside the eyeball is high, an eye specialist (ophthalmologist) will probably give you eye drops and perhaps oral medicines. The aim of both is to reduce the pressure inside the eye.

- Take the medicines your doctor prescribes. (These are given for life for acute glaucoma.)

- Do not take any medicine–even a nonprescription one–without your doctor or pharmacist's okay. Most cold medications and sleeping pills, for example, can cause the pupil in the eye to dilate. This can lead to increased eye pressure.

If medicines do not control the pressure, other options exist:

- Ultrasound, which uses sound waves to reduce the pressure in the eye.

- Laser beam surgery and other surgical procedures that can widen the drainage channels within the eye. These relieve fluid buildup.

There are also some things you can do on your own:

- Avoid getting upset and fatigued. This can increase pressure in the eye.

- Don't smoke cigarettes. Smoking causes blood vessels to constrict, which reduces blood supply to the eye.

(See "Places to Get Information & Help" under "Visual Problems" on page 377.)

137 Gout

Gout is a form of arthritis and is most common in men older than 30. It is less common in women. In women it usually comes after menopause. It is caused by increased blood levels of uric acid, which is made by the breakdown of protein in the body. When blood levels of uric acid rise above a critical level, thousands of hard, tiny uric acid crystals collect in the joints. These crystals act like tiny, hot, jagged shards of glass, resulting in pain and inflammation. Crystals can collect in the tendons and cartilage, in the kidneys (as kidney stones), and in the fatty tissues beneath the skin. {*Note:* Crystals other than uric acid can cause some acute attacks of gout.}

Gout can strike any joint, but often affects those in the feet, such as the big toe, and those in the legs. A gout attack can last several hours to a few days. Persons who have gout can be symptom-free for years between attacks. Gout can be triggered by:

- Mild trauma or blow to the joint

- Drinking alcohol (beer and wine more than distilled alcohol)

- Taking certain medications (e.g., aspirin, diuretics, and nicotinic acid)

Signs and Symptoms

- Excruciating pain and inflammation in a joint or joints that strike suddenly and peak quickly

- Affected area that is swollen, red or purplish in color, feels warm, and is very tender to the touch

- Feeling of agonizing pain after even the slightest pressure, such as rubbing a sheet against the affected area

- Sometimes a low-grade fever

- Sometimes chills and fever

Treatment and Care

Never assume you have gout without consulting a physician. Many conditions can mimic an acute attack of gout. These include infection, injury, and rheumatoid arthritis. Only a doctor can diagnose the problem.

If you do have gout, treatment will depend on the reasons behind your high levels of uric acid. Your doctor can conduct a simple test to tell if your kidneys aren't clearing uric acid from the blood the way they should or to find out if your body simply makes too much uric acid.

The first goal is to relieve the acute gout attack. The second goal is to prevent future attacks.

- For immediate relief, your doctor will prescribe colchicine, a nonsteroidal anti-inflammatory medication and/or other pain reliever (not aspirin) and tell you to rest the affected joint.

- For long-term relief, your doctor will probably recommend that you lose excess weight, limit your intake of alcohol, drink lots of liquids, and take medication, if necessary. One type of medication (allopurinol) decreases uric acid production. Another (probenecid) increases the excretion of uric acid from the kidneys.

(See "Places to Get Information & Help" under "Arthritis" on page 375.)

138 High Blood Pressure

High blood pressure (hypertension) happens when your blood moves through your arteries at a higher pressure than normal. The heart is actually straining to pump blood through the arteries. This isn't healthy because:

- It promotes hardening of the arteries (atherosclerosis). Hardened, narrowed arteries may not be able to carry the amount of blood the body's organs need.

- Blood clots can form or lodge in a narrowed artery. (This could cause a stroke or heart attack.)

- The heart can become enlarged. (This could result in congestive heart failure.)

- Kidney failure or vision loss can result from uncontrolled high blood pressure

More than half of all older adults have high blood pressure. About 50% of all people who have it don't know it. They usually feel no discomfort or outward signs of trouble. For this reason you should get your blood pressure checked at every office visit or at least every 2 years. Directly or indirectly, high blood pressure accounts for nearly a million deaths a year. Many people who know their blood pressure is dangerously high are doing nothing to try to control it. And for 90% of those affected, there is no known cause. When this is the case, it is called primary or essential hypertension. When high blood pressure results from another medical disorder or a medicine, it is known as secondary hypertension. In these cases (about 10% of total), when the root cause is corrected, blood pressure usually goes back to normal.

Detection

How's your blood pressure? Blood pressure is normally measured with a blood pressure cuff placed on the arm. The numbers on the gauge measure your blood pressure in millimeters of mercury (mmHg). The first (higher) number measures the systolic pressure. This is the maximum pressure exerted against the arterial walls while the heart is beating. The second (lower) number records the diastolic pressure. This is the pressure between heartbeats, when the heart is resting. The results are then recorded as systolic/diastolic pressure (120/80 mmHg, for example). Blood pressure is considered high in adults if it is consistently a reading of 140–160 mmHg systolic and/or 90 mmHg diastolic or higher.

To get an accurate finding of your blood pressure, an average of 2 or more readings should be taken at 2 or more separate times. If your blood pressure is generally pretty good and suddenly reads high, don't be alarmed. Anxiety and other strong emotions, physical exertion, drinking a large amount of coffee, or eating recently can temporarily raise normal blood pressure with no lasting effects. If, after several readings, your doctor is convinced you do indeed have high blood pressure, follow his or her advice. The risk of stroke, heart attack, and kidney disease increases when high blood pressure is not under control.

High Blood Pressure, *Continued*

Treatment and Care

Blood pressure is one of the easiest health problems to control. Here's a multipoint plan to control high blood pressure:

- If you're overweight, lose weight.

- Don't smoke. If you smoke, quit.

- Limit alcohol to 2 drinks or less a day.

- Reduce your intake of salt and foods high in salt. (This is helpful for many people.) Use salt substitutes if your doctor says it's okay.

- Get regular exercise at least 3 times a week.

- Learn to handle stress by practicing relaxation techniques and rethinking stressful situations.

- Take any prescribed blood pressure medicine as directed. Tell your doctor if you have any side effects such as dizziness, faintness, skin rash, or even a dry cough in the absence of a cold. Another medicine can be prescribed. Don't stop taking your prescribed medicine unless your doctor tells you to.

- Talk to your physician or pharmacist before you take antihistamines that contain ephendrine and decongestants. An ingredient in some of these can raise your blood pressure.

- Don't eat black licorice.

(See "Places to Get Information & Help" under "Heart Disease/High Blood Pressure" on page 376.)

24. Chronic Illnesses

139 HIV/AIDS

HIV stands for human immunodeficiency virus. AIDS, acquired immune deficiency syndrome, is thought to be caused by HIV. HIV destroys the body's immune system, leaving the person unable to fight certain types of infection or cancer. The virus also attacks the central nervous system, causing mental and neurological problems.

The virus is carried in body fluids such as semen, vaginal secretions, breast milk, and blood (including menstrual blood).

Certain activities are likely to promote contracting HIV. High-risk activities include:

- Unprotected* anal, oral and/or vaginal sex except in a monogamous relationship in which neither partner is infected with HIV. Particularly high-risk situations are having sex:

  • When drunk or high

  • With multiple or casual sex partners

  • With a partner who has had multiple or casual sex partners

  • With a partner who has used drugs by injection or is bisexual

  • When you or your partner have signs and symptoms of a genital tract infection

* "Unprotected" means without using condoms alone or with other latex or polyurethane barriers. When used correctly every time and for every sex act, these provide protection from HIV. Though not 100% effective, they will reduce the risk. Male latex condoms are preferred. The Reality female condom may also offer protection.

- Sharing needles and/or "the works" when injecting any kind of drugs

- Pregnancy and delivery if the mother is infected with HIV. This can put the child at risk. (The use of the drug AZT can lower this risk a great deal. See "Treatment and Care" in this section on page 358.)

- Having had blood transfusions, especially before 1985, unless you have tested negative for HIV

There is some concern about the risk of getting HIV from an infected doctor, dentist, or patient. There are almost no cases of health workers passing HIV to a patient. Patient-to-health-workers transmission has been more noted. Measures are required by medical and dental associations to decrease these possible risks. The risks are extremely low, though.

Blood screening tests are also done on donated blood. This makes it highly unlikely that you'd get HIV from current blood transfusions. You cannot get HIV from:

- Donating blood

- Casual contact such as touching, holding hands, or hugging

- A cough, sneeze, tears, or sweat

- An animal or insect bite

- A toilet seat

- Using a hot tub or swimming

HIV/AIDS, *Continued*

You can get screening tests for HIV at doctors' offices, clinics, and health departments. A small sample of your blood is tested for HIV antibodies. If these antibodies are present, you test positive for and are considered infected with HIV. It could take as long as 6 months from exposure to the virus for these antibodies to show up. The most common reason for a false negative test is when a person gets tested before HIV antibodies have formed. If you test positive for HIV, a second type of blood test is done to confirm it. HIV/AIDS symptoms may not show up for as long as 8 to 11 years after a person is infected with the virus.

You can also use a home collection test and counseling service called *Home Access*. Look for this test kit in drug stores, national retail stores, public health clinics and on college campuses. You can also buy a *Home Access* test kit by phone. Call: 1-800-HIV-TEST (448-8378). Follow the products' instructions. With the product, you get information on HIV, anonymous counseling services by phone, and test materials to find out your HIV status. Test materials include a lancet to get a few drops of blood from a fingertip; a card or special paper to put the blood sample on; and mailing materials to send the test back to the company. The sample is identified by number, not by name. You call the kit's 800 number for test results. This means the results are kept anonymous and confidential.

Signs and Symptoms

Early symptoms of HIV/AIDS:

- Fatigue
- Loss of appetite
- Chronic diarrhea
- Weight loss
- Persistent dry cough
- Fever
- Night sweats
- Swollen lymph nodes

Persons with AIDS fall prey to many diseases such as skin infections, fungal infections, tuberculosis, pneumonia, and cancer. These "opportunistic" infections are what lead to death in an AIDS victim. When HIV invades the brain cells, it leads to forgetfulness, impaired speech, trembling, and seizures.

Prevention

Someday a cure for AIDS may exist. For now, prevention is the only protection. Take these steps to avoid contracting HIV:

- Unless you are in a long-term, monogamous relationship, use male latex condoms every time you have sex. The spermicide, Nonoxynol-9 may inactivate HIV. But this was only shown in laboratory studies, not in studies on humans. Using a latex condom is most important. Don't use Nonoxynol-9 spermicide alone.

HIV/AIDS, *Continued*

- Don't have sex with people who are at high risk for contracting HIV. These have been noted to be:

  - Homosexual or bisexual persons, especially with multiple sex partners or who inject illegal drugs

  - Heterosexual partners of persons infected or exposed to HIV

  - Persons who have had multiple blood transfusions, especially before 1985, unless tested negative for HIV

- Don't have sex with more than one person.

- Ask specific questions about your partner's sexual past, i.e., have they had many partners or unprotected (no condom) sex? Do not be afraid to ask if they have been tested for HIV and if the results were positive or negative.

- Don't have sex with anyone who you know or suspect has had multiple partners. (If you've had sex with someone you suspect is HIV-positive, see your doctor).

- Don't share needles and/or "the works" with anyone. This includes not only illegal drugs such as heroin but steroids, insulin, etc. Don't have sex with people who use or have used injected illegal drugs.

- Don't share personal items that have blood on them, such as razors.

Treatment and Care

Current treatments for HIV/AIDS include:

- Medications. Older drugs are AZT, DDI, DDC, D4T, and 3TC with AZT. These slow the virus but do not destroy it. A newer class of medicines called protease inhibitors may help keep the AIDS virus from growing. The newer drugs are now given with older ones in combinations called "cocktails". {*Note:* The medicine AZT has been shown to greatly reduce the risk of a pregnant woman passing HIV to her unborn baby. AZT is given to the mother at certain times during pregnancy and delivery. It is also given to the baby after it is born.}

- Taking measures to reduce the risk of getting infections and diseases. Get adequate rest, proper nutrition, and take vitamin supplements as suggested by your doctor.

- Emotional support

- Treating infections. For example, giving antibiotics such as Bactrim or Septra for pneumonia

- Radiation therapy and surgery have been used in the treatment of some patients.

AIDS is under intensive study and research. Better forms of treatment are being researched worldwide. One example for women is vaginal foams, gels, or creams that have a chemical that could kill HIV on contact.

(See "Places to Get Information & Help" under "AIDS" on page 374.)

140 Kidney Stones

Kidney stones are hard masses of mineral deposits (e.g., calcium) or other organic substances (e.g., uric acid) that form in the kidneys or urinary tract. They can be found in the kidney itself or anywhere in the duct (ureter) that carries urine from the kidney to the bladder. Kidney stones can be as small as a tiny pebble or an inch or more in diameter. They are more common in men (especially between 30 and 50 years old) than in women or children.

Signs and Symptoms

Kidney stones can be present for many years without causing symptoms. When a stone becomes large enough to produce problems, the following symptoms may occur:

- Blocked flow of urine

- Frequent and painful urination

- Blood in the urine

- Nausea and vomiting

- Fever, chills

- Severe pain and tenderness over the affected area. This is usually felt in the lower abdomen on the right or left side.

- Pain that travels down the side of the abdomen and into the groin area when the stone becomes lodged in the ureter

{*Note:* If these symptoms are severe, emergency care may be needed.}

Treatment, Care, and Prevention

Treatment will depend on the size, symptoms, location and cause of the kidney stone(s). If the stone is small and can be passed, treatment may be just drinking plenty of fluids. For kidney stones too large to be passed, a procedure known as lithotripsy is used in most cases.

Lithotripsy causes little or no pain and costs less than invasive surgery. In lithotripsy, shock waves are directed to the areas where the stone is located. The shock waves break it into fragments. After the treatment, the patient drinks a lot of water to flush the stone fragments from his or her system. Lithotripsy is usually done in an outpatient setting.

Kidney stones can and do recur. If you're prone to developing stones, heed these guidelines:

- Save any stones you pass so your doctor can have them analyzed.

- Follow your doctor's dietary advice. If you tend to form calcium stones, he or she will probably advise you not to take calcium in excess. If you form uric acid stones, your doctor may recommend that you eat less protein and take sodium bicarbonate.

- Drink plenty of fluids – at least 8 glasses of water a day, 8 or more ounces each.

- See your doctor as often as needed to be sure your kidneys are working as they should.

(See "Places to Get Information & Help" under "Kidney Diseases" on page 376.)

141 Lung Cancer

Today lung cancer is the leading cause of death from cancer in men and women. About 150,000 Americans die from lung cancer each year, and 85 percent of them can thank cigarettes for the disease. In less than a decade, lung cancer deaths for white females have increased 60 percent, replacing breast cancer as the most common cause of cancer-related deaths in women. Besides cigarette smoke, the risk for getting lung cancer increases with exposure to asbestos or other carcinogens (cancer-causing agents). One of these is radon, a radioactive gas. High levels of radon are found in underground uranium mines. Much lower levels can build up in some homes.

Lung cancer is especially deadly because the rich network of blood vessels that deliver oxygen from the lungs to the rest of the body can also spread cancer very quickly. By the time it's diagnosed, other organs may be affected.

Signs and Symptoms

Symptoms of lung cancer include:

- Chronic cough
- Blood-streaked sputum
- Shortness of breath
- Wheezing
- Chest discomfort with each breath
- Weight loss
- Fatigue

Prevention and Treatment

Lung cancer is difficult to detect in its early, more treatable stages, so the best way to combat the disease is to prevent it. To help prevent lung cancer:

- Don't smoke. The risk of developing lung cancer is proportional to the number of cigarettes smoked per day. Also, the longer a person smokes and the more deeply the smoke is inhaled, the greater the risk of getting lung cancer. Avoid secondhand smoke.

- Avoid or limit exposure to environmental pollutants and asbestos

- Have your home tested for radon. This can be done with a home testing kit, or by a professional.

Treatment for lung cancer includes one or more of the following:

- Tests to determine the type of lung cancer present and the stage of the disease

- Surgery to remove a small part of the lung, an entire lobe of the lung, or the entire lung. Respiratory therapy is generally given after surgery.

- Radiation therapy

- Chemotherapy

(See "Places to Get Information & Help" under "Cancer" on page 375.)

142 Multiple Sclerosis

The nervous system carries messages to and from the rest of your body. Normally, delicate nerves are protected with a covering called myelin. With multiple sclerosis (MS), the myelin becomes inflamed and eventually dissolves. Over time, scar tissue (sclerosis) forms where the myelin used to be, in scattered locations in the brain and spinal cord. Nerve impulses, which normally travel at a speed of 225 miles per hour, either slow down considerably or come to a complete halt. People most prone to MS are:

- White adults between 20 and 40 years of age
- Those with a family history of the disease
- Women (at a ratio of 3 women to every 2 men)
- Residents of the northern United States, Canada, and northern Europe

Causes

No one knows what causes MS. Some theories point to a virus or other infectious agent and/or an autoimmune problem. With an autoimmune problem, the immune system attacks the body's own cells instead of foreign invaders. Toxins, trauma, nutritional deficiencies, and other factors that lead to the destruction of myelin are also possible causes. Things known to precede the onset of MS include overwork, fatigue, the postpartum period for women, acute infections, and fevers.

Signs and Symptoms

Early signs and symptoms may be mild and present for years before the diagnosis is made for multiple sclerosis. Once diagnosed, the symptoms may last for hours or weeks, vary from day to day, and come and go with no predictable pattern. Symptoms include:

- Fatigue that can be extreme
- Weakness
- Feelings of pins and needles
- Muscle spasms
- Poor coordination (trembling of the hand, for example)
- Bladder problems (frequent urination, urgency, infection, as well as incontinence)
- Blurred vision, double vision, or the loss of vision in one eye
- Emotional mood swings, irritability, depression, anxiety, euphoria

Treatment and Care

While no cure exists for multiple sclerosis, several steps can be taken to make living with the disease easier. These include:

- Getting plenty of rest
- Treating bacterial infections and fever as soon as they occur

Multiple Sclerosis, *Continued*

- Minimizing stressful situations, especially physically demanding ones, since physical stress may aggravate the symptoms

- Staying out of the heat and sun, since an increased body temperature can aggravate MS symptoms

- Avoiding hot showers or baths, since they, too, can aggravate symptoms. In fact, cool baths or swimming in a pool may improve symptoms by lowering body temperature.

- Maintaining a normal routine at work and at home if activities aren't physically demanding

- Getting regular exercise (physical therapy may be helpful)

- Having body massages to help maintain muscle tone

- Getting professional, supportive psychological counseling

- Taking prescribed medication. This may include:

  - Interferon beta 1-a (Avonex)

  - Interferon beta 1-b (Betaseron)

  - Copolymer 1 (Copaxone)

  - Short-term courses of cortisonelike drugs such as intravenous (IV) or oral steroids

  - Antispasmodics

  - Muscle relaxants

  - Antidepressants

  - Antianxiety drugs

  - Antibiotics (to treat any bacterial infections)

  - Medications to control urinary function

(See "Places to Get Information & Help" under "Multiple Sclerosis" on page 376.)

143 Osteoporosis

Osteoporosis is a major health problem for Americans. Seven to 8 million Americans have the disease. Seventeen million are at an increased risk for developing it. Eighty percent of those affected are women. Persons with osteoporosis suffer from a loss in bone mass and bone strength. Their bones become weak and brittle, which makes them more prone to fracture. Any bone can be affected by osteoporosis, but the hips, wrists, and spine are the most common sites. Peak bone mass is reached between the ages of 25 and 35. After age 35, everyone's bones lose density.

Causes

The actual causes of osteoporosis are unknown. Certain risk factors increase the likelihood of developing osteoporosis, however:

■ Being female. Women are 4 times more likely to develop osteoporosis than men. The reasons are as follows:

- Female bones are generally thinner and lighter

- Women live longer on average than men

- Women have rapid bone loss at menopause due to a sharp decline of estrogen. The risk also increases for women who:

  – Go through menopause before age 45. This could be natural menopause or one that results from surgical removal of both ovaries.

  – Experience a lack of or irregular menstrual flow

■ Having a thin, small-framed body

■ Being Caucasian or Asian, although African Americans and Hispanic Americans are at significant risk as well.

■ Lack of physical activity, especially activities such as walking, running, tennis, and other weight-bearing exercises. Or, exercising too much to the point where menstrual periods cease.

■ Lack of calcium. Adequate calcium intake throughout life helps to insure that calcium deficiency does not contribute to a weakening of bone mass.

■ Heredity factors. The risk increases if there is a history of osteoporosis and/or bone fractures in your family.

■ Smoking cigarettes

■ Alcohol consumption. Regularly consuming alcoholic beverages may be damaging to bones. Heavy drinkers often have poor nutrition and may be more prone to fractures because they are more prone to falls.

■ Taking certain medications such as: cortico-steroids (anti-inflammatory medicines used to treat a variety of conditions such as asthma, arthritis, lupus, etc.); some antiseizure medi-cines; overuse of thyroid hormones; and aluminum-containing antacids

■ Other disorders such as hyperthyroidism, hyperparathyroidism, and certain forms of bone cancer

Osteoporosis, *Continued*

Prevention

To prevent or slow osteoporosis, take these steps now:

■ Be sure to eat a balanced diet. Plan to get your recommended Adequate Intake (AI) for calcium every day. AIs are the Dietary Reference Intakes that have been set by the Food and Nutrition Board of National Academy of Sciences. These are the set intakes of calcium that appear to provide the amount of calcium needed for good health for different ages.

AIs (Adequate Intakes) for Calcium:	
Age	Milligrams (Mgs.) Calcium/Day
0–6 months	210
6 months – 1 year	270
1 year – 3 years	500
4–8 years	800
9–18 years	1,300
Pregnant and breast feeding women:	
• 18 years and younger	1,300
• Over 18 years	1,000
19–50 years	1,000
51+ years	1,200

To get your recommended calcium:

■ Choose high-calcium foods daily:

   • Soft-boned fish and shellfish, such as salmon, sardines, or shrimp

   • Skim and low-fat milks, yogurts, and cheeses. {*Note:* If you are lactose intolerant, you may need to use dairy products that are treated with the enzyme lactase, or you can add this enzyme using over-the-counter drops or tablets.}

   • Vegetables, especially broccoli, kale, and collard greens

   • Beans and bean sprouts as well as tofu (soybean curd), if processed with calcium

   • Calcium-fortified foods such as some orange juices, apple juices, and ready-to-eat cereals

   • Calcium supplements, if necessary and advised by your doctor

■ Follow a program of regular, weight-bearing exercise at least 3 or 4 times a week. Examples include walking, jogging or low-impact or non-impact aerobics. (A person with osteoporosis should follow the exercise program outlined by his or her doctor.)

■ Do not smoke. Smoking makes osteoporosis worse and may negate the beneficial effects of estrogen replacement therapy.

■ Limit alcohol consumption.

■ Check with your doctor regarding medical management to prevent further bone loss and/ or osteoporosis fractures, especially if you are at high risk for getting these. He or she may prescribe:

   • Estrogen replacement therapy, if you are female

   • Calcitonin

   • Alendronate sodium (Fosamax)

Osteoporosis, *Continued*

Signs and Symptoms

Osteoporosis is a "silent disease" because it can progress without any noticeable signs or symptoms. Often the first sign is when a bone fracture of the hip, wrist, or spine occurs. Symptoms include:

- Gradual loss of height
- Rounding of the shoulders
- Back pain
- Stooped posture or dowager's hump

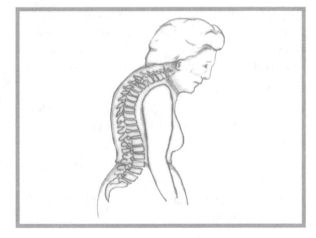

Treatment and Care

Special X-rays, such as dual energy X-ray absorptiometry (DEXA) can measure bone mass in various sites of the body. They are safe and painless. These tests can help doctors decide if and what kind of treatment is needed. Treatment for osteoporosis includes:

- Medication therapy: Estrogen replacement therapy (ERT), calcitonin, or alendronate sodium (Fosamax)

- Dietary measures: A balanced diet rich in calcium, and calcium supplementation if necessary

- Daily exercises approved by your doctor

- Proper posture

- Fall-prevention strategies:
  - Use grab bars and safety mats or nonskid tape on your tub or shower.
  - Use handrails on stairways.
  - Don't stoop to pick up things. Pick things up by bending your knees and keeping your back straight.
  - Wear flat, sturdy, nonskid shoes.
  - If you use throw rugs, make sure they have nonskid backs.
  - Use a cane or walker if necessary.
  - See that halls, stairways, and entrances are well lit. Use night lights in hallways, bathrooms, etc.

There is no cure for osteoporosis. The focus of treatment is to prevent the disease (see prevention measures on page 364), prevent further bone loss, and build new bone.

(See "Places to Get Information & Help" under "Osteoporosis" on page 377.)

144 Parkinson's Disease

Parkinson's disease is a nervous system disorder. It causes tremors (involuntary shaking in the limbs and head) a shuffling gait, and a gradual, progressive stiffness of muscles. Parkinson's disease is found equally in men and women of all races and ethnic groups. It most often strikes people over 45 years of age.

Causes

The exact cause of Parkinson's disease is not known. What is known, though, is that certain cells in the lower part of the brain can't produce dopamine, a substance nerves need for coordination of body movement.

{*Note:* Some medications may bring on Parkinsonian symptoms. These medicines include major tranquilizers and Reglan, which is usually prescribed for digestive tract problems.}

Signs and Symptoms

The signs and symptoms of Parkinson's disease include:

- Slow or stiff movement
- Stooped posture
- Shuffling or dragging of the feet
- Tremors and shaking of the head or hands
- Monotonic voice, weak and high-pitched
- Blinking less often than normal
- Lack of spontaneity in facial expression
- Problems in swallowing
- Difficulty in changing positions
- Depression and anxiety
- Dementia (in advanced stages)

Treatment and Care

Parkinson's disease is not yet curable. For the most part, though, symptoms can be relieved or controlled.

The main method of treatment is medication. Medicines used include Levodopa and Sinemet, which increase the dopamine level in the brain. Another medicine, Eldepryl, sometimes used with Levodopa or Carbidopa to enhance their effects, may help to slow the progression of the disease.

Other treatments try to make the person with Parkinson's more comfortable. Warm baths and massages, for example, can help prevent muscle rigidity. Here are some other helpful hints:

- Take care to maintain a safe home environment. (Examples: Replace razor blades with electric shavers; use nonskid rugs and handrails to prevent falls.)
- Simplify tasks. Replace tie shoes with loafers, for instance, and wear clothing that can be pulled on or that has zippers or Velcro closures instead of buttons.
- Include high-fiber foods in the diet and drink lots of fluids to prevent constipation.
- Get expert physical therapy. Speech therapy may also be helpful.
- Remain as active as possible.
- Get professional help to relieve depression, if necessary.

(See "Places to Get Information & Help" under "Parkinson's Disease" on page 377.)

145 Peptic Ulcers

An ulcer is a sore or break in one of the body's protective tissue layers. Ulcers located in the stomach (gastric ulcers) and ulcers in the first section of the small intestine (duodenal ulcers) are grouped under the label "peptic ulcers." They afflict men, women, and children.

Causes

Persons with a family history of peptic ulcers tend to be at greater risk for getting them. A bacteria called *Heliobacter pylori* may cause about 80% of peptic ulcers. About 20% of peptic ulcers may be caused by the repeated use of aspirin and other nonsteroidal anti-inflammatory drugs (NSAIDs) such as ibuprofen, ketoprofen, and naproxen sodium.

Signs and Symptoms

Common symptoms of peptic ulcers are:

- A gnawing or burning feeling just above the navel within $1\frac{1}{2}$–3 hours after eating
- Pain that feels like indigestion, heartburn, or hunger. The pain often awakens the person at night. Pain relief comes within minutes with food or antacids
- Bloody, black, or tarry-looking stools
- Nausea or vomiting blood or material that looks like coffee grounds
- Weight loss without trying or loss of appetite
- Paleness and weakness if anemia is present

Treatment and Care

Doctors can diagnose peptic ulcers with an analysis of gastric acids, X-rays, and/or endoscopy. Endoscopy is done by passing a long tube through the mouth and into the stomach and small intestine. It is the most accurate way to diagnose a peptic ulcer.

For treatment, your doctor may prescribe:

- An antibiotic (Example: Biaxin) and a medicine that blocks acid (Example: Prilosec) if *Heliobacter pylori* is present
- Prescription medicines to decrease or stop the stomach's production of hydrochloric acid
- Over-the-counter antacids, or acid controllers or reducers
- Surgery to cut the nerves that stimulate acid production or to remove part of the stomach. This may be needed if other treatment methods fail.

If you have an ulcer, you can soothe the pain in various ways. Under a doctor's care:

- Eat smaller, lighter, more frequent meals for a couple of weeks. Big, heavy lunches and dinners can spell trouble for people with ulcers. Frequent meals tend to take the edge off pain.
- Avoid things that stimulate excess stomach acid. That includes coffee, tea, and soft drinks containing caffeine. Even decaffeinated coffee should be avoided.
- Limit alcohol or avoid it, if necessary
- Discontinue use of aspirin and other NSAID's, which irritate the stomach lining.
- Try antacids (with your physician's okay) on a short-term basis. (Don't try to self-medicate an ulcer. You may soothe the symptoms without treating the problem itself.)
- Don't smoke. Smokers get ulcers more often than nonsmokers. No one is sure why.
- Try to minimize stress in your life. Stress doesn't cause ulcers. But for some people, stress may trigger the release of stomach acid, which can result in ulcer flare-ups.

146 Phlebitis & Thrombosis

Phlebitis is inflammation in a vein. Thrombosis is when a blood clot forms. When both of these occur together it is called thrombophlebitis. Phlebitis is usually caused by infection, injury, or poor blood flow in a vein. It is more common in women over age 50.

Signs and Symptoms

- Superficial Phlebitis (SP) occurs just under the skin's surface. The affected area is swollen and feels warm and tender. At times a hard ropy vein is felt. This type seldom showers clots into the bloodstream.

- Deep-Vein Thrombosis (DVT) occurs within a muscle mass (commonly the leg). It is apt to release showers of clots (emboli) that often go to the lung (pulmonary emboli). The symptoms may resemble those of SP; the limb may swell and/or the muscle involved may ache. Often, DVT symptoms are silent and invisible. In silent DVT, the first symptoms may be from the pulmonary emboli. These include breathlessness, sudden chest pain, and/or collapse.

Conditions that can lead to SP and/or DVT include:

- Inactivity (from a sedentary job); a long trip, especially in a cramped space (Example: economy class section of a plane); prolonged bed rest

- Heart failure or heart attack

- Being overweight, in poor physical condition, or older aged

- Trauma to an arm or leg (a fall) or injury to the vein (from injections or IV needles)

- Some cancers

- Varicose veins, pregnancy or estrogen therapy

Prevention

- Avoid sitting or standing for long periods without moving around.

- Inform your doctor if you have a history of varicose veins, SP, or DVT and take estrogens. Avoid tobacco.

- Don't sit with your legs crossed or wear tight garments below the waist (Examples: garters, knee-high hosiery). These restrict blood flow.

- On trips, drink a lot of fluids (no alcohol) and move about at least every hour. Exercise the legs in place.

- If you're confined to a bed or a chair, stretch often. Push with the feet, pretending you're pressing on a gas pedal and then release it. Do this with one foot, then the other.

Treatment and Care

Only a physician can tell the difference between SP with or without DVT and DVT alone. At times multiple tests are needed. These include ultrasound or X-rays called venograms. Always see your physician and seek emergency care for any chest symptoms.

- SP alone can be treated with resting the affected part and pain relievers. See "Pain relievers" in "Your Home Pharmacy" on pages 22 and 23.

- DVT will require hospitalization, blood thinning medicine, etc.

- DVT with pulmonary emboli may require surgery to tie off the vein, etc.

147 Pneumonia

Pneumonia is lung inflammation. It is one of the leading causes of death in the United States. Pneumonia can develop when the lungs are infected by bacteria, viruses, fungi, or toxins, causing inflammation. Certain people are at a greater risk for pneumonia than others. They include:

- Elderly people, because the body's ability to fight off disease lessens with age

- People who are hospitalized for other conditions

- Individuals with suppressed cough reflex following a stroke

- Smokers, because tobacco smoke paralyzes the tiny hairs in the lungs that help to expel germ-ridden mucus from the lungs

- People who suffer from malnutrition, alcoholism, or viral infections

- Anyone with a recent respiratory infection

- People with emphysema or chronic bronchitis

- People with sickle cell anemia

- People getting radiation treatments or chemotherapy, or people taking any medications which wear down the immune system. (Example: corticosteroids)

- People with HIV/AIDS

Signs and Symptoms

Pneumonia symptoms may include:

- Chest pain when breathing in

- Fever and chills

- Coughing, usually with bloody, dark yellow, or rust-colored sputum

- Difficulty in breathing, rapid breathing

- General fatigue, headache, nausea, vomiting

- Bluish lips and fingertips

Treatment, Care, and Prevention

Treatment for pneumonia will depend on its type (viral, bacterial or chemical, for example) and location. Blood tests, X-rays, and sputum analysis can help identify these. Treatment includes:

- Getting plenty of bed rest

- Using a "cool-mist" humidifier in the room or rooms in which you spend most of your time

- Drinking plenty of fluids

- Taking an over-the-counter medicine for pain and/or fever. {*Note:* See "Pain relievers" in "Your Home Pharmacy" on pages 22 and 23.}

- Taking any medications your doctor prescribes: antibiotics to treat bacterial pneumonia or to fight a secondary bacterial infection; antiviral medications if indicated.

- Nose drops, sprays, or oral decongestants to treat congestion in the upper respiratory tract

- Cough medicines as needed: a cough suppressant for a dry, nonproductive cough; an expectorant type for a mucus-producing cough

- Removing fluid from the lungs by suction, anti-inflammatory medications, and oxygen therapy may be used for some pneumonias such as ones caused by chemical irritants

- Getting vaccines for influenza and pneumonia. They are recommended for persons aged 65 and older and for some persons younger than 65 who have certain medical conditions. Ask your doctor about them. (See "Immunization Schedule" on page 18.)

- Not smoking

148 Sickle Cell Anemia

Red blood cells are normally round. In sickle cell anemia, the red blood cells take on a sickle shape. This makes the blood thicker and affects the red blood cells' ability to carry oxygen to the body's tissues. The result is a chronic disease that affects many systems in the body.

Causes

Sickle cell anemia is inherited. It mostly affects blacks. About 1 in 12 African Americans carries the gene for the sickle cell trait (that is, they have the ability to produce children with sickle cell anemia, but have no symptoms of the disease). If both parents carry the trait, the chance of having a child with sickle cell anemia is 1 out of 4, or 25%. About 1 in every 400 African Americans is born with sickle cell anemia.

The disease usually doesn't become apparent until the end of the child's first year. The average life expectancy with proper medical care is now between the ages of 40 and 50.

Signs and Symptoms

A blood test can detect sickle cell anemia. Signs and symptoms include the following:

- Pain, ranging from mild to severe, in the chest, joints, back, or abdomen

- Swollen hands and feet

- Jaundice

- Repeated infections, particularly pneumonia or meningitis

- Kidney failure

- Gallstones (at an early age)

- Strokes (at an early age)

Treatment, Care, and Prevention

For now, no medicines exist to effectively treat sickle cell anemia. At best, treatment aims to prevent complications. Painful episodes are treated with painkillers, fluids, and oxygen. The diet is supplemented with folic acid, a B-vitamin. Because people with sickle cell anemia are prone to developing pneumonia, they should be vaccinated against pneumonia.

To prevent sickle cell anemia in offspring, couples, especially African American couples, should have a blood test to determine if they are carriers for the sickle cell trait. Genetic counseling can help them decide what to do.

After conception, sickle cell anemia can be diagnosed by amniocentesis in the second trimester of pregnancy. If the fetus has sickle cell anemia, the parents may elect to terminate the pregnancy.

{*Note:* Recently, some persons have been cured of sickle cell anemia with chemotherapy drugs and a bone marrow transplant. The transplant used bone marrow from a sibling with similar genetic makeup. This new form of treatment is risky and may not be suited for all persons with sickle cell anemia.}

(See "Places to Get Information & Help" under "Sickle Cell Anemia" on page 377.)

149 Strokes

Strokes, also called cerebrovascular accidents, are the third leading cause of death in the United States. A stroke is caused by lack of blood (and therefore lack of oxygen) to the brain, usually due to either clogged arteries or a ruptured blood vessel in the brain. In either case, the end result is brain damage (and possible death). Persons who suffer from both high blood pressure and hardening of the arteries are most prone to having a stroke. A stroke can happen suddenly, but it often follows years of the slow buildup of fatty deposits inside the blood vessels.

Some people experience a temporary lack of blood supply to the brain, or a transient ischemic attack (TIA). The symptoms mimic a stroke (see next column), but clear within 24 hours. TIAs can be a warning that a stroke may follow.

Prevention

To reduce the risks of a stroke:

- Control your blood pressure. Have it checked regularly. Take medication if your doctor prescribes it.
- Reduce blood levels of cholesterol to below 200 milligrams per deciliter (measured by a blood test).
- Get regular exercise.
- Keep your weight down.
- Don't smoke.
- Keep blood sugar levels under control if you have diabetes.
- Use alcohol in moderation, if at all.
- Learn to manage stress.
- Ask your doctor about taking daily aspirin (low-dose, such as a baby aspirin).

- Ask your doctor to evaluate you for a surgical procedure that scrapes away fatty deposits in one or both of the main arteries in the neck.
- Take the medication your doctor has prescribed to help prevent strokes. An example is blood-thinning medicine for atrial fibrillation (a heart condition).

Signs and Symptoms

- Sudden numbness or weakness of the face, arm or leg, especially on one side of the body
- Sudden confusion, trouble speaking or understanding
- Sudden trouble seeing in one or both eyes
- Sudden trouble walking, dizziness, loss of balance or coordination
- Sudden severe headache with no known cause

Treatment and Care

Tests can be done to find if there is a blood flow problem to the brain. The doctor may then prescribe medicines and/or surgery. When an actual stroke occurs, it is crucial to get emergency treatment. Treatment includes:

- Medications that reduce brain tissue swelling, inhibit the normal clotting of the blood, or prevent existing clots from getting bigger
- Surgery, if warranted
- Rehabilitation as needed by speech, physical, and occupational therapists

(See "Places to Get Information & Help" under "Heart Disease/High Blood Pressure" on page 376.)

150 Thyroid Problems

The thyroid is a small, butterfly-shaped gland located just in front of the windpipe (trachea) in your throat. Its normal function is to produce L-thyroxine and L-thyronine, hormones that influence a variety of metabolic processes in the body. These include converting food to energy, regulating growth and fertility, and maintaining body temperature. Thyroid problems occur when conditions exist that cause too much or too few thyroid hormones.

Signs and Symptoms

Hyperthyroidism (two common forms of which are Graves' disease and toxic multinodular goiter) occurs when the thyroid produces too much thyroid hormone. Some signs and symptoms are:

- Tremors
- Mood swings
- Weakness
- Diarrhea
- Heart palpitations
- Heat intolerance
- Shortened menstrual periods
- Unexplained weight loss
- Fine hair (or hair loss)
- Rapid pulse
- Nervousness
- Bulging eye or eyes
- Enlarged thyroid gland

Hypothyroidism occurs when the thyroid gland does not make enough thyroid hormone to meet the body's needs. Some signs and symptoms are:

- Fatigue and excessive sleeping
- Dry, pale skin
- Deepening of the voice
- Weight gain
- Dry hair that tends to fall out
- Decrease in appetite
- Frequently feeling cold
- Puffy face (especially around the eyes)
- Heavy and/or irregular menstrual periods
- Poor memory
- Constipation
- Enlarged thyroid gland

Treatment

Treatment for thyroid problems depends on which condition is present. Hypothyroidism is generally treated with iodine and/or medicine to supplement thyroid hormones. A person may require lifelong supplementation and follow-up care to monitor treatment. Hyperthyroidism treatment varies with its cause, but generally includes one or more of the following:

- Surgical removal of the thyroid
- Radioactive iodine
- Medicine to stop overproduction of thyroid hormones

Surgical removal and radioactive iodine treatments frequently result in the need to take thyroid supplementation thereafter.

SECTION V
Health Resources

Introduction

You can get information for health related topics by calling or writing to organizations in this section. The organizations for specific concerns are listed from A to Z by subject area. When calling the numbers, consider the tips below to make your time as productive as possible.

- Call early in the day when the telephone lines are not as busy.

- Check the time zone of the location that you are calling to see how it corresponds to your time. Most organizations staff their phones from 9:00 a.m. – 5:00 p.m. (their time), Monday through Friday.

- Write down the specific questions you want to ask before you call.

- Ask if written materials are available and can be sent to you.

- Some places offer a prerecorded message or will take your name and phone number and call you back. Others may ask for your address to send you written material.

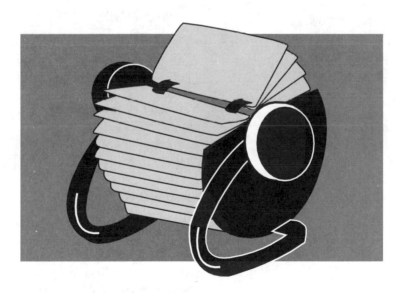

Places to Get Information & Help

General Health Information

American Academy of Family Physicians
8880 Ward Pkwy.
Kansas City, MO 64114
1-800-274-2237

National Health Information Center
P.O. Box 1133
Washington, DC 20013-1133
1-800-336-4797

For Specific Concerns

AIDS

AIDS Information Hotline
U.S. Public Health Service
American Social Health Association
P.O. Box 13827
Research Triangle Park, NC 27709
1-800-342-AIDS (2437)
1-800-344-7432 (in Spanish)
1-800-243-7889 (for hearing impaired)

Alcohol/Drug Abuse

Al-Anon Family Group Headquarters
(includes Alateen)
P.O. Box 862
Midtown Station
New York, NY 10018-0862
1-800-356-9996

Alcoholics Anonymous (AA)
General Service Office
475 Riverside Drive
New York, NY 10115
212-870-3400
To find an AA group in your area, call:
Intergroup 212-647-1680

Children of Alcoholics Foundation (COAF)
555 Madison Ave. 20th Floor
New York, NY 10022
1-800-359-COAF (2623)
212-754-0656

Cocaine Anonymous World Services, Inc.
3740 Overland Ave., Suite G
Los Angeles, CA 90034
1-800-347-8998
213-554-2554

Men for Sobriety (MFS) and Women for Sobriety (WFS) Inc.
P.O. Box 618
Quakertown, PA 18951-0618
1-800-333-1606
215-536-8026

Narcotics Anonymous (NA)
NA World Services
P.O. Box 9999
Van Nuys, CA 91409
818-773-9999

National Cocaine Hotline
c/o Phoenix House
164 West 74th St.
New York, NY 10023
1-800-COCAINE (262-2463)
1-800-662-HELP (4357)

National Institute on Drug Abuse
Drug Treatment Helpline
107 Lincoln St.
Worcester, MA 01605
1-800-662-HELP (4357) (English)
1-800-66-AYUDA (Spanish)
Drug-Free Workplace Hotline: 1-800-843-4571

Rational Recovery (RR)
Rational Recovery Self-Help Network (RRSN)
Box 800
Lotus, CA 95651
916-621-2667

Alzheimer's Disease

Alzheimer's Association
919 North Michigan Ave., Suite 1000
Chicago, IL 60601-1676
1-800-272-3900

Anxiety/Phobias

Agoraphobics in Motion (A.I.M.)
1729 Crooks
Royal Oak, MI 48067
810-547-0400

Anxiety Disorders Association of America
(ADAA)
6000 Executive Blvd., Suite 513
Rockville, MD 20852
301-231-9350

National Center for the Treatment of Phobias,
Anxiety and Depression
1755 S. Street, NW
Washington, DC 20009
202-363-7792

Arthritis

Arthritis Foundation
P.O. Box 7669
Atlanta, GA 30357-0669
1-800-238-7000

Cancer

Cancer Information Service
(National Cancer Institute)
900 Rockville Pike
Bethesda, MD 20892
1-800-4-CANCER (422-6237)

Depression

Depression Awareness Recognition & Treatment
(DART)
5600 Fishers Lane, Room 10-85
Parklawn Building
Rockville, MD 20857
1-800-421-4211 (to request information)
301-443-4140 (to talk to someone)

Diabetes

American Diabetes Association
1660 Duke St.
Alexandria, VA 22314
1-800-232-3472

Juvenile Diabetes Foundation International
432 Park Ave. S.
New York, NY 10016
1-800-223-1138

Domestic Violence

Child Help U.S.A.
Independent Order of Foresters (IOF)
National Child Abuse Hotline
1-800-4-A-CHILD (422-4453)

National Domestic Violence Hotline
1-800-799-SAFE (7233)

Eating Disorders

National Association of Anorexia Nervosa and
Associated Disorders (ANAD)
P.O. Box 7
Highland Park, IL 60035
708-831-3438

National Eating Disorders Organization (NEDO)
6655 South Yale Avenue
Tulsa, OK 74136-3329
918-481-4044

25. Places to Get Information & Help

25. Places to Get Information & Help

Epilepsy

Epilepsy Foundation of America
4351 Garden City Dr., 4th Floor
Landover, MD 20785
1-800-332-1000

Grief

The Compassionate Friends National Support Group
900 Jorie Blvd.
Oakbrook, IL 60521
708-990-0010

Grief Recovery Helpline
1-800-445-4808

Headaches

National Headache Foundation
5252 N. Western Ave.
Chicago, IL 60625
1-800-843-2256

Hearing and Speech Problems

Better Hearing Institute – Hearing Help Line
P.O. Box 1840
Washington, DC 20013
1-800-327-9355

Heart Disease/High Blood Pressure

American Heart Association
7272 Greenville Ave.
Dallas, TX 75231-4596
1-800-242-8721

National Heart Lung and Blood Institute (NHLBI)
Information Center
P.O. Box 30105
Bethesda, MD 20824-0105
1-800-575-WELL (9355)
301-251-1222

Kidney Diseases

American Kidney Fund
6110 Executive Blvd., Suite 1010
Rockville, MD 20852
1-800-638-8299

Liver Diseases

American Liver Foundation
1425 Pompton Avenue
Cedar Grove, NJ 07009
1-800-223-0179

Lung Diseases

National Jewish Center for Immunology
and Respiratory
Medicine – Lung Line
1400 Jackson St.
Denver, CO 80206
1-800-222-LUNG

See also NHLBI listing under "Heart Disease/
High Blood Pressure"

Medical Identification

MedicAlert Foundation International
2323 Colorado Ave.
Turlock, CA 95380
1-800-344-3226

Mental Health

National Mental Health Association
1021 Prince Street
Alexandria, VA 22314-2971
1-800-969-NMHA (6642)

Multiple Sclerosis

National Multiple Sclerosis Society
733 Third Ave.
New York, NY 10017-3288
213-986-3240

Nutrition

National Center for Nutrition and Dietetics
American Dietetic Association
216 West Jackson Blvd., Suite 800
Chicago, IL 60606
Consumer Nutrition
Information Hotline
1-800-366-1655

Osteoporosis

National Osteoporosis Foundation
1150 17th Street N.W., Suite 500
Washington, D.C. 20036
202-223-2226

Osteoporosis and Related Bone Diseases
National Resource Center
1150 17th Street, NW, Suite 500
Washington, DC 20036
1-800-624-BONE (2663)

Parkinson's Disease

National Parkinson Foundation
1501 N.W. 9th Ave.
Bob Hope Rd.
Miami, FL 33136
1-800-327-4545

Reyes Syndrome

National Reye's Syndrome Foundation
P.O. Box 829
Bryan, OH 43506
1-800-233-7393

Safety

National Safety Council
1121 Spring Lake Drive
Itasca, Illinois 60143-3201
1-800-621-7619

Senior Citizen Health

American Association of Retired Persons (AARP)
601 E St. N.W.
Washington, DC 20049
1-800-424-2277

ElderCare Locator
1-800-677-1116
A public service of the National Association of
Area Agencies on Aging.

Healthy Older People
National Health Information Center
P.O. Box 1133
Washington, DC 20013-1133
1-800-336-4797

Sickle Cell Anemia

Sickle Cell Disease Association of America
200 Corporate Pointe, Suite 495
Culver City, California 90230
1-800-421-8453

Suicide

American Suicide Foundation
1045 Park Ave., Suite 3C
New York, NY 10028
1-800-531-4477 (For information. Not a crisis hotline)

Arlington Heights, IL 60005
1-800-635-0635

Visual Problems

American Council for the Blind
1155 15th Street N.W., Suite 720
Washington, DC 20005
1-800-424-8666

Prevent Blindness America
500 E. Remington Rd.
Schaumberg, IL 60173
1-800-221-3004

25. Places to Get Information & Help

Index

Index

Index

Index

Index

Index